Atlas of
GLAUCOMA

Atlas of GLAUCOMA

Second Edition

Edited by

Neil T Choplin, MD
Glaucoma Specialist,
Eye Care of San Diego
Captain, Medical Corps,
United States Navy, Retired
Former Chairman and Residency Director
Naval Medical Center
San Diego, CA
USA

Diane C Lundy, MD
Captain, Medical Corps,
United States Navy, Retired
Former Director of Glaucoma Services and
Residency Directory
Naval Medical Center
San Diego, CA
USA

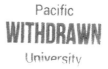
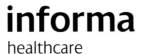
informa
healthcare

First edition published in the United Kingdom in 1998 by Martin Dunitz Ltd. Second edition published by Informa Healthcare, 4 Park Square, Milton Park, Abingdon, Oxon OX14 4RN. Informa Healthcare is a trading division of Informa UK Ltd. Registered office, 37/41 Mortimer Street, London W1T 3JH. Registered in England and Wales number 1072954.

Tel: +44(0)20 7017 6000
Fax: +44 (0)20 7017 6336
Email: info.medicine@tandf.co.uk
Website: www.informahealthcare.com

A CIP record for this book is available from the British Library.
Library of Congress Cataloging-in-Publication Data

Data available on application

ISBN-10: 1 84184 518 3
ISBN-13: 978 1 84184 518 0

Distributed in North and South America by
Taylor & Francis
6000 Broken Sound Parkway, NW, (Suite 300)
Boca Raton, FL 33487, USA

Within Continental USA
Tel: 1 (800) 272 7737; Fax: 1 (800) 374 3401
Outside Continental USA
Tel: (561) 994 0555; Fax: (561) 361 6018
Email: orders@crcpress.com

Distributed in the rest of the world by
Thomson Publishing Services
Cheriton House
North Way
Andover, Hampshire SP10 5BE, UK
Tel: +44 (0)1264 332424
Email: tps.tandfsalesorder@thomson.com

Composition by Exeter Premedia Services Pvt Ltd, Chennai, India
Printed and bound in India by Replika Press Pvt Ltd

Dedication

This book is warmly dedicated to George L Spaeth, MD, Director of the Glaucoma Service of the Wills Eye Hospital in Philadelphia, Pennsylvania and Professor of Ophthalmology at Thomas Jefferson University, and to Donald S Minckler, MD, former Director of the Glaucoma Service of the Doheny Eye Institute of the University of Southern California and Professor of Ophthalmology at the University of Southern California (now with the University of California, Irvine), and their associates, who taught us what there is to know and what there is to learn about glaucoma, and how to learn.

Contents

Contributors

Iqbal Ike Ahmed, MD, FRCSC
Department of Ophthalmology
University of Toronto
Toronto, ON
Canada

Rupert RA Bourne, MBBS, BSc, FRCOphth, MD
Glaucoma Service
Department of Ophthalmology
Hinchingbrooke Hospital
Huntingdon, Cambs
UK

Christopher Bowd, PhD
Hamilton Glaucoma Center
Department of Ophthalmology
University of California San Diego
La Jolla, CA
USA

Graziano Bricola, MD
Clinica Oculistica
Di N.O.G University di Genova
Azienda Ospedaliera Universitaria San Martino
Genova
Italy

Louis B Cantor, MD
Professor, Director of Glaucoma Service
Department of Ophthalmology
Indiana University School of Medicine
Indianapolis, IN
USA

Neil T Choplin, MD
Glaucoma Specialist, Eye Care of San Diego
Captain, Medical Corps,
United States Navy, Retired
Former Chairman and Residency Director
Naval Medical Center
San Diego, CA
USA

Anne L Coleman, MD, PhD
Jules Stein Eye Institute
University of California
Los Angeles, CA
USA

James W Doyle
Department of Ophthalmology
University of Florida School of Medicine
Gainesville, FL
USA

Robert D Fechtner, MD
Director, Glaucoma Service
University of Medicine and Dentistry of
New Jersey
Newark, NJ
USA

Fabio De Feo
Clinica Oculistica
Di N.O.G University di Genova
Azienda Ospedaliera Universitaria San Martino
Genova
Italy

Ronald Fellman
Glaucoma Associates of Texas
Dallas, TX
USA

Maher M Fanous, MD
North Florida Eye Center
Gainesville, FL
USA

Donna J Gagliuso, MD
Department of Ophthalmology
Mount Sinai School of Medicine
New York, NY
USA

Gustavo E Gamero, MD
St. Luke's Cataract & Laser Institute
Tarpon Springs, FL
USA

JoAnn A Giaconi, MD
Clinical Assistant
Professor of Ophthalmology
Jules Stein Eye Institute
Veterans Administration of Greater Los Angeles,
Los Angeles, CA
USA

David S Greenfield, MD
Associate Professor Clinical Ophthalmology
Bascom Palmer Eye Institute
University of Miami School of Medicine
Miami, FL
USA

Alon Harris, PhD
Department of Ophthalmology
Indiana University School of Medicine
Indianapolis, IN
USA

Jeffrey D Henderer, MD
Assistant Professor of Ophthalmology
Thomas Jefferson University School of Medicine
Assistant Surgeon
Wills Eye Hospital Glaucoma Service
Philadelphia, PA
USA

Richard A Hill, MD
Orange County Glaucoma
Santa Ana, CA
USA

Christian P Jorescu-Cuypers, MD, PhD
University of Saarland/Homburg
Homburg/Saar
Germany

L Jay Katz, MD
Professor of Ophthalmology
Thomas Jefferson Medical College
Attending Surgeon
Wills Eye Hospital Glucoma Service
Philadelphia, PA
USA

Baseer U Khan, MD FRCS
Department of Ophthalmology
University of Toronto
Toronto, ON
Canada

Paul P Lee, MD, JD
Professor of Ophthalmology
Duke University Medical Center
Durham, NC
USA

Paul S Lee, MD
James J. Peters Veteran Affairs Medical Center
Bronx, NY
USA

Jeffrey M Liebmann, MD
Professor, Clinical Ophthalmology
Director, Glaucoma Service
Manhattan Eye, Ear and Throat Hospital
New York University School of Medicine
New York, NY
USA

Diane C Lundy, MD
Captain, Medical Corps
United States Navy, Retired
Former Director of Glaucoma Services and
Residency Directory
Naval Medical Center
San Diego, CA
USA

Jonathan Myers
Associate Professor
Thomas Jefferson Medical College
Associate Attending Surgeon
Wills Eye Hospital Glaucoma Service
Philadelphia, PA
USA

Arvind Neelakantan, MD, FRCOphth
Bascom Palmer Eye Institute
Miami, FL
USA

Robert Ritch, MD
Professor, Clinical Ophthalmology
Director, Glaucoma Service
New York Eye and Ear Infirmary
New York Medical College
New York, NY
USA

Janet B Serle, MD
Professor
Department of Ophthalmology
Mount Sinai School of Medicine
New York, NY
USA

Mark B Sherwood, MD
Department of Ophthalmology
University of Florida College of Medicine
Gainesville, FL
USA

Mary Fran Smith, MD
Department of Ophthalmology
University of Florida College of Medicine
Gainesville, FL
USA

Richard Tamesis, MD
Department of Ophthalmology
University of Nebraska Medical Center
Omaha, NE
USA

Celso Tello, MD
Associate Professor Clinical Ophthalmology
Associate Director of Glaucoma Service
The New York Eye and Ear Infirmary
New York, NY
USA

Carol B Toris, PhD
Department of Ophthalmology
University of Nebraska Medical Center
Omaha, NE
USA

Carlo E Traverso, MD
Director of Centro di Ricerca Clinica e Laboratorio
per il Glaucoma e lacornea
Clinica Oculistica
Di N.O.G University di Genova
Azienda Ospedaliera Universitaria San Martino
Genova
Italy

Robert N Weinreb, MD
Hamilton Glaucoma Center
Department of Ophthalmology
University of California San Diego
La Jolla, CA
USA

Jennifer S Weizer, MD
Assistant Professor
Ophthalmology and Visual Sciences
Kellogg Eye Center
University of Michigan
Ann Arbor, MI
USA

Richard Wilson, MD
Professor
Wills Eye Hospital
Philadelphia, PA
USA

Darrell WuDunn, MD, PhD
Associate Professor
Department of Ophthalmology
Indiana University School of Medicine
Indianapolis, IN
USA

Michael E Yablonski, MD
Department of Ophthalmology
University of Nebraska Medical Center
Omaha, NE
USA

Linda M Zangwill, PhD
Hamilton Glaucoma Center
Department of Ophthalmology
University of California San Diego
La Jolla, CA
USA

Foreword

Since 'glaucoma' encompasses a wide variety of clinical findings, diagnostic techniques, and treatment options, we thought it best to assemble a book like this one from many parts, each manufactured by someone who is an expert in that particular subject matter. Although at times it felt like we were trying to herd mercury, this project has come together in a way that has exceeded our expectations.

Editing a project like this can be trying; the big benefit comes from having the material to read as part of the editorial process. We learned a lot about glaucoma as we went through the individual chapters, and trust that the readers will likewise benefit. The chapters were written by authors recognized for their clinical and research expertise, particularly in their subject areas: Drs Toris and Yablonski (two of the world's experts in fluorophotometry) from the University of Nebraska (with wonderful artwork by Richard Temesis) on aqueous humor dynamics, Ron Fellman on gonioscopy, Gustavo Gamero from Tarpon Springs, Florida with Rob Fechtner from the University of Medicine and Dentistry of New Jersey, Newark, New Jersey on the optic nerve (Rob was one of the first people in the world to work with scanning laser polarimetry), Jennifer Weizer and Paul Lee from Duke University (an expert in epidemiology as well as glaucoma) on primary open angle glaucoma, Jonathan Meyers and L Jay Katz from the Wills Eye Hospital in Philadelphia, Pennsylvania, on secondary glaucoma, Jeff Liebman and the group from the New York Eye and Ear Infirmary on the angle closure glaucomas (pioneering experts on ultrasound biomicroscopy), Lou Cantor and the group from the University of Indiana on normal tension glaucoma, Alon Harris on ocular blood flow, Carlo Traverso from the University of Genoa, Italy, on developmental glaucoma and its treatment (Carlo's experience with the subject while in Saudi Arabia is staggering, where he saw something like 300 cases of congenital and developmental glaucoma in a three-year period!), Paul S Lee, Donna Gagliuso, and Janet Serle from Mount Sinai School of Medicine, New York, NY on medical treatment (new to the Second Edition, welcome!), Rick Hill from the University of California, Irvine (who has done outstanding work in laser sclerostomy and ciliodestruction), on laser therapy, Jeffrey Henderer and Rick Wilson from the Wills Eye Hospital in Philadelphia on filtering surgery (Rick was one of Dr Choplin's mentors on the art of trabeculectomy), Anne Coleman and JoAnn Giaconi from the University of California, Los Angeles on aqueous shunts (Anne was one of the original investigators for the Ahmed Glaucoma Valve, and was the senior author on the first published paper dealing with the device), and Mark Sherwood and co-workers from the University of Florida, Gainesville (superb clinicians and experienced glaucoma researchers), on the co-management of cataract and glaucoma. As times have changed since the publication of the First Edition, we have added two new very exciting chapters in this Second Edition: Ike Ahmed on non-penetrating filtering surgery, and Chris Bowd, Lindal Zangwill, and Bob Weinreb from the University of California, San Diego, on scanning laser imaging. It was in Dr Weinreb's laboratory that scanning laser polarimetry was 'born'.

Having a diversity of authors makes for a diversity of styles. Although the editors wielded a broad editorial pen, attempting to maintain a consistent style throughout the book, the reader will note that each chapter has its own unique character. Some chapters have much text and few illustrations, while others are almost exclusively graphical, with extensive legends written to bring out the teaching point of the picture. Hopefully, the material, no matter how it is presented, will add to the readers' knowledge of glaucoma, as it has for ours.

Disclaimer

The editors are former active duty medical officers in the United States Navy, now both retired from active service. Neither of us have any further official relationship with the United States Navy (except as 'retirees'), and this book, as the First Edition, was not written as part of any official duties.

Notwithstanding, the views and opinions expressed in this work are ours or those of the individual authors, and should not be construed as official opinions of the Department of the Navy, the Department of Defense, or of the United States government. Dr Lundy has no financial or proprietary interest in any company, product, drug, machine, or device mentioned in this book, while Dr Choplin is a paid consultant to Carl Zeiss Meditec, Inc., and has received travel funds and honoraria from most of the major ophthalmic pharmaceutical companies.

Neil T Choplin
Diane C Lundy

Preface

It was once said to me that there is no specialty in the field of medicine that deals with only one disease. I suppose there are endocrinologists who specialize in treating only patients with diabetes mellitus, making them 'diabetologists', but there may not be any other 'one disease doctors' except for the ophthalmologists who specialize in the diagnosis and management of patients with glaucoma, and these specialists may be termed 'glaucomologists'. However, if it is true that 'diabetologists' treat only one disease, it is not true that 'glaucomologists' treat only one disease, simply because glaucoma is not one disease. In fact, at this point in time, it is hard to say exactly what glaucoma is. What is becoming clear is that glaucoma is a spectrum of clinical entities that encompasses many ocular and systemic conditions. It may be a primary eye disease, or a manifestation of some other ocular or systemic disease.

It was while contemplating some aspect of a lecture to be given (or thinking about one just given, I can't remember which) that it occurred to me that in my day-to-day clinical practice I'm really not doing anything the way I was trained over 20 years ago. As I continued to reflect on this it became apparent that nothing in glaucoma is what it was. Indeed, this gave way to a lecture called 'Current Concepts in Glaucoma: Nothing is What it Was'. Indeed, the change in the definition of glaucoma from a pressure disease to an optic neuropathy, intraocular pressure as a risk factor rather than the cause of glaucoma, new methods for early detection and diagnosis of glaucoma ('pre-perimetric'), and a solid scientific basis for approaches to treatment (based upon a number of landmark clinical studies) are all different from what they were when I was a glaucoma fellow.

Around the time of the publication of the First Edition, ophthalmologists had begun to recognize that glaucoma is an optic nerve disease, with 'characteristic' progressive structural changes leading to loss of visual function in a 'characteristic' way. The use of intraocular pressure levels to define the disease has pretty much gone away, and now pressure is used to gauge the risk of having, or developing, glaucoma. Does that mean that the 65-year-old patient with 'cupped out' optic nerves, central and temporal islands in the visual fields, and an untreated intraocular pressure of 12 mmHg has glaucoma, while the 45-year-old myopic male with pigment dispersion syndrome and an initial intraocular pressure of 52 mmHg in each eye with normal optic nerves and visual fields doesn't? The former patient may be in the 'burned out' stage of glaucoma or may have suffered visual loss from anterior ischemic optic neuropathy, while the latter may be in the early stages of glaucoma or may have simply had a transient rise in pressure following a brisk walk. To try to describe multiple disease, conditions, and scenarios in a widely disparate group of patients with a single term 'glaucoma' is subject to frustration. 'Glaucomologists' do not deal with a single disease.

Comprehension of glaucoma's pathophysiology is improving, but there is much we don't know. We are well into a new era in glaucoma research, focusing on the cellular mechanisms responsible for the death of optic nerve axons. The research is proceeding on many different fronts: genetic, biochemical, and cellular biological, to name but a few. New ideas are emerging. Perhaps intraocular pressure (in some people) is the initiating event that damages a handful of neurons, with the bulk of the damage then done by the propagation of environmental toxins released when those cells die. Perhaps glaucoma is the genetically predetermined self-destruction of the optic nerve, with similar genetically determined mechanisms in the trabecular meshwork responsible for the observed increase in intraocular pressure, with no causal relationship between intraocular pressure and optic nerve damage. Perhaps glaucoma is a condition in which the blood flow to the optic nerve is insufficient for its nutritional requirements, leading to its ultimate demise. How different these ideas are from the concept that 'glaucoma is a disease in which the intraocular pressure rises and this causes optic nerve damage'.

This book illustrates what we know about 'glaucoma' today. It encompasses a wide variety of subjects, as one would expect for a disease that encompasses a wide variety of clinical conditions, syndromes, and findings.

Neil T Choplin, MD

Acknowledgments

Thank you to our co-workers, spouses, and families, and to our residents and former residents for keeping us on our toes and advancing our knowledge as we attempted to advance theirs. We would also like to acknowledge the hard work and effort put forth by the contributors and their co-workers, without whom this book would not have been possible. We remain extremely grateful to Alan Burgess, the commissioning editor for the First Edition, for his help, advice, and constant encouragement. Lastly, this project might not have been seen through to completion were it not for the diligence, persistence, badgering (always in a nice way), and encouragement of Oliver Walter, whose names we have finally got in the correct order. Thank you, Oliver.

1 Introduction to glaucoma

Diane C Lundy, Neil T Choplin

INTRODUCTION

Glaucoma is a diagnosis that may be readily and perhaps too frequently made, based upon a variety of clinical findings by different eye-care professionals. It is not a single disease, but rather a group of diseases with some common characteristics (see Chapter 2). The hallmarks of glaucoma are typical, often progressive, optic nerve head changes and visual field loss (Figure 1.1) or the potential for them. Optic nerve damage (discussed in Chapters 6 and 7), and its corresponding visual field loss (discussed in Chapter 8), is often, but not always, reached in the setting of intraocular pressure deemed to be too high for the affected eye (Chapters 3, 4, 9 and 12). All glaucomatous disease may have a common end point, that being irreversible loss of visual function and even blindness. Since 'glaucoma' is not a single disease, there is no typical 'glaucoma patient' or single best 'glaucoma treatment'.

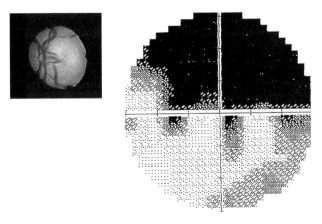

Figure 1.1 Optic disc and corresponding visual field from a patient with glaucoma. Note the thinning of the temporal rim of this left optic disc with extension of the cup to the inferior rim. The visual field shows a superior altitudinal hemianopia, corresponding to the loss of the inferior rim.

THE SPECTRUM OF GLAUCOMA

The manifestations of glaucoma are protean regardless of which parameter is considered. At one end of the clinical spectrum is the white, quiet, painless eye of a patient with primary open-angle glaucoma (POAG) who may, in fact, be unaware of the presence of the disease (Chapter 9). At the other extreme is the patient with acute angle closure glaucoma who is distraught with eye pain, decreased vision, and possibly even systemic symptoms such as nausea and vomiting (Chapter 11). The age of the glaucoma patient at the time of clinical presentations is likewise variable. Congenital glaucoma (Chapter 14) presents in the newborn, while typical patients with glaucoma due to the exfoliation syndrome (Chapter 10) are usually in their seventh or eighth decade of life. Although the glaucomas share a common end point, their proximal etiologies range from acute macroscopic mechanical closure of the outflow structures, as in acute angle closure, to a macroscopically open angle with increased resistance to outflow at the microscopic and cellular level, as in POAG. In some patients with glaucoma, intraocular pressure may have nothing to do with the observed damage. Newer evidence points towards a possible role of neurotoxins as a distal part of the route to glaucomatous optic neuropathy and field loss.

The differing manifestations of glaucoma are reflected in the clinical examination findings, which can range from the normal-appearing anterior segment of the POAG patient to the markedly abnormal findings in the patient with uveitic glaucoma or iridocorneal endothelial syndrome (ICE). (Consider the appearance of the eye of a patient with Rieger's syndrome shown in Figure 1.2.) Intraocular pressure may be quite elevated, as in the case of acute angle closure, or well within the 'average' range (Chapter 12). The visual field examination of the glaucoma patient may likewise represent a spectrum

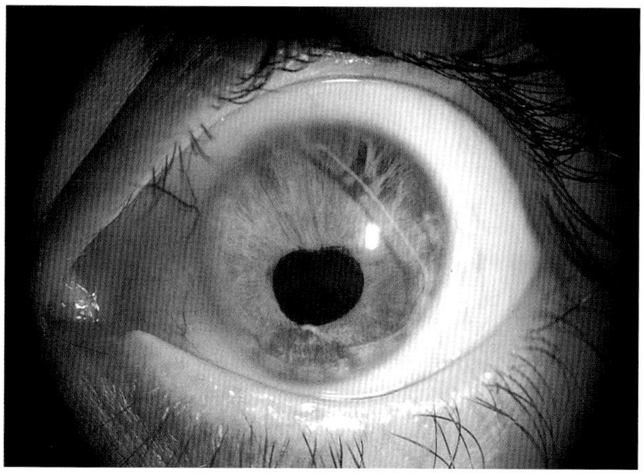

Figure 1.2 Rieger's syndrome. This eye shows many of the structural abnormalities of anterior segment dysgenesis affecting the iris, cornea, anterior chamber angle, and pupil. See Chapter 14 for a complete discussion of this syndrome and other developmental glaucomas.

of findings (Chapter 8). At one extreme is the mild diffuse loss of early POAG while the patient with advanced normal tension glaucoma (NTG) may demonstrate focal defects which are deep and close to fixation (Chapter 12). Evidence of structural damage to the optic nerve or dysfunction of the retinal nerve fibers will usually precede the functional damage seen in the visual field, and may sometimes be detectable by newer diagnostic modalities (Chapter 7).

Befitting such a diverse group of diseases, treatment of the glaucomas ranges from careful observation in some patients with ocular hypertension (Chapter 9) to cyclodestructive surgery and tube shunts (Chapter 19) for neovascular glaucoma. Medical therapy (Chapter 15), the mainstay of treatment for most types of glaucoma at this time, ranges from topical prostaglandin analogues in POAG to oral calcium channel blockers in NTG to intravenous carbonic anhydrase inhibitors in acute angle closure. Laser surgery (Chapter 16) may be offered to the glaucoma patient: laser peripheral iridotomy (LPI) for primary angle closure glaucoma, laser trabeculoplasty for exfoliation glaucoma, iridoplasty for plateau iris, or ciliary body destruction as an end-stage procedure in all types of glaucoma. Surgery may be the primary treatment modality as in goniotomy for congenital glaucoma (Chapter 21), or an end-stage procedure as in enucleation for the patient with a blind painful eye as the result of a central retinal vein occlusion and recalcitrant neovascular glaucoma. More often, surgery such as a trabeculectomy or a tube shunt is offered after medical and laser treatment fail to adequately control progression of optic nerve damage (Chapters 17–20).

In spite of the broad range of treatment modalities available, the prognosis of the glaucomas is variable and reflects the broad scope of underlying etiologies. The typical myopic male patient with onset of pigment dispersion glaucoma in his forties

has a much better prognosis than the patient with absolute glaucoma as the result of an ischemic central retinal vein occlusion and complete angle closure from iris neovascularization. POAG is the most common type of glaucoma and has a fairly good prognosis in most cases once the diagnosis is made. However, delay in diagnosis can lead to blindness or significant visual disability. The risk of functional visual loss is of even greater concern, given the ever lengthening average life expectancy of our patients.

The diagnosis of glaucoma may be difficult to make, particularly on a single examination. Considering the progressive nature of the disease, observation of its progression may be necessary to confirm the diagnosis. Consider the patient whose photograph of the right optic disc is shown in Figure 1.3a. This patient is an African-American male in his mid-fifties with elevated intraocular pressure (mid-twenties) in both eyes. His visual field examination was entirely within normal limits, and the other eye was identical, i.e. symmetrical. He was started on medical therapy to lower his pressure, and followed at regular intervals. Figures 1.3b and c are disc photographs of the same eye taken 7 and 9 years later, respectively. Each time the visual field remained normal, although there was a very subtle but steady decrease in mean sensitivity. The optic discs remained symmetrical. Taken as a series, these photographs demonstrate concentric enlargement of the cup over time, corresponding to the diffuse loss of sensitivity in the visual field. Each individual time period, viewed independently of the rest, is consistent with 'ocular hypertension' and might be treated by periodic follow-up visits, as with this patient. Viewed as a series, however, this patient clearly has progressive open-angle glaucoma. Glaucoma, therefore, may be like a movie depicting the destruction of the optic nerve, with each examination but one frame from the movie.

Further difficulty in making a diagnosis arises when the patient's examination is seemingly normal. The photograph in Figure 1.4a was obtained because the fellow eye had a congenital optic nerve pit. Additional photographs were obtained when the patient developed giant cell arteritis (biopsy proven), but without any evidence of acute anterior ischemic optic neuropathy. Figures 1.4b–d were obtained 6, 7 and 8 years after Figure 1.4a, respectively. There is a steady concentric enlargement of the cup, with extension inferiorly, eventually reaching the inferior disc rim. Intraocular pressure in this eye was never greater than 18 mmHg. This would most likely be termed 'normal tension glaucoma', and in this case may be due to chronic ischemia. Again, it is the observed progression over time that leads to the diagnosis, not the individual examinations.

Observation of progression is really the key to diagnosing the optic nerve disease of glaucoma.

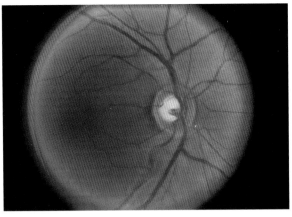
(a)

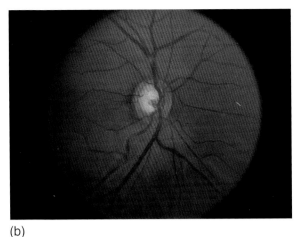
(b)

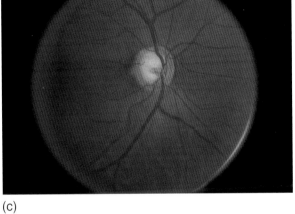
(c)

Figure 1.3 Progressive glaucoma. This series of disc photographs demonstrates concentric enlargement of the cup in a patient initially thought to have ocular hypertension. The baseline photograph is (a), with follow-up photographs taken 7 (b) and 9 (c) years later.

There are hundreds of optic nerve diseases, many of which comprise a single event leading to damage and never progress or change over the remainder of the patient's lifetime. A good example would be non-arteritic anterior ischemic optic neuropathy. It thus becomes the important but often difficult task to identify those who truly have disease as early as possible to prevent loss of visual function, while avoiding treatment in those who do not need it.

Glaucoma has to start at some point in a person's life. The progression of the disease from 'normal' to axonal dysfunction to death of axons to visual dysfunction to blindness has been termed by Dr Robert Weinreb from the University of California in San Diego the 'glaucoma continuum' and is illustrated in Figure 1.5. The concept of glaucoma as a disease characterized by progressive loss of retinal nerve fibers at a rate greater than expected for age, along with the rationale for 'early' diagnosis and institution of therapy, is illustrated in Figure 1.6.

RISK FACTORS FOR GLAUCOMATOUS DISEASE

One could debate what the concept of 'glaucoma treatment' actually means. All current treatment for glaucoma consists of lowering intraocular pressure.

But, in reality, glaucoma is a disease of the optic nerve and retinal nerve fiber layer. Lowering intraocular pressure reduces the risk of glaucoma developing (in the case of ocular hypertension) or progressing (in the case of established open angle glaucoma) (Table 1.1). Therefore, until we can repair the damage to the optic nerve, we are really treating *risk*. A useful summary of risk evaluation as determined from a host of recent clinical trials was presented by Dr Graham Trope from Canada at the International Glaucoma Symposium held in Cape Town, South Africa in March of 2005, and is shown in Table 1.2.

POAG is the most common of the glaucomas and affects an estimated two million Americans, half of whom are unaware that they have the disease. Since it is often asymptomatic in the early to moderately advanced stages, patients may suffer substantial irreversible vision loss prior to diagnosis and treatment. Therefore, considerable effort has been made to identify at-risk populations and develop accurate screening tests to make the diagnosis in order that sight-preserving treatment can begin early in the disease process. Several population-based studies have been carried out to determine the prevalence of POAG as well as identifying risk factors for the disease (Chapter 9). Some of the information from these studies is conflicting, but

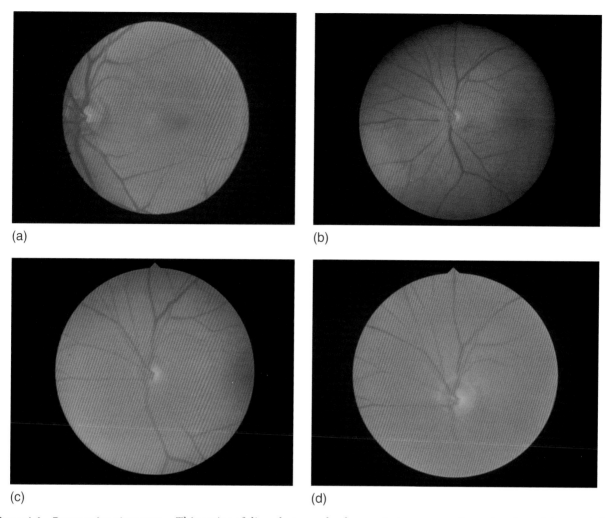

(a)

(b)

(c)

(d)

Figure 1.4 Progressive glaucoma. This series of disc photographs demonstrates progressive extension of the cup inferiorly and temporally, with eventual loss of rim. The baseline photograph (a) was taken because of a congenital optic nerve pit in the fellow eye. Follow-up photographs were obtained 6 (b), 7 (c), and 8 (d) years following the baseline after the patient developed giant cell arteritis.

race and intraocular pressure consistently appear as risk factors. In one US urban population, the age-adjusted prevalence of POAG was four times greater for African-Americans as opposed to Caucasians. Elevated intraocular pressure (> 22 mmHg) was also associated with a greater incidence of glaucoma. However, in this same group, 16% of persons with glaucomatous nerve changes and field loss never had an intraocular pressure greater than 20 mmHg on multiple examinations. Unfortunately, intraocular pressure, while easy to measure in a mass-screening setting, is a much poorer predictor of disease than visual field or optic nerve examination. Visual fields and dilated optic nerve examinations, while more sensitive and specific, are time and labor intensive, and therefore not conducive to screening large numbers of people. Newer methods of optic nerve examination, which can be performed rapidly through the non-dilated pupil, may offer better means of screening for POAG (Chapter 7).

Myopia, systemic hypertension, diabetes mellitus, or a family history of glaucoma have long been associated with an increased risk for POAG, although results of recent studies have questioned the strength of these associations. Many still consider these as risk factors, although to a lesser degree than race and elevated intraocular pressure. There may also be an association between angle-recession (post-traumatic) glaucoma and POAG in the non-recession eye as well as central vein occlusion (CRVO) and POAG in the non-CRVO eye. In addition, there is good evidence that patients who demonstrate steroid responsiveness (elevated intraocular pressure with chronic steroid use) have a higher incidence of POAG than non-responders. Identifying pertinent risk factors and accurate screening criteria for glaucoma are complex issues complicated by the fact that we are dealing with a heterogeneous collection of diseases rather than a single entity. However, the asymptomatic nature of the majority

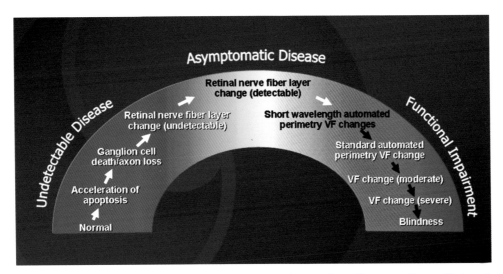

Figure 1.5   The glaucoma continuum.   (Courtesy of Dr Robert N Weinreb, Hamilton Glaucoma Center, University of California San Diego). Prior to the onset of glaucoma, a person would be expected to have a full complement of normally functioning retinal nerve fibers for his or her age. The disease is conceptualized as beginning with axon dysfunction at a presently undetectable sub-cellular level. This proceeds to frank axonal dysfunction and accelerated rate of axonal loss beyond what is expected for age, which may or may not be detectable with currently available diagnostic tests. As further axonal loss occurs, visual dysfunction occurs, first manifest with tests of axon subsets and eventually on standard white-on-white perimetry. At the far end of the continuum, loss of functional vision and blindness occur. VF, visual field.

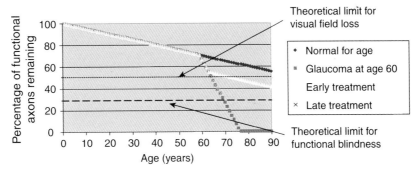

Figure 1.6   Glaucoma progression.   A person starts out in life with 100% of their retinal nerve fibers, and loses some over the course of his or her lifetime. This rate can only be estimated from cross-sectional studies, and is thought to be around 5000 axons per year. People without glaucoma live out their lives without developing visual dysfunction related to not having 'enough' nerve fibers (dark blue line). The person with glaucoma, on the other hand, begins to lose nerve fibers at a rate greater than expected from aging alone, and, if untreated, eventually has insufficient nerve fibers to maintain normal visual function, manifest first as visual field defects and later as functional blindness as more fibers are lost (pink line). If the glaucoma is detected after visual field loss has occurred, it is assumed that institution of sufficient pressure-lowering therapy will restore the rate of axonal loss back to what is expected from aging alone, and the person may still develop functional blindness if he or she lives long enough (light blue line). Ideally, glaucoma should be detected prior to the onset of visual field loss, and even if the visual field loss shows some progression, the person should still have sufficient fibers left to avoid functional blindness (yellow line).

of glaucomas and the irreversible nature of the resulting vision loss demand effective screening strategies if we are to make early vision-preserving interventions.

Glaucoma thus comprises a group of diseases encompassing a broad spectrum of clinical presentations, etiologies, and treatment modalities. The pathophysiology of the glaucomas remains uncertain and research efforts are hindered by the fact that we are dealing with a heterogeneous group of diseases rather than a single entity, but one that results in a common end point. However, as we learn more about the differing routes to their common end point, we hope to be better able to classify and treat this group of vision-threatening diseases.

Table 1.1   Risk factors for glaucoma (other than POAG)

Risk factor	Associated glaucoma
Race	
Caucasian	Exfoliation syndrome
Asian	Primary angle closure, normal tension
Refractive error	
Myopia	Pigmentary glaucoma
Hyperopia	Primary angle closure
Family history	Anterior segment dysgenesis syndromes (Axenfeld's, Rieger's)
Vasospastic conditions (migraine, Raynaud's phenomenon)	Normal tension glaucoma

Table 1.2   Evidence-based assessment of risk in glaucoma

	Risk of progression		
Diagnosis	Without treatment	With treatment	Risk factors for progression
Ocular hypertension (1)	9.5%	4.4%	Thin cornea, large c/d, baseline IOP, age
Normal tension glaucoma (2)	60%	20%	Female, migraine, disc hemorrhage
Early glaucoma (3)	62%	45%	Exfoliation, IOP, vf loss, age, disc hemorrhage
Advanced glaucoma (4)	?	30% (14% w/IOP<15)	IOP, age, fluctuation in IOP (> 3 mmHg)

(1) Ocular Hypertension Treatment Study (OHTS)
(2) Collaborative Normal Tension Glaucoma Study (CNTGS)
(3) Early Manifest Glaucoma Trial (EMGT)
(4) Advanced Glaucoma Intervention Study (AGIS)
c/d, cup/disc; IOP, intraocular pressure; vf, visual field

Further reading

Gordon MO, Beiser JA, Brandt JD, et al., for the Ocular Hypertension Treatment Study Group. The Ocular Hypertension Treatment Study: baseline factors that predict the onset of primary open angle glaucoma. Arch Ophthalmol 2002; 120: 714–20

Hollows FC, Graham PA. Intraocular pressure, glaucoma, and glaucoma suspects in a defined population. Br J Ophthalmol 1966; 50: 570–86

Kahn HA, Milton RC. Alternative definitions of open angle glaucoma; effect on prevalence and associations in the Framingham Eye Study. Arch Ophthalmol 1980; 98: 2172–7

Klein BEK, Klein R, Sponsel WE, et al. Prevalence of glaucoma: the Beaver Dam Eye Study. Ophthalmology 1992; 99: 1499–504

Mason RP, Kosoko O, Wilson R, et al. National survey of the prevalence and risk factors of glaucoma in St Lucia, West Indies. Ophthalmology 1989; 96: 1363–8

Quigley HA, Enger C, Katz J, et al. Risk factors for the development of glaucomatous visual field loss in ocular hypertension. Arch Ophthalmol 1994; 112: 644–9

Sheffield VC, Stone EM, Alward WLM, et al. Genetic linkage of familial open single glaucoma to chromosome 1q21–q31. Nat Genet 1993; 4: 47–50

Singh SS, Zimmerman MB, Podhajsky P, et al. Nocturnal arterial hypotension and its role in optic nerve head and ocular ischemic disorders. Am J Ophthalmol 1994; 177: 603–24

Sommer A, Tielsch JM, Katz J, et al. Relationship between intraocular pressure and primary open angle glaucoma among white and black Americans: the Baltimore Eye Survey. Arch Ophthalmol 1991; 109: 1090–5

Tielsch JM, Katz J, Singh K, et al. A population-based evaluation of glaucoma screening: the Baltimore Eye Survey. Am J Epidemiol 1991; 134: 1102–10

Tielsch JM, Sommer A, Katz J, et al. Racial variations in the prevalence of primary open angle glaucoma: the Baltimore Eye Study. J Am Med Assoc 1991; 266: 369–74

2 Classification of glaucoma

Neil T Choplin

INTRODUCTION

As discussed in Chapter 1, the term 'glaucoma' encompasses a wide variety of diseases and conditions. In order to arrive at a working diagnosis and institute appropriate therapy, the patient's history must be obtained and an examination performed. Classification of diseases such as glaucoma into various categories, each distinguished from the other by some essential characteristic or set of characteristics, allows us to deal with a patient's disease appropriately. For example, the initial treatment of a patient with a pressure of 48 mmHg due to angle-closure glaucoma is very different from that of a patient with the same pressure presenting for the first time with open-angle glaucoma. Similarly, the therapeutic goal set for a patient with extensive visual field loss and optic nerve cupping may be very different if the presenting intraocular pressure was 40 as opposed to 21. Thus, the approach to diagnosis often looks along some sort of classification scheme in which the subcategories have common diagnostic or therapeutic characteristics. Various classification schemes exist, and almost all glaucomatous disease falls somewhere in all of them. Most of the entities will be discussed in other chapters of this atlas.

CLASSIFICATION OF GLAUCOMA BY MECHANISM

The mechanistic classification is probably the most common scheme for sorting out the various glaucomatous diseases (Figure 2.1). The main division of this classification is between open-angle and angle-closure glaucoma. This type of division emphasizes the importance of gonioscopy (Chapter 5) for arriving at the correct diagnosis. It would be impossible to differentiate between primary open-angle glaucoma

and primary chronic angle-closure glaucoma (where the patient never had an acute attack) without gonioscopy. The other important differentiation in this classification scheme is between primary (primary disease of the eye with no associated conditions or diseases) and secondary glaucomas (where the glaucoma is attributed to some underlying condition or disorder). This differentiation may be important for therapeutic considerations. For example, primary open-angle glaucoma may respond well to miotics such as pilocarpine while inflammatory glaucoma may be worsened by treatment with miotics. Iridotomy is appropriate for treating pupillary block angle closures, but not non-pupillary block angle closure. Note that the classification scheme as presented here does not mention 'narrow angle' glaucoma. The term 'angle closure' is preferred, since 'narrowing' of the anterior chamber angle is really of no significance until the angle becomes closed (partially or completely).

CLASSIFICATION BY AGE OF ONSET

Table 2.1 illustrates a classification of glaucoma by age of onset. The developmental glaucomas are discussed in Chapter 14.

CLASSIFICATION BY INTRAOCULAR PRESSURE

The main subdivisions in this classification are 'hyperbaric' and 'normal or low tension' glaucoma. Table 2.2 lists some distinguishing characteristics. The term 'hyperbaric' is not often used except to distinguish 'garden variety' open-angle glaucoma from normal-tension glaucoma. Open-angle glaucoma is discussed in Chapter 9, while normal-tension glaucoma is discussed in Chapter 12.

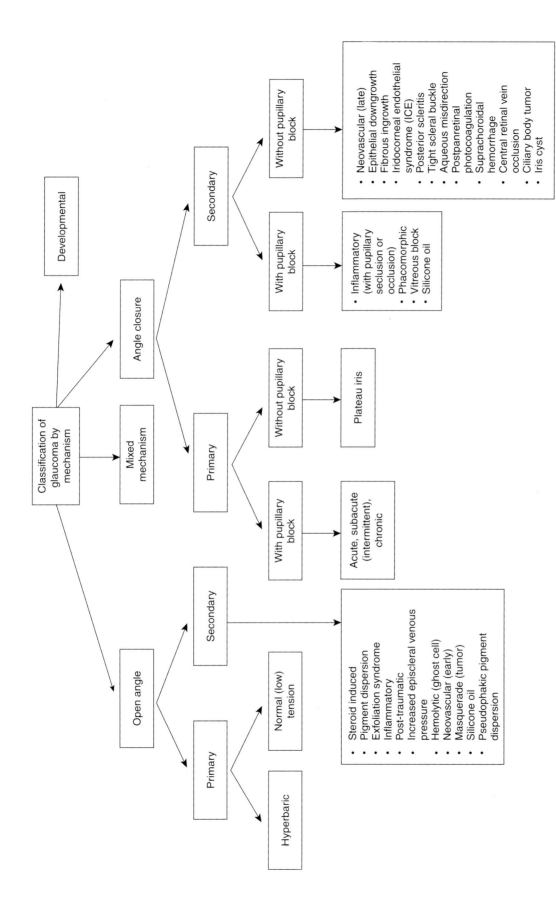

Figure 2.1 Classification of glaucoma by mechanism. Note the main subdivisions are open angle and angle closure.

Table 2.1 Classification of glaucoma by age of onset

Age of onset	Distinguishing characteristics
Congenital	Present at birth, related to developmental abnormalities, almost always requires surgical treatment
Infantile	Glaucoma not present at birth but developing before 2 years of age
Juvenile	Onset after age 2, often having identifiable angle abnormalities (such as absence of ciliary body band) that distinguish the condition from adult open-angle glaucoma
Adult	Typical open-angle glaucoma, onset usually in mid-to-late adulthood (after age 35), no identifiable structural abnormalities in the angle

Table 2.2 Classification of glaucoma by level of intraocular pressure. Hyperbaric glaucoma is usually synonymous with open-angle glaucoma as the term is usually used. The division between normal-tension and low-tension glaucoma is somewhat arbitrary

Level of intraocular pressure (IOP)	Name of condition	Distinguishing characteristics
Low	Low-tension glaucoma	IOP less than 21 mmHg, focal loss of optic disc rim, dense nerve-fiber bundle defects with loss close to fixation; may require very low IOP for stabilization
Normal	Normal-tension glaucoma	Similar to low-tension glaucoma with slightly higher IOP levels
High	Hyperbaric glaucoma (but usually just referred to as 'open-angle glaucoma')	Elevated IOP consistently greater than 22 mmHg and frequently much higher, concentric enlargement of the cup over time, diffuse loss of sensitivity may precede focal loss of visual field, treatment directed at 'normalizing' IOP

CLASSIFICATION BY STAGE OF DISEASE

Classification by stage may be important for setting therapeutic goals, for prognosis, or for disability determinations. Table 2.3 illustrates stages of glaucoma.

CLASSIFICATION BASED UPON THE INTERNATIONAL CLASSIFICATION OF DISEASES (ICD-9)

The International Classification of Diseases, Ninth Revision, Clinical Modification (ICD-9-CM) is derived from a classification of diseases from the World Health Organization. It uses codes to classify all diseases and disorders, originally intended for indexing of hospital records by disease and operations for the purpose of data storage and retrieval. Coding is used for such things as billing and database management. Codes 360–379 cover the eye and adnexa, and the 365 codes include the glaucomas. Table 2.4 lists the ICD-9 codes for glaucoma.

Table 2.3 Classification of glaucoma by stage of disease

Stage	Potential characteristics	Possible optic nerve findings	Possible visual field findings
Glaucoma suspect with borderline findings	Borderline intraocular pressure	Borderline cupping	Normal
Ocular hypertension	Intraocular pressure >21 mmHg	Normal	Normal
Mild	Early changes of glaucomatous disease	Mild cup-to-disc asymmetry, vertical cupping with intact rims, concentric enlargement of the cup, mild nerve-fiber layer loss	Normal or mild diffuse loss of sensitivity, defects generally <10 dB in depth, early nasal step or paracentral depressions, increasing short-term fluctuation
Moderate	Definite disease with minimal functional impairment	Extension of cup to rim, disc hemorrhage, bared vessels, diffuse thinning of neuroretinal rim	Loss of sensitivity 10–20 dB diffusely or at isolated points or small clusters, well defined nasal steps, focal defects from loss of nerve-fiber bundles
Advanced	Significant disease	Cup to disc >0.8, segmental loss of rim	Loss on both sides of the horizontal, large nerve-fiber bundle defects or altitudinal loss, areas of absolute loss
Far advanced	May be symptomatic with reduced visual acuity; may be aware of visual field loss	Cup to disc >0.9, pallor, undermining of the rim	Requires change to larger stimulus size to measure, temporal and central islands remaining
End stage	Legally or totally blind	Total cup, 4+ pallor	Unmeasurable

Table 2.4 Classification of glaucoma in the International Classification of Diseases, Ninth Revision, Clinical Modification

365.0 Borderline glaucoma (glaucoma suspect)

365.00	Preglaucoma, unspecified
365.01	Open angle with borderline findings
	Open angle with: borderline intraocular pressure, cupping of optic discs
365.02	Anatomical narrow angle
365.03	Steroid responders
365.04	Ocular hypertension

365.1 Open-angle glaucoma

365.10	Open-angle glaucoma, unspecified
365.11	Primary open-angle glaucoma
365.12	Low-tension glaucoma
365.13	Pigmentary glaucoma

365.14	Glaucoma of childhood, infantile or juvenile glaucoma
365.15	Residual stage of open-angle glaucoma

365.2 Primary angle-closure glaucoma

365.20	Primary angle-closure glaucoma, unspecific
365.21	Intermittent angle-closure glaucoma
365.22	Acute angle-closure glaucoma
365.23	Chronic angle-closure glaucoma
365.24	Residual stage of angle-closure glaucoma

365.3 Corticosteroid-induced glaucoma

365.31	Glaucomatous stage
365.32	Residual stage

(cont'd)

Table 2.4   Classification of glaucoma in the International Classification of Diseases, Ninth Revision, Clinical Modification (cont'd)

365.4   Glaucoma associated with congenital anomalies, dystrophies, and systemic syndromes

365.41   Glaucoma associated with chamber-angle anomalies, Axenfeld's anomaly (743.44), Reiger's anomaly or syndrome (743.44)

365.42   Glaucoma associated with anomalies of iris aniridia (743.45), essential iris atrophy (364.51)

365.43   Glaucoma associated with other anterior segment anomalies, microcornea (743.41)

365.45   Glaucoma associated with systemic syndromes, neurofibromatosis (237.7), Sturge–Weber syndrome (759.6)

365.5   Glaucoma associated with disorders of the lens

365.51   Phacolytic glaucoma

365.52   Pseudoexfoliation glaucoma

365.59   Glaucoma associated with other lens disorders

365.6   Glaucoma associated with other ocular disorders

365.60   Glaucoma associated with unspecified ocular disorder

365.61   Glaucoma associated with pupillary block

365.62   Glaucoma associated with ocular inflammation

365.63   Glaucoma associated with vascular disorders

365.64   Glaucoma associated with tumors or cysts

365.65   Glaucoma associated with ocular trauma

365.8   Other specified forms of glaucoma

365.81   Hypersecretion glaucoma

365.82   Glaucoma associated with increased episcleral venous pressure

365.83   Other specific glaucoma

365.9   Unspecified glaucoma

Note: The codes for some of the associated disorders have not been included in the table.

Further reading

Hoskins HD Jr, Kass M. Becker–Shaffer's Diagnosis and Therapy of the Glaucomas, 6th edn. St Louis, MO: CV Mosby, 1989

Jones MK, Castillo LA, Hopkins CA, Aaron WS, eds. ICD-9-CM Code Book for Physician Payment. Reston, VA: St Anthony Publishing, 1995

3 Aqueous humor dynamics

Carol B Toris, Michael E Yablonski, Richard Tamesis

Normal visual function requires the shape of the globe to remain fixed and the optical pathway from the cornea to the retina to remain clear. This requires that the nutrition of the intraocular tissues in the optical pathway must occur with a minimum number of blood vessels. All of this is accomplished very efficiently by the production of the clear aqueous humor, its circulation into the anterior chamber and its drainage from the anterior chamber angle through tissues with high resistance (trabecular meshwork and uvea). The intraocular pressure thus is maintained, the shape of the eye is preserved, the refracting surfaces are kept in place and the avascular cornea and lens are provided with nourishment and waste removal.

FLOW OF AQUEOUS HUMOR

Aqueous humor is produced by the ciliary body and is secreted into the posterior chamber. Most of this fluid then flows into the anterior chamber and drains out of the chamber angle via one of two outflow pathways, through the trabecular meshwork or through the ciliary muscle. Trabecular outflow is pressure dependent and flow through the ciliary muscle (often called uveoscleral outflow) is relatively pressure independent (Figure 3.1).

AQUEOUS PRODUCTION MECHANISMS

The primary function of the ciliary processes is to produce ocular aqueous humor. These processes constitute the internal aspect of the pars plicata of the ciliary body. The anterior portions of the larger processes have many capillary fenestrations and epithelial mitochondria, indicating specialization for aqueous humor production. Ciliary processes have a highly vascularized core (Figures 3.2 and 3.3) and their perfusion directly regulates the volume

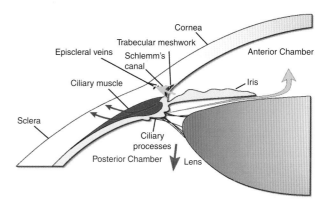

Figure 3.1 Circulation and drainage of aqueous humor. Ocular aqueous humor is secreted by the ciliary processes of the ciliary body into the posterior chamber. Some fluid circulates between the lens and the iris through the pupil into the anterior chamber (large green arrow). It drains from the anterior chamber by passive bulk flow via two pathways. Trabecular outflow is the drainage of aqueous humor sequentially through the trabecular meshwork, Schlemm's canal, collector channels, episcleral veins, anterior ciliary veins and into the systemic circulation (small green arrow). Uveoscleral outflow is the drainage of aqueous humor from the chamber angle into the tissue spaces of the ciliary muscle and on into the suprachoroidal space. From there some fluid percolates through the scleral substance and emissarial canals and some fluid is reabsorbed by uveal blood vessels (blue arrows). Although the bulk of the posterior chamber aqueous humor exits the eye through the pupil, some drains across the vitreous into the retina and retinal pigment epithelium (red arrow). The active transport of fluid out of the eye by the retinal pigment epithelium utilizes a mechanism similar to that of the non-pigmented ciliary epithelium.

of capillary ultrafiltration and indirectly influences active secretion by controlling the supply of blood-borne nutrients to the ciliary epithelium.

The first step in the formation of aqueous humor is the development of a stromal pool of

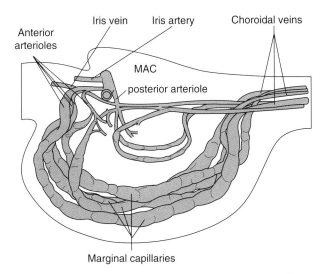

Figure 3.2 Ciliary process vasculature. One ciliary process of a monkey is shown in lateral view. The vasculature consists of a complex anastomotic system supplied by anterior and posterior arterioles radiating from the major arterial circle (MAC). The anterior arterioles supply the anterior aspect of the process and drain posteriorly into the choroidal veins. The posterior arterioles provide posteriorly draining capillaries generally confined to the base of the process. The choroidal veins drain blood from the iris veins, ciliary processes and the ciliary muscle. (Redrawn from Morrison JC, Van Buskirk EM. Ciliary process microvasculature of the primate eye. Am J Ophthalmol 1984; 97: 372–83.)

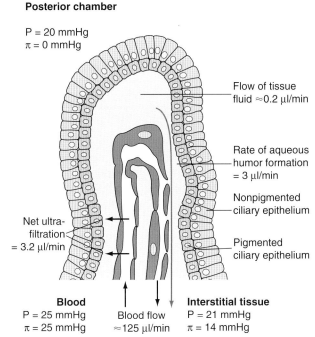

Figure 3.3 Production of aqueous humor. The ciliary process consists of a core containing capillaries and interstitial tissue surrounded by two epithelial layers oriented apex to apex. The innermost layer consists of non-pigmented ciliary epithelial cells which are connected to each other by tight junctions and desmosomes. The outer layer consists of pigmented ciliary epithelial cells connected to each other by gap junctions. The production of aqueous humor by the ciliary processes involves both ultrafiltration and active secretion. Plasma filtrate enters the interstitial space through capillary fenestrations (ultrafiltration). The net filtration of fluid from the capillaries (3.2 μl/min) has to correspond to the formation of the aqueous humor (3 μl/min) plus any loss of tissue fluid from the processes (0.2 μl/min). The net filtration of filtrate from the capillaries corresponds to about 4% of plasma flow. The capillary wall is a major barrier for the plasma proteins but the most significant barrier is in the non-pigmented ciliary epithelium where tight junctions occlude the apical region of the intercellular spaces. The outcome of this design is a high protein concentration in the tissue fluid. This causes a high oncotic pressure in the tissue fluid and a reduction in the transcapillary difference in the oncotic pressure. The hydrostatic pressure (P) and colloid osmotic pressure (π) of the blood, interstitial tissue and posterior chamber are listed for the rabbit. The effect of hydrostatic and oncotic pressure differences across the ciliary epithelium is a pressure of about 13 mmHg tending to move water into the processes from the posterior chamber. Therefore, under normal conditions the movement of fluid into the posterior chamber requires secretion. Because the π is zero in the posterior chamber, the only way to secrete fluid into this chamber is via active transport across the ciliary epithelial layers. (Modified from Bill A. Blood circulation and fluid dynamics in the eye. Physiol Rev 1975; 55: 383–417.)

plasma filtrate by ultrafiltration through the ciliary process capillary wall (Figure 3.3). Active transport of ions out of the cell establishes an osmotic gradient in the intercellular spaces of the ciliary epithelium (Figure 3.4). Finally, water moves into the posterior chamber along the osmotic gradient (Figures 3.4 and 3.5). The posterior chamber aqueous humor is modified by diffusion of molecules into or out of the surrounding tissue. A small percentage of the modified aqueous humor flows posteriorly through the vitreous and across the retina and retinal pigment epithelium, but most flows through the pupil into the anterior chamber (Figure 3.1). The flow of aqueous humor into the anterior chamber is easily measured giving a reasonable estimation of the aqueous production rate.

The rate at which aqueous humor enters the anterior chamber in the normal human eye averages about 2.5 μl/min. There is a circadian fluctuation in aqueous flow such that the rate is lowest during sleep at night and highest around noon to 1 p.m. (Figure 3.6). The circadian rhythm is not affected by eyelid closure, supine posture, sleep deprivation, sleep in a lighted room or short naps. The factors mediating the reduction in aqueous flow are unclear, but corticosteroids and catecholamines may play a role.

Intraocular pressure can be reduced by administering drugs that reduce aqueous production.

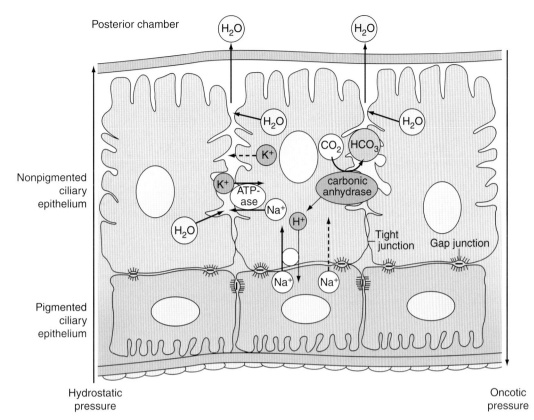

Figure 3.4 **Active transport of aqueous humor.** Active transport is the work required for the continuous formation of a fluid that is not in thermodynamic equilibrium with the blood plasma. This secretion is accomplished in the ocular anterior segment by the active transport of ions from the non-pigmented ciliary epithelium (NPE) cells into the intercellular clefts. There are indications that the active transport of Na^+ across the NPE is the key process in aqueous humor formation. The active transport of HCO_3^- and Cl^- also plays a role. Enzymatic inhibitors of these transport processes can significantly reduce aqueous flow. Examples include the carbonic anhydrase inhibitor, acetazolamide, and the inhibitor of $Na^+ - K^+$ ATPase, ouabain. The osmotic pressure in the clefts increases as ions are pumped in. The presence of apical tight junctions connecting adjacent NPE cells necessitates the movement of water and its solutes out into the posterior chamber.

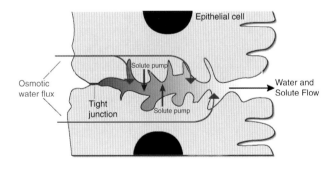

Figure 3.5 **Cole's hypothesis of fluid production.** A standing gradient osmotic flow system is represented by this diagram. The system consists of a long, narrow channel with a restriction at the apical end (tight junction). Solute pumps line the walls of the channel and solute is continuously and actively transported from the cells into the intercellular channel (blue arrows). This makes the channel fluid hyperosmotic. As water flows along the path of least resistance towards the open end of the channel (black arrow), more water enters across the walls because of the osmotic differential (red arrows). In the steady state a standing gradient is maintained. The relative osmolarity is depicted by the blue color. Volume flow is directed towards the open end of the channel. (Modified from Cole DF. Secretion of the aqueous humour. Exp Eye Res 1977; 25 (Suppl): 161–76.)

Clinically available drugs with this ocular hypotensive mechanism of action are listed in Table 3.1.

AQUEOUS HUMOR OUTFLOW PATHWAYS

In the anterior chamber, some of the aqueous humor may be lost via the cornea and iris or gained from iridial blood vessels, but these gains or losses are very small so that, in a steady state, the rate of drainage of aqueous humor through the chamber angle is nearly equal to the rate of inflow of aqueous humor through the pupil. Thus, aqueous flow (F_a) can be defined as the sum of aqueous humor

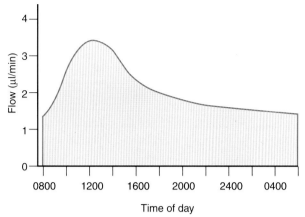

Figure 3.6   Aqueous flow versus time of day.   In humans, aqueous humor flow into the anterior chamber is highest between 1200 and 1300 hours peaking at a rate of about 3.2 μl/min. It decreases through the afternoon and into the night to a rate of about 1.6 μl/min at 0400 hours. This represents a 45% reduction in aqueous flow. The magnitude of reduction is greater than that produced by pharmacological aqueous humor suppressants. (Data from Reiss GR, Lee DA, Topper JE, Brubaker RF. Aqueous humor flow during sleep. Invest Ophthalmol Vis Sci 1984; 25: 776–8.)

drainage through two outflow pathways, the trabecular meshwork (F_{trab}) and the uvea (F_u):

$$F_a = F_{trab} + F_u \qquad (1)$$

Trabecular outflow

In the primary trabecular outflow pathway, the aqueous humor drains sequentially through the trabecular meshwork, Schlemm's canal, collector channels, episcleral veins, anterior ciliary veins and into the systemic circulation (Figure 3.1). It is generally agreed that the tissues between the anterior chamber and Schlemm's canal provide the major portion of normal resistance to aqueous drainage. Which tissue constitutes the greatest resistance is somewhat controversial. To exit the eye via Schlemm's canal, aqueous humor must traverse three layers of trabecular meshwork and the inner wall of Schlemm's canal (Figure 3.7). The resistance to fluid flow increases along this pathway. The outer layer contains a delicate meshwork of elastic-like fibers which are connected at one end with the endothelium of Schlemm's canal, and at the other end with tendons of the ciliary muscle. Contraction of the ciliary muscle may increase spaces between the plates of the meshwork and reduce resistance to flow. Pilocarpine may reduce

Table 3.1   Effects of clinically available IOP-lowering drugs on aqueous humor dynamics in humans

Class	Generic name	Trade name	Aqueous flow Day	Aqueous flow Night	C	F_u	P_{ev}
Beta blockers	timolol maleate[1–3]	TIMOPTIC	↓	–	–	–	–
	levobunolol HCl[4]	BETAGAN	↓		–		–
	carteolol HCl[5]	OCUPRESS	↓				
	betaxolol HCl[6]	BETOPTIC	↓		–		
Topical CAIs	brinzolamide HCl[7]	AZOPT	↓	↓			
	dorzolamide HCl[7]	TRUSOPT	↓	↓			
Prostaglandins	bimatoprost[8,9]	LUMIGAN	↑ – a	↑ – a	↑	↑	
	latanoprost[10–12]	XALATAN	–	–	↑ – a	↑	–
	travoprost (Camras et al., presented at the 2004 AAO annual meeting)	TRAVATAN	–	–	↑	↑	–
	unoprostone[13]	RESCULA	–		↑	–	–
Muscarinics	pilocarpine HCl[14,15]	PILOCAR	–		↑	–	–
Alpha₂ agonists	apraclonidine HCl[16,17]	IOPIDINE	↓		↑	–	–
	brimonidine tartrate[18–21]	ALPHAGAN	↓b –c		–	↑c	–
Sympathomimetics	epinephrine HCl[22–25]	GLAUCON	↓↑ a		↑	↑ –a	–

a, inconsistent effect; b, effect of 1 week of treatment or less; c, effect of 1 month of treatment

C, outflow facility; CAI, carbonic anhydrase inhibitor; F_u, uveoscleral outflow; IOP, intraocular pressure; P_{ev}, episcleral venous pressure; ↓, decreased; ↑, increased; –, no effect.

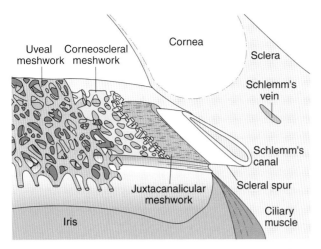

Figure 3.7   Three layers of the trabecular meshwork. Aqueous humor first passes through the inner layer or the uveal meshwork. This layer is a forward extension of the ciliary muscle. It consists of flattened sheets which branch and interconnect in multiple planes. The uveal meshwork does not offer any significant resistance to aqueous drainage because of the presence of large overlapping holes in these sheets. The middle layer, the corneoscleral meshwork, includes several perforated sheets of connective tissue extending between the scleral spur and Schwalbe's line. Relative to the openings in the uveal meshwork, the openings in these sheets are small and do not overlap. The sheets are connected to each other by tissue strands and endothelial cells. The result of this architectural design is a circuitous path of high resistance to the flow of aqueous humor. The outer layer, the juxtacanalicular meshwork, lies adjacent to the inner wall of Schlemm's canal. It contains collagen, a ground substance of glycosaminoglycans and glycoproteins, fibroblasts and endothelium-like juxtacanalicular cells. It also contains elastic fibers that may provide support for the inner wall of Schlemm's canal. This meshwork contains very narrow, irregular openings providing high resistance to fluid drainage.

trabecular outflow resistance (increase trabecular outflow facility) by this mechanism. The inner wall of Schlemm's canal consists of a monolayer of endothelial cells interconnected by tight junctions. It has been hypothesized that this wall serves as the major barrier to aqueous humor drainage. One possible means for fluid to traverse this barrier is via transcellular channels within the endothelial cells (Figure 3.8).

In humans, trabecular outflow accounts for 5 to 95% of aqueous drainage depending on the health of the eye, while in healthy monkeys the rate is about 50%. This flow is pressure dependent, meaning that the flow is proportional to the difference between IOP and the hydrostatic pressure in the canal.

Uveoscleral outflow

Anterior chamber aqueous humor that does not drain through the trabecular meshwork, flows from

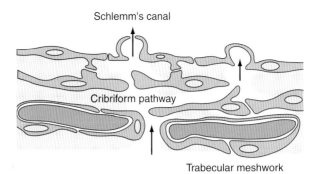

Figure 3.8   Inner wall of Schelmm's canal and the juxtacanalicular meshwork (also called cribriform meshwork). This wall contains a monolayer of spindle-shaped endothelial cells interconnected by tight junctions. One theory is that fluid may move through this area in transcellular channels. These channels may form and recede in a cyclic fashion, beginning as invaginations on the meshwork side of the endothelial cell and progressing to a transcellular channel into Schlemm's canal. Only a few channels appear to open at a time, providing the major resistance to trabecular outflow. One channel is drawn as a vacuole and one is shown opened to Schlemm's canal. The arrows indicate the direction of fluid flow. (Modified from Rohen JW. Why is intraocular pressure elevated in chronic simple glaucoma? Anatomical considerations. Ophthalmology 1983; 90: 758–65.)

the chamber angle into the supraciliary space and ciliary muscle, and then seeps through the scleral substance or flows through emissarial canals or is absorbed into uveal blood vessels (Figure 3.1). This is called 'uveoscleral' outflow. Other names for this drainage include 'unconventional', 'pressure independent' and 'uveovortex' outflow. These names arose from attempts to describe a relatively undefined seepage route. It would be more accurate to refer to this drainage as simply 'uveal' outflow, to include all anterior chamber aqueous humor egress from the uvea. The term appearing most often in the literature is 'uveoscleral outflow' hence its use in this chapter.

In contrast to trabecular outflow, uveoscleral outflow is effectively pressure independent. At IOPs greater than about 5 mmHg this outflow remains relatively constant and the facility of uveoscleral outflow is very low (approximately 0.02 µl/min per mmHg). Uveoscleral outflow reportedly accounts for anywhere from 4 to 45% of total aqueous drainage in humans. It can be increased by drugs that relax the ciliary muscle and be reduced by drugs that contract it (Figure 3.9). In general, topical prostaglandin (PG)-$F_{2\alpha}$ analogs reduce IOP predominantly by increasing uveoscleral outflow. The mechanism of the flow reduction appears to be a relaxation of the ciliary muscle causing the acute effect and the biochemical modification of its intercellular matrix, causing a more chronic effect. The mechanism for the pressure reduction in clinically

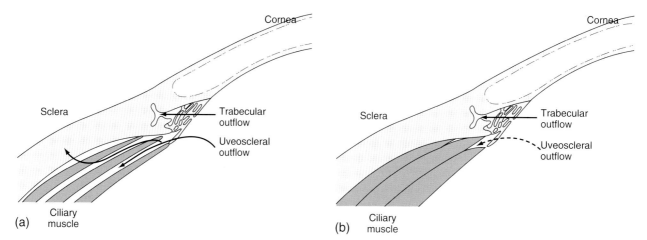

Figure 3.9   Ciliary muscle effects on uveoscleral outflow.   (a) A depiction of the ciliary muscle in the relaxed state. The spaces between muscle bundles are substantial and aqueous humor can easily pass through the tissue. Drugs that relax the ciliary muscle can increase uveoscleral outflow. Examples include the cholinergic agonist, atropine, and prostaglandin $F_{2\alpha}$ analogs. (b) The ciliary muscle in the contracted state. The spaces between muscle bundles are obliterated and uveoscleral outflow is greatly reduced. Drugs that severely contract the ciliary muscle reduce uveoscleral outflow. An example is the high doses of cholinergic antagonist, pilocarpine. (From Bill A. Blood circulation and fluid dynamics in the eye. Physiol Rev 1975; 55: 383–417.)

available topical ocular drugs is summarized in Table 3.1.

TECHNIQUES FOR MEASURING AQUEOUS FLOW

Aqueous flow was first measured by injecting a tracer such as para-aminohippuric acid or fluorescein into the blood stream, allowing it to enter the anterior chamber, and then sampling the aqueous humor to determine the rate of its disappearance. The relationship between aqueous humor tracer concentration and plasma tracer concentration was monitored to determine aqueous flow. Subsequently, oral administration of fluorescein was used for the same purpose. Injecting a large-molecular-weight tracer such as albumin or fluorescein isothiocynate dextran directly into the anterior chamber and collecting aqueous samples over time provided a more direct measure of aqueous flow. The rate of disappearance of the tracer from the aqueous humor is a function of aqueous flow.

Another method to determine aqueous flow in humans was a non-invasive photogrammetric technique. With the anterior chamber filled with fluorescein, freshly secreted aqueous humor appeared as a clear bubble in the pupil. The increase in volume of this bubble was determined by geometric optics and was an indication of the rate of aqueous flow.

Currently the method of choice to assess aqueous flow is fluorophotometry. Fluorescein is administered to the eye either topically (Figure 3.10) or by corneal iontophoresis. Fluorescein traverses the cornea, enters the anterior chamber and drains through the chamber angle (Figure 3.11). When an

equilibrium has been established, the concentrations of fluorescein in the cornea (C_c) and the anterior chamber (C_a) decrease over time. A fluorophotometer (Figure 3.12) is used to monitor these changes. The instrument can focus separately on the cornea and then on the anterior chamber, thus allowing a discrete measurement of each region.

The rate of aqueous flow determines the cornea and anterior chamber fluorescein decay curves. The typical time course of the tracer in the corneal stroma and anterior chamber is illustrated in Figure 3.13. The magnitude of the anterior chamber aqueous humor flow (F_a) is a function of the anterior chamber volume (V_a), the absolute value of the slope of the decay curve (A) and the ratio of the mass of fluorescein in the cornea to that in the anterior chamber (M_c/M_a) (Equation 2):

$$F_a = V_a A[1 + M_c/M_a] \qquad (2)$$

M_c can be rewritten as V_c/C_c where V_c is the corneal stroma volume and C_c is the corneal stroma fluorescein concentration. Similarly, M_a can be rewritten as V_a/C_a where C_a is the anterior chamber concentration of fluorescein. Equation 2 then becomes

$$F_a = V_a A[1 + V_c C_c /V_a C_a] \qquad (3)$$

Assuming that V_c and V_a remain constant in the steady state, then F_a is a function of the slope of the decay curve (A) and C_c/C_a. The logarithm of C_c/C_a is represented by the distance between the parallel decay curves (Figure 3.13). Equation 3 shows that the more rapid the rate of aqueous humor flow (F_a) the steeper will be the decay curves and the larger the magnitude of the distance between the two

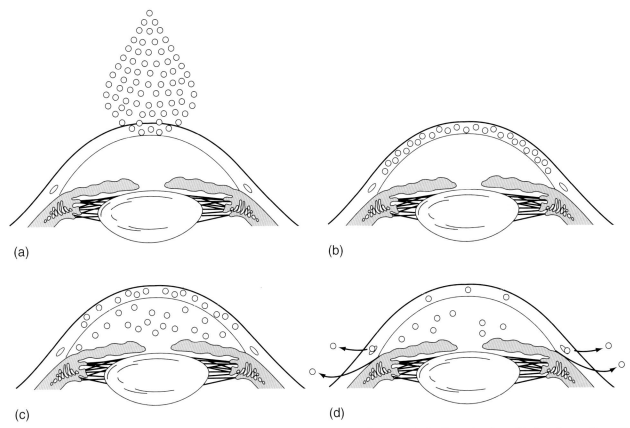

Figure 3.10 Ocular distribution of topically administered fluorescein. Fluorescein (yellow dots) applied to the surface of the cornea (a), penetrates the epithelium and fills the corneal stroma (b). The epithelium is approximately 1000-fold less permeable than the endothelium, hence, once in the stroma, effectively all the fluorescein diffuses into the anterior chamber (c). Diffusional loss into limbal or iridial vessels is very small; hence, once in the anterior chamber, approximately 95% of the fluorescein leaves with the bulk flow of aqueous humor through the two anterior chamber drainage routes (arrows) (d). The rate of disappearance of the fluorescein is used to determine aqueous flow.

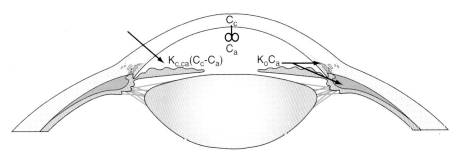

Figure 3.11 The dynamics of topically administered fluorescein. This figure demonstrates some of the important assumptions which are the basis for the fluorophotometric determination of the anterior chamber aqueous humor flow, F_a. The anterior chamber, by virtue of normal thermoconvective streams, is a well mixed compartment of uniform fluorescein concentration. The net flux of fluorescein into the anterior chamber is given by $K_{c.ca}$ ($C_c–C_a$) multiplied by the volume of the anterior chamber. $K_{c.ca}$ is the transfer coefficient for fluorescein between the cornea and anterior chamber per unit volume of the anterior chamber. C_c and C_a are the fluorescein concentrations of the corneal stroma and anterior chamber, respectively. The net flux of fluorescein out of the anterior chamber is given by K_oC_a multiplied by the volume of the anterior chamber. K_o is the fraction per minute of anterior chamber volume turned over by aqueous flow.

decay curves. At the other extreme, if F_a becomes zero, the fluorescein concentrations in the anterior chamber and corneal stroma will equalize by diffusion and the decay curves will be flat (A = 0).

Several assumptions are included in the fluorophotometric measurement of aqueous flow. The fluorescein is evenly distributed in the anterior chamber, there is minimal diffusional loss of fluorescein into limbal or iridial vessels or into the vitreous cavity, and there are no obstructions causing light scatter. The method does not work in eyes that are aphakic, are pseudophakic, have undergone iridectomy or have any condition in which fluorescein can exit the eye by means other than through the physiological chamber angle outflow pathways. The method is also invalid in eyes with cornea opacity, or severe uveitis because of the light scatter.

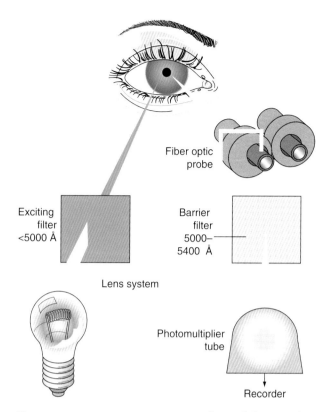

Figure 3.12 The fluorophotometer. Several hours after fluorescein is applied topically to the cornea, a vertical beam of blue light is projected into the eye. The blue light is produced by placing an excitation filter in the light path. The blue light excites the fluorescein, causing it to fluoresce. Simultaneously, a detector filtered for fluoresced light is focused on the same point in the eye. The fluorescence signal at the intersection of the two light paths is detected by the fluorophotometer and is transformed to an electrical impulse by a photomultiplier tube. The intersection of the two light paths can be moved, providing discrete measurements of the fluorescence from the cornea through the anterior chamber. The signal is sent to a recorder and converted into units of ng/ml by referencing a standard curve.

TECHNIQUES FOR MEASURING AQUEOUS DRAINAGE

Trabecular outflow

The trabecular outflow pathway is IOP dependent because flow into the canal of Schlemm is passive in response to the hydrostatic pressure driving force, which is equal to IOP minus the hydrostatic pressure in the canal. This pressure difference, for practical purposes, can be assumed to be equal to the episcleral venous pressure, P_{ev}, although the actual pressure in the canal is slightly greater than P_{ev}.

There are three ways to measure facility of trabecular outflow: tonography, perfusion, and fluorophotometry. Tonography has been the most widely used method and, although it is no longer used as a routine clinical test, its use has provided a large body of information about the pathophysiology of glaucoma and the mechanism of action of

treatment modalities. It is still used in the research setting. Tonography is accomplished by placing a Schiotz tonometer (Figure 3.14) or electronic tonometer on the cornea of the supine patient for 2 or 4 minutes. The calibrated weight of the tonometer increases IOP and hence, aqueous drainage. The IOP declines over the time interval and with the aid of the Friedenwald tables, the change in the IOP allows one to infer the volume of aqueous humor displaced from the eye. If it is assumed that the displacement of fluid from the eye across the trabecular meshwork by the weight of the tonometer, ΔV, is the only factor to account for the IOP decrease, then

$$\Delta V/t = \text{rate of fluid outflow caused by the increase in IOP above normal} \qquad (4)$$

Outflow facility, C, is calculated from Grant's equation,

$$C = (\Delta V/t)/(P_t - P_o) \qquad (5)$$

P_o is the IOP before the weighted tonometer is applied and P_t is the average IOP at the end of the test. Tonography rests on a number of assumptions that have been debated for years. Two include pseudo-facility and scleral rigidity. Tonography is visually depicted in Figure 3.15.

In experimental work, the method of choice to determine outflow facility has been the constant-pressure perfusion technique (Figure 3.16). The eye is cannulated and the pressure is set by the height of an external reservoir. The inflow of fluid from the reservoir into the anterior chamber (F_1 and F_2) is measured at each of two different pressures (P_1 and P_2). The assumption is made that the aqueous production rate and the venous pressure do not change during the measurement. Also assumed is that the tissue fluid volume and the blood volume do not change except within a few seconds after the change in the IOP. Under these conditions, outflow facility is calculated from the formula:

$$C = (F_2 - F_1)/(P_2 - P_1) \qquad (6)$$

In a variation of the constant-pressure perfusion method, the flow of fluid from the reservoir into the anterior chamber is set with the constant rate of infusion by a syringe pump. At each of two different flows (F_1 and F_2), a resulting pressure is recorded (P_1 and P_2) and formula 6 is used again. This is the constant-flow perfusion method.

Two major problems exist with the perfusion method. One is the need to insert needles in the eye which can cause trauma and breakdown of the blood–aqueous barrier in some animals. Also, this precludes its use in humans. The other is the 'washout' phenomenon. When an eye is perfused experimentally, the flow resistance of the eye decreases progressively, probably from the depletion of proteins in the trabecular meshwork.

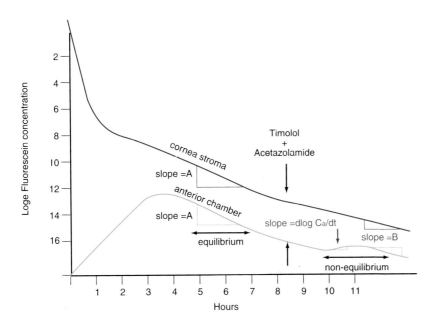

Figure 3.13 Time course of fluorescein concentration in the corneal stroma and anterior chamber after topical administration. At equilibrium, the absolute value of the slope of the fluorescein decay curves for both the cornea and anterior chamber is A. If the volumes of the cornea and anterior chamber remain constant in the steady state, then the magnitude of the anterior chamber aqueous humor flow is a function of A and C_c/C_a, the ratio of the fluorescein concentrations in the cornea and anterior chamber. At equilibrium, this ratio does not change over time. Baseline aqueous flow is calculated from the equilibrium data when the cornea and anterior chamber decay curves are parallel. Aqueous flow suppressants will change the slope of the curve, after a period of non-equilibrium, to a new slope, B. Two quick-acting aqueous flow suppressants that do not have any effect on outflow are oral acetazolamide and topical timolol. They are used to determine trabecular outflow facility by fluorophotometry and equation 6.

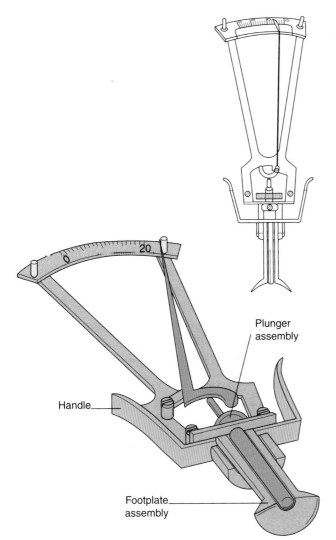

Figure 3.14 The Schiotz tonometer. The tonometer weighs 16.5 g when a 5.5-g weight is applied to the central plunger assembly. From the indentation of the cornea, one can infer the IOP (the higher the IOP the less the cornea indentation caused by the plunger). For higher pressures, higher plunger weights should be applied. The relationship between corneal indentation and IOP assumes a 'normal' scleral rigidity and corneal curvature.

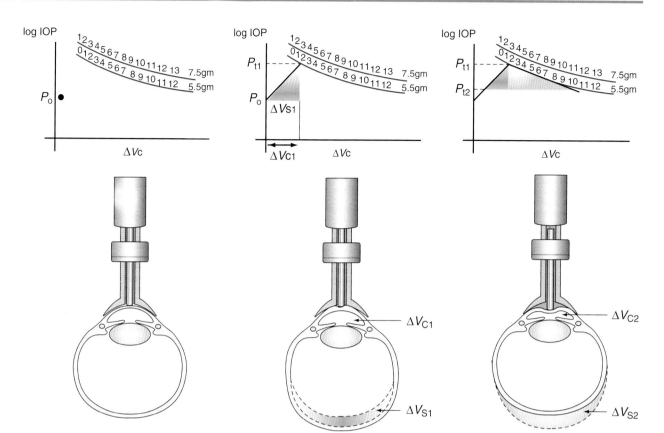

Figure 3.15 Tonography. Tonography exploits the fact that the 16.5-g weight of the Schiotz tonometer raises IOP while it is being applied to the cornea. This increase in IOP causes an increase in the rate of outflow of aqueous humor across the trabecular meshwork. The ratio of the increase in flow across the trabecular meshwork to the increase in IOP is the trabecular outflow facility, $C_{trab} = \Delta F_{trab}/\Delta IOP$.

The figure on the left shows the eye just before the weight of the tonometer is applied. The baseline IOP, P_o, before application of the tonometer, is shown on the graph by the dot indicating that, when measured by the applanation tonometer, the cornea was only slightly indented (about 0.5 μl). Therefore, the applanation tonometer does not change the IOP during its measurement. In contrast, as shown in the middle figure and graph, the Schiotz tonometer, when applied to the eye, indents the cornea to appreciably decrease the anterior chamber volume by ΔV_{C1} which pushes fluid posteriorly to expand the sclera by ΔV_{S1}. ΔV_{C1} equals $-\Delta V_{S1}$. The IOP correspondingly rises, with the above changes in intraocular volumes, to P_{t1} along the line shown in the graph whose slope equals the scleral rigidity, defined as $\Delta logIOP/\Delta V_{S1}$. This line connects the point representing the applanation IOP, P_o, to the number on the appropriate nomogram curve for the Schiotz plunger weight used, which gives the reading of corneal indentation on the Schiotz scale. The figure and graph on the right show the situation after t minutes of tonography. The cornea has further indented to decrease anterior chamber volume by ΔV_{C2}. ΔV_{C2} is caused by fluid exiting through the trabecular meshwork, in excess of normal trabecular flow, during the period of the tonography measurement. In addition, because IOP has decreased from P_{t1} to P_{t2}, during the period t of tonography, scleral volume contracts along the same scleral rigidity slope as shown in the middle graph, yielding ΔV_{S2}. This contraction of scleral volume also represents fluid loss from the eye during the tonography period. Total fluid forced out across the trabecular meshwork, above that which normally flows across the trabecular meshwork, therefore is equal to $\Delta V_{C2} + \Delta V_{S2}$. This value is given by the length of the horizontal line connecting the final reading on the nomogram to the scleral rigidity line, as shown in the graph. Dividing this volume by t gives the rate of this excess outflow during tonography. The average IOP during the period of tonography is assumed to equal $(P_{t1} + P_{t2})/2$ and the increase in IOP causing the increase in trabecular flow, above normal flow, is equal to $(P_{t1} + P_{t2})/2 - P_o$. Inserting these values into the above equation yields:

$$C_{trab} = \Delta F_{trab}/\Delta IOP = (\Delta V_{C2} + \Delta V_{S2})/((P_{t1} + P_{t2})/2 - P_o)t$$

Some of the assumptions that go into the calculation of outflow facility from tonography are that the rate of aqueous humor production during tonography remains at the normal rate and that the change from P_{t1} to P_{t2} is due to fluid being forced out of the eye only across the trabecular meshwork. Any decrease in the rate of aqueous humor formation or, if fluid is forced out of the eye by non-trabecular routes, for example decreased blood volume or extracellular fluid volume, are the term included in 'pseudofacility'. Pseudofacility is an inherent part of tonography. Therefore, the outflow facility measured by tonography equals the true trabecular outflow facility plus pseudofacility.

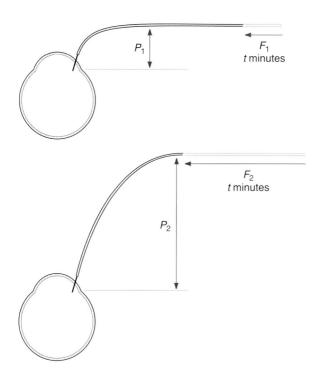

Figure 3.16   Measurement of outflow facility by the two-level constant pressure perfusion method (C_{tot}). A cannula connected to a reservoir filled with mock aqueous humor is inserted into the anterior chamber. The end of the cannula is placed at an exact height above the eye to establish a specific pressure (P_1) above the spontaneous intraocular pressure. The amount of fluid flowing into the eye during time t to maintain P_1 is F_1. The cannula end is raised to a new height to establish a new pressure (P_2) and, during the next time interval, t, the flow of fluid into the eye to maintain P_2 is F_2. C_{tot} is calculated as $(F_2 - F_1)/(P_2 - P_1)$.

The consequence of this is an artifactual increase over time in the experimentally measured outflow facility.

Circumventing the problems of the perfusion method is a non-invasive fluorophotometric method to assess C. This method has been used productively in humans. After measuring the intraocular pressure (P) with tonometry and aqueous flow (F) with fluorophotometry, the patient is given either a carbonic anhydrase inhibitor or a β-blocker to reduce F and hence reduce P. These drugs are known to reduce intraocular pressure solely by reducing aqueous flow (Figure 3.17) so they are the pharmacological equivalent of lowering the reservoir and slowing the infusion pump. One to three hours after administering the aqueous flow suppressants, intraocular pressure is remeasured and formula 6 is used to calculate C. This method avoids the problems of pseudofacility and scleral rigidity, and it can detect changes in trabecular outflow facility that are missed by tonography. This method does not work well in subjects with low IOPs because an IOP and aqueous flow reduction is difficult to achieve.

Uveoscleral outflow

One technique for measuring uveoscleral outflow is to infuse a large-molecule tracer, in which the flux can be assumed to be entirely by solvent drag, into the anterior chamber at a predetermined pressure. Usually radioactive-labeled protein or fluorescein-labeled dextran are used as tracers. At a specified time, usually 30 to 60 minutes, the eye is enucleated and dissected. All of the tracer collected from the ocular tissues and ocular fluids (minus the anterior chamber fluid) within the given time period is considered to be uveoscleral outflow (Figure 3.18). If the time of tracer infusion exceeds the time needed to saturate the tissues then there is a risk of loss of tracer from the globe. Some research laboratories handle this problem by collecting periocular and periorbital tissues, but they run the risk of collecting tracer exiting the eye via the trabecular meshwork and thus overestimating F_u. Without collecting these extraocular tissues however, underestimating F_u is a distinct possibility.

The second technique to determine uveoscleral outflow is an indirect assessment. By measuring all other components of aqueous humor dynamics, one can calculate F_u with the formula:

$$F_u = F_a - (C(\text{IOP} - P_{ev})) \quad (7)$$

This provides a means of evaluating F_u without sacrifice of the animal and it can be used repeatedly in animals and humans. The drawback is that mean F_u measured in this way has a large standard deviation. This is because of the variability of each of the components defining F_u (equation 7). This can be overcome by the use of a large number of subjects to minimize the standard error of the mean.

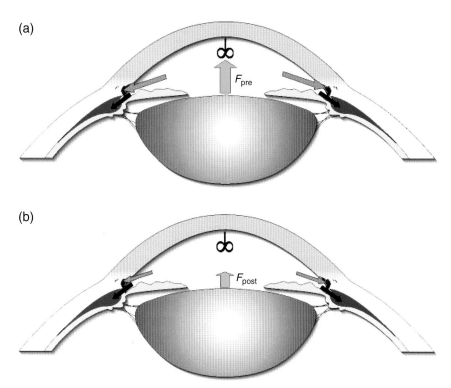

Figure 3.17 Measurement of outflow facility by fluorophotometry. The measurement of outflow facility by fluorophotometry is like that of tonography and of the two-level constant pressure method, in that it also attempts to measure a change in flow across the trabecular meshwork caused by a known change in IOP. After measuring the baseline flow of aqueous humor, F_{pre} (green arrow in a), from the equilibrium data, the eye is treated with a topical β-blocker and/or systemic carbonic anhydrase inhibitor, causing a decrease in anterior chamber aqueous humor flow to F_{post} (green arrow in b). It is assumed that the entire difference between F_{pre} and F_{post} causes an equal decrease in trabecular outflow, F_{trab} (blue arrow into canal of Schlemm). In other words, it is assumed that the magnitude of uveoscleral flow F_{u} (black arrow) is unchanged by the administration of topical β-blocker and/or systemic carbonic anhydrase inhibitor. Therefore, unlike tonography or the two-level constant pressure method, pseudofacility does not contaminate the measurement, since the change in flow across the trabecular meshwork is measured more directly. Dividing this change in flow, ΔF_{trab} by the corresponding change in IOP yields the fluorophotometrically determined outflow facility: $C_{trab} = \Delta F_{trab}/\Delta IOP$. It can be assumed that the outflow facility measured by this technique is closer to the true outflow facility, since pseudofacility is bypassed by this method. To determine the magnitude of uveoscleral flow, F_{trab} is calculated by multiplying C_{trab} by outflow pressure (IOP – P_{ev}), using the baseline IOP and episcleral venous pressure (P_{ev}) measured by venomanometry: $F_{trab} = C_{trab}$ (IOP – P_{ev}). Subtracting F_{trab} from baseline F_{pre} yields baseline uveoscleral flow, F_{u}: $F_{u} = F_{pre} - F_{trab}$.

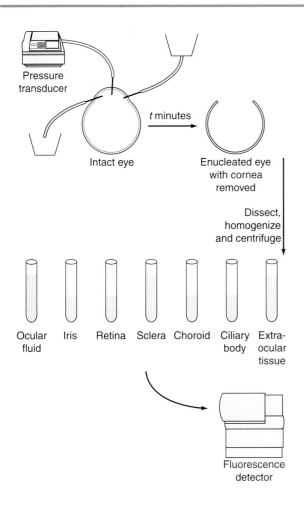

Ocular fluid | Iris | Retina | Sclera | Choroid | Ciliary body | Extra-ocular tissue

Fluorescence detector

Figure 3.18 Measurement of uveoscleral outflow with infusion of intracameral tracer. A large-molecular-weight tracer such as fluorescein isothiocynate dextran is infused into the anterior chamber of an anesthetized animal at a pressure of around spontaneous intraocular pressure (IOP). IOP is monitored with a pressure transducer. After a 30–60-min time interval (t), infusion is stopped, the eye is enucleated, the cornea is removed and the surface of the iris and lens are rinsed to remove all intracameral tracer. The eye is dissected into the tissues as shown. The supernatant from each homogenized and centrifuged sample is measured with a fluorescence detector. Uveoscleral outflow (F_u) is calculated by dividing the sum of all the tissue tracer values, expressed as equivalent volumes of aqueous (ΣV), by the infusion time (t), $F_u = \Sigma V/t$.

REFERENCES

1. Yablonski ME, Zimmerman TJ, Waltman SR, Becker B. A fluorophotometric study of the effect of topical timolol on aqueous humor dynamics. Exp Eye Res 1978; 27: 135–42

2. Coakes RL, Brubaker RF. The mechanism of timolol in lowering intraocular pressure in the normal eye. Arch Ophthalmol 1978; 96: 2045–8

3. Topper JE, Brubaker RF. Effects of timolol, epinephrine, and acetazolamide on aqueous flow during sleep. Invest Ophthalmol Vis Sci 1985; 26: 1315–19

4. Yablonski ME, Novack GD, Burke PJ, et al. The effect of levobunolol on aqueous humor dynamics. Exp Eye Res 1987; 44: 49–54

5. Araie M, Takase M. Effects of S-596 and carteolol, new beta-adrenergic blockers, and flurbiprofen on the human eye: a fluorophotometric study. Graefes Arch Clin Exp Ophthalmol 1985; 222: 259–62

6. Reiss GR, Brubaker RF. The mechanism of betaxolol, a new ocular hypotensive agent. Ophthalmology 1983; 90: 1369–72

7. Ingram CJ, Brubaker RF. Effect of brinzolamide and dorzolamide on aqueous humor flow in human eyes. Am J Ophthalmol 1999; 128: 292–6

8. Brubaker RF, Schoff EO, Nau CB, et al. Effects of AGN 192024, a new ocular hypotensive agent, on aqueous dynamics. Am J Ophthalmol 2001; 131: 19–24

9. Christiansen GA, Nau CB, McLaren JW, Johnson DH. Mechanism of ocular hypotensive action of bimatoprost (Lumigan) in patients with ocular hypertension or glaucoma. Ophthalmology 2004; 111: 1658–62

10. Dinslage S, Hueber A, Diestelhorst M, Krieglstein GK. The influence of Latanoprost 0.005% on aqueous humor flow and outflow facility in glaucoma patients: a double-masked placebo-controlled clinical study. Graefes Arch Clin Exp Ophthalmol 2004; 242: 654–60

11. Toris CB, Camras CB, Yablonski ME. Effects of PhXA41, a new prostaglandin F_{2a} analog, on aqueous humor dynamics in human eyes. Ophthalmology 1993; 100: 1297–304

12. Ziai N, Dolan JW, Kacere RD, Brubaker RF. The effects on aqueous dynamics of PhXA41, a new prostaglandin F_{2a} analogue, after topical application in normal and ocular hypertensive human eyes. Arch Ophthalmol 1993; 111: 1351–8

13. Toris CB, Zhan G, Camras CB. Increase in outflow facility with unoprostone treatment in ocular hypertensive patients. Arch Ophthalmol 2004; 122: 1782–7

14. Gaasterland D, Kupfer C, Ross K. Studies of aqueous humor dynamics in man. IV. Effects of pilocarpine upon measurements in young normal volunteers. Invest Ophthalmol 1975; 14: 848–53

15. Toris CB, Zhan G-L, Zhao J, et al. Potential mechanism for the additivity of pilocarpine and latanoprost. Am J Ophthalmol 2001; 131: 722–8

16. Gharagozloo NZ, Relf SJ, Brubaker RF. Aqueous flow is reduced by the alpha-adrenergic agonist, apraclonidine hydrochloride (ALO 2145). Ophthalmology 1988; 95: 1217–20

17. Toris CB, Tafoya ME, Camras CB, Yablonski ME. Effects of apraclonidine on aqueous humor dynamics in human eyes. Ophthalmology 1995; 102: 456–61

18. Larsson L-I. Aqueous humor flow in normal human eyes treated with brimonidine and timolol, alone and in combination. Arch Ophthalmol 2001; 119: 492–5

19. Maus TL, Nau C, Brubaker RF. Comparison of the early effects of brimonidine and apraclonidine as topical ocular hypotensive agents. Arch Ophthalmol 1999; 117: 586–91

20. Toris CB, Camras CB, Yablonski ME. Acute versus chronic effects of brimonidine on aqueous humor dynamics in ocular hypertensive patients. Am J Ophthalmol 1999; 128: 8–14

21. Toris CB, Gleason ML, Camras CB, Yablonski ME. Effects of brimonidine on aqueous humor dynamics in human eyes. Arch Ophthalmol 1995; 113: 1514–17

22. Kupfer C, Gaasterland D, Ross K. Studies of aqueous humor dynamics in man. II. Measurements in young normal subjects using acetazolamide and L-epinephrine. Invest Ophthalmol 1971; 10: 523–33

23. Schenker HI, Yablonski ME, Podos SM, Linder L. Fluorophotometric study of epinephrine and timolol in human subjects. Arch Ophthalmol 1981; 99: 1212–16

24. Townsend DJ, Brubaker RF. Immediate effect of epinephrine on aqueous formation in the normal human eye as measured by fluorophotometry. Invest Ophthalmol Vis Sci 1980; 19: 256–66

25. Wang Y-L, Hayashi M, Yablonski ME, Toris CB. Effects of multiple dosing of epinephrine on aqueous humor dynamics in human eyes. J Ocul Pharmacol Ther 2002; 18: 53–63

Further reading

Araie M, Sawa M, Takase M. Physiological study of the eye as studied by oral fluorescein. I. Oral administration of fluorescein and its pharmacokinetics. J Jpn Ophthalmol Soc 1980; 84: 1003–11

Bárány EH, Kinsey VE. The rate of flow of aqueous humor: I. The rate of disappearance of para-aminohippuric acid, radioactive Rayopake, and radioactive Diodrast from the aqueous humor of rabbits. Am J Ophthalmol 1949; 32: 177–88

Bárány EH. Simultaneous measurement of changing the intraocular pressure and outflow facility in the vervet monkey by constant pressure infusion. Invest Ophthalmol 1964; 3: 135–43

Bill A. The aqueous humor drainage mechanism in the cynomolgus monkey (Macaca irus) with evidence for unconventional routes. Invest Ophthalmol 1965; 4: 911–19

Bill A, Bárány EH. Gross facility, facility of conventional routes, and pseudofacility of aqueous humor outflow in the cynomolgus monkey. Arch Ophthalmol 1966; 75: 665–73

Bill A. Conventional and uveo-scleral drainage of aqueous humour in the cynomolgus monkey (Macaca irus) at normal and high intraocular pressures. Exp Eye Res 1966; 5: 45–54

Bill A. Further studies on the influence of the intraocular pressure on aqueous humor dynamics in cynomolgus monkeys. Invest Ophthalmol 1967; 6: 364–72

Bill A. Aqueous humor dynamics in monkeys (Macaca irus and Cercopithecus ethiops). Exp Eye Res 1971; 11: 195–206

Bill A, Phillips CI. Uveoscleral drainage of aqueous humour in human eyes. Exp Eye Res 1971; 12: 275–81

Bill A. Blood circulation and fluid dynamics in the eye. Physiol Rev 1975; 55: 383–417

Bill A. Basic physiology of the drainage of aqueous humor. Exp Eye Res 1977; 25: 291–304

Brubaker RF. Flow of aqueous humor in humans. Invest Ophthalmol Vis Sci 1991; 32: 3145–66

Cole DF. Secretion of the aqueous humour. Exp Eye Res 1977; 25: 161–76

Diamond JM, Bossert WH. Standing-gradient osmotic flow. A mechanism for coupling of water and solute transport in epithelia. J Gen Physiol 1967; 50: 2061–83

Friedenwald JS. Some problems with the calibration of tonometers. Am J Ophthalmol 1948; 31: 935–44

Goldmann H. Abflussdruck, minutenvolumen und widerstand der kammerwasser-strömung des menschen. Doc Ophthalmol 1951; 5–6: 278–356

Grant WM. Tonographic method for measuring the facility and rate of aqueous flow in human eyes. Arch Ophthalmol 1950; 44: 204–14

Grant WM. Clinical measurements of aqueous outflow. AMA Arch Ophthalmol 1951; 46: 113–31

Hayashi M, Yablonski ME, Mindel JS. Methods for assessing the effects of pharmacologic agents on aqueous humor dynamics. In: Tasman W, Jaeger EA, eds. Duane's Biomedical Foundations of Ophthalmology. Philadelphia: JB Lippincott, 1990: 1–9

Hayashi M, Yablonski ME, Novack GD. Trabecular outflow facility determined by fluorophotometry in human subjects. Exp Eye Res 1989; 48: 621–5

Holm O, Krakau CET. Measurements of the flow of aqueous humor according to a new principle. Experientia 1966; 22: 773–4

Holm O. A photogrammetric method for estimation of the pupillary aqueous flow in the living human eye. Acta Ophthalmol 1968; 46: 254–77

Jacob E, FitzSimon JS, Brubaker RF. Combined corticosteroid and catecholamine stimulation of aqueous humor flow. Ophthalmology 1996; 103: 1303–8

Johnson M, Gong H, Freddo TF, Ritter N, Kamm R. Serum proteins and aqueous outflow resistance in bovine eyes. Invest Ophthalmol Vis Sci 1993; 34: 3549–57

Jones RF, Maurice DM. New methods of measuring the rate of aqueous flow in man with fluorescein. Exp Eye Res 1966; 5: 208–20

Kaufman PL. Aqueous humor dynamics. In: Duane TD, ed: Clinical Ophthalmology. Philadelphia. Harper & Row, 1985: 1–24

Langham ME, Taylor CB. The influence of superior cervical ganglionectomy on intraocular dynamics. J Physiol 1960; 152: 447–58

Linnér E, Friedenwald JS. The appearance time of fluorescein as an index of aqueous flow. Am J Ophthalmol 1957; 44: 225–9

Mäepea O, Bill A. The pressures in the episcleral veins, Schlemm's canal and the trabecular meshwork in monkeys: effects of changes in intraocular pressure. Exp Eye Res 1989; 49: 645–63

Nagataki S. Effects of adrenergic drugs on aqueous humor dynamics in man. J Jpn Ophthalmol Soc 1977; 81: 1795–800

O'Rourke J, Macri FJ. Studies in uveal physiology. II. Clinical studies of the anterior chamber clearance of isotopic tracers. Arch Ophthalmol 1970; 84: 415–20

Reiss GR, Lee DA, Topper JE, Brubaker RF. Aqueous humor flow during sleep. Invest Ophthalmol Vis Sci 1984; 25: 776–8

Sperber GO, Bill A. A method for near-continuous determination of aqueous humor flow; effects of anaesthetics, temperature and indomethacin. Exp Eye Res 1984; 39: 435–53

Toris CB, Pederson JE. Effect of intraocular pressure on uveoscleral outflow following cyclodialysis in the monkey eye. Invest Ophthalmol Vis Sci 1985; 26: 1745–9

Toris CB, Wang Y-L, Chacko DM. Acetazolamide and the posterior flow of aqueous humor. Invest Ophthalmol Vis Sci 1995; 36(4): S724 (Abstract)

Toris CB, Yablonski ME, Wang Y-L, Hayashi M. Prostaglandin A_2 increases uveoscleral outflow and trabecular outflow facility in the cat. Exp Eye Res 1995; 61: 649–57

Wang Y-L, Toris CB, Zhan G, Yablonski ME. Effects of topical epinephrine on aqueous humor dynamics in the cat. Exp Eye Res 1999; 68: 439–45

4 Intraocular pressure and its measurement

Neil T Choplin

INTRODUCTION

Intraocular pressure is determined by the relative balance between the production and drainage of aqueous humor, discussed in Chapter 3. The range of intraocular pressures in the normal population is fairly wide, showing a quasi-normal distribution with a skew to the right (Figure 4.1). In the non-glaucomatous population (defined as having normal-appearing optic nerves and without detectable visual field loss) the average intraocular pressure is approximately 16 mmHg with a standard deviation of 2.5. The 'statistical' normal range, defined as the mean ± two standard deviations, would therefore be approximately 11–21 mmHg. Two to three per cent of the normal population would be expected to have pressures above the statistical upper limit, and it is this segment of the population that is said to have 'ocular hypertension'.

Intraocular pressure in a given eye is subject to a certain degree of variability from day to day and hour to hour. This 'diurnal variation' in pressure is usually no more than 4 mmHg in normal eyes, with the majority of eyes having their highest pressure during the late morning. Furthermore, intraocular pressure in the supine position is higher at all times compared to the upright position, and in many patients the highest intraocular pressure may actually occur in the very early morning hours while sleeping (supine). Eyes with glaucoma may show much greater variability in measurement during the course of a day, sometimes spiking very high pressures while measuring within the normal range at other times (Figure 4.2). Some of this variability has been attributed to, among other things, serum cortisol levels which are also subject to diurnal variation. Diurnal variation is one of the factors that makes intraocular pressure measurement a poor screening tool for glaucoma, since a pressure reading within the normal range does not rule out glaucoma. The measurement of the 'diurnal curve', with particular attention to uncovering pressure

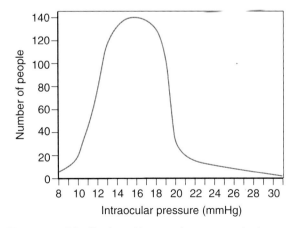

Figure 4.1 Distribution of intraocular pressure in the normal population. The pressure approximates normal distribution around a mean of 16 ± 2.5 mmHg. The tail to the right (above 21 mmHg) represents the segment of the population with 'ocular hypertension'.

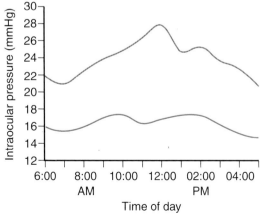

Figure 4.2 Diurnal variation in intraocular pressure. Normal pressure shows limited variation during the course of a day (bottom curve), while eyes with glaucoma may show considerably more variation (top curve).

spikes, should be considered in any patient with apparent glaucomatous optic neuropathy in whom the pressure has been measured within the normal range, or in any glaucoma patient who appears to be progressing despite normal pressure readings.

Since intraocular pressure is determined by the relative balance between aqueous humor inflow and outflow, any factors which increase inflow and/or decrease outflow will raise intraocular pressure, while factors decreasing aqueous formation and/or increasing outflow will lower pressure. Some of these factors are listed in Table 4.1.

using manometric techniques is obviously impractical, and so indirect measurements have been devised. These techniques rely upon the determination of the eye's response to an externally applied force. Tonometers developed for the purpose of measuring intraocular pressure fall into two categories: indentation, in which the amount of corneal or globe deformation in response to an externally applied weight is determined, and applanation, in which the force necessary to flatten a known surface area of cornea is determined. In both cases it is the intraocular pressure that resists the externally applied force.

MEASUREMENT OF INTRAOCULAR PRESSURE

The measurement of intraocular pressure should be part of any eye examination. Direct measurement of pressure by cannulation of the anterior chamber

ESTIMATION OF INTRAOCULAR PRESSURE BY PALPATION

In the absence of an instrument to measure eye pressure, an estimation can be made by palpation.

Table 4.1   Factors affecting intraocular pressure

Site of action	Increased inflow (raising pressure)	Decreased inflow (lowering pressure)	Decreased outflow (raising pressure)	Increased outflow (lowering pressure)
Ciliary body	Increased fluid load Increased blood flow Beta agonists	Decreased body fluid (dehydration) Reduced blood flow Beta blockers Digitalis Cyclitis Age Carbonic anhydrase inhibitors Alpha$_2$ agonists Choroidal detachment, uveal effusion Surgical destruction		
Conventional outflow pathways			Age Prostaglandin E$_1$ Pigment, debris Anticholinergics, e.g. atropine Corticosteroids	Cholinergics, e.g. pilocarpine Laser trabeculoplasty
Non-conventional outflow pathways			Cholinergics, e.g. pilocarpine	Anticholinergics, e.g. atropine Alpha$_2$ agonists Prostaglandin F$_{2alpha}$ analogs, e.g. latanoprost
Blood–aqueous barrier	Breakdown, e.g. uveitis Osmotic gradients, e.g. protein Cholinergics, e.g. phospholine iodide	Stabilization, e.g. anti-inflammatories Anticholinergics, e.g. atropine		
Other			Angle closure Increased episcleral venous pressure	Sclerostomy Rhegmatogenous retinal detachment Cyclodialysis cleft

Although palpation is not highly accurate, it is usually easy to differentiate between very low and very high pressure. Obviously, this technique should not be employed in cases of suspected globe rupture. It is useful in emergency-room settings when faced with a patient with a red painful eye, and acute glaucoma is in the differential diagnosis. To estimate intraocular pressure by palpation, the patient should close the eye and look down. The examiner uses the index finger of both hands, gently alternating pressure to the superior part of the eye through the closed lids, to determine the force necessary to indent the eye wall (Figure 4.3). It is usually obvious whether the eye is rock hard or very soft. If palpation is applied after determining pressure by another technique, the examiner may become quite capable of estimating intraocular pressure to within 2–3 mmHg.

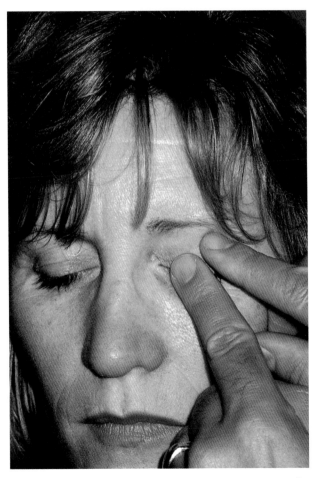

Figure 4.3 Estimation of intraocular pressure by palpation. The patient is instructed to close the eye and look down. The examiner uses the index fingers of both hands, alternately applying slight pressure to estimate the force necessary to indent the globe. The resistance to indentation is provided by the intraocular pressure. By correlating 'finger tension' with applanation readings obtained just prior to palpation, the examiner can learn how much force correlates with varying levels of intraocular pressure, and may be able to estimate intraocular pressure to within 2–3 mmHg.

SCHIOTZ TONOMETRY

The Schiotz tonometer is an indentation instrument which measures intraocular pressure by registering the depth of indentation of the cornea produced when the instrument, carrying a known weight, is applied to the anesthetized eye. The instrument is illustrated schematically in Figure 4.4. The weight is carried on a plunger which should move freely within the holder. When the weight is applied to the eye, the intraocular pressure provides a counterbalancing force which pushes back up on the plunger. This causes a deflection of the pointer along the inclined scale transmitted through the convex hammer. Each unit on the scale, which ranges from 1 to 20, corresponds to an indentation of 1/20 of a millimeter in the cornea. High intraocular pressure resists indentation, resulting in low scale readings, while low intraocular pressure allows for easy indentation, manifested by high scale readings. In cases with elevated intraocular pressure (scale readings of less than 4 with any weight), the next higher weight should be placed on top of the standard 5.5 g weight until a scale reading greater than 4 is obtained. The intraocular pressure is determined by referring to the calibration chart (Figure 4.5) and reading the pressure that corresponds to the scale reading for the plunger load applied.

In order to perform a measurement, the patient must be supine (Figure 4.6). Topical anesthetic is applied. Calibration of the instrument is tested by placing the plunger on the test block provided in the case; a scale reading of zero should be obtained (a set screw is provided on the handle for any necessary adjustments). The examiner then gently holds the patient's lids open (without exerting pressure on the globe), instructs the patient to look straight ahead, and places the instrument on the cornea. The handle is then lowered to a position midway between the top and bottom of the cylinder. The scale reading is determined by lining up the pointer with its mirror image on the inclined scale, thus providing a reading free of parallax. The intraocular pressure is then determined by reading from the chart as above.

Although the Schiotz tonometer is generally accurate, it has largely been replaced by other forms of tonometry. First, the positioning of the patient that is required makes the instrument somewhat awkward to use. More importantly, measurements may be subject to fairly large errors induced by scleral rigidity. For example, myopic eyes are more elastic than other eyes. When an external weight is applied (such as a Schiotz tonometer), some of the weight may be dissipated through the sclera (which lacks resistance to distension), resulting in less resistance to corneal indentation and underestimation of intraocular pressure. The opposite is true of hyperopic (and more rigid) eyes.

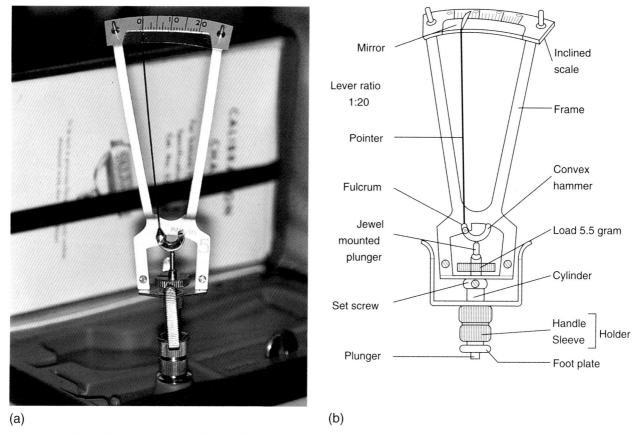

(a)   (b)

Figure 4.4   The Schiotz tonometer.   (a) A Schiotz tonometer resting on the calibration block. Since the block resists indentation, the scale should read zero. (b) Schematic diagram of a Schiotz tonometer. The various parts of the tonometer are labeled.

APPLANATION TONOMETRY

Applanation tonometry is the procedure of choice in most clinical situations, and tonometers have been developed for use both at the slit lamp and hand-held for use outside the examining lane. Included in this category are the Goldmann tonometer, the Perkins tonometer, the Mackay–Marg tonometer, the pneumatic tonometer, and the Tonopen. The underlying principle is similar for each instrument. Intraocular pressure is determined by measuring the force necessary to applanate, or flatten, a known surface area of the cornea.

Complete descriptions and instructions for use of each of the following instruments should be found in the manufacturer's documentation provided with the instrument.

GOLDMANN TONOMETER

The Goldmann tonometer (Figure 4.7) is probably the most widely used tonometer and is the international standard for measuring intraocular pressure. In developing this tonometer, a number of assumptions had to be made. The first was that the human eye could be approximated to a per-

fectly elastic and infinitely thin sphere, and that its internal pressure could be measured by applying an external force that would be resisted by that pressure. It was assumed also that the cornea had a central thickness of approximately 520 μm. However, human corneas vary considerably in thickness among individuals, and this is now known to affect the accuracy of Goldmann tonometry in measuring intraocular pressure. As early as 1975 it was shown, by measuring intraocular pressure manometrically at the time of cataract surgery, that eyes with thicker corneas measured higher than actual, and eyes with thinner corneas measured lower than actual. Measurements of intraocular pressure following laser vision correction are usually lower than the preoperative levels, now correctly attributed to the thinning of the cornea by laser ablation. Applying this principle to ocular hypertension, it has been demonstrated that eyes with ocular hypertension tend to have corneas that are thicker than average, and that eyes with thinner corneas are at higher risk for 'converting' to glaucoma at a given level of pressure. For example, in the Ocular Hypertension Treatment Study, eyes with pressures greater than 26 mmHg and central corneal thickness greater than 588 μm had a 6% chance of converting to glaucoma within 5 years, while those with central

Scale reading	Plunger load (in grams)			
	5.5	7.5	10.0	15.0
0	41	59	82	127
.5	38	54	75	118
1.0	35	50	70	109
1.5	32	46	64	101
2.0	29	42	59	94
2.5	27	39	55	88
3.0	24	36	51	82
3.5	22	33	47	76
4.0	21	30	43	71
4.5	19	28	40	66
5.0	17	26	37	62
5.5	16	24	34	58
6.0	15	22	32	54
6.5	13	20	29	50
7.0	12	19	27	46
7.5	11	17	25	43
8.0	10	16	23	40
8.5	9	14	21	38
9.0	9	13	20	35
9.5	8	12	18	32
10.0	7	11	16	30
10.5	6	10	15	27
11.0	6	9	14	25
11.5	5	8	13	23
12.0		8	11	21
12.5		7	10	20
13.0		6	10	18
13.5		6	9	17
14.0		5	8	15
14.5			7	14
15.0			6	13
15.5			6	11
16.0			5	10
16.5				9
17.0				8
17.5				8
18.0				7

Figure 4.5 Calibration chart for Schiotz tonometers. The amount of corneal indentation is read from the column on the left (corresponding to the scale reading). The intraocular pressure is listed under the load weight used to take the measurement.

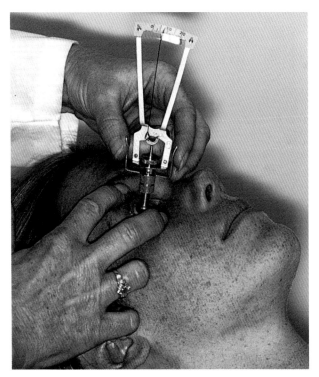

Figure 4.6 Measurement of intraocular pressure with a Schiotz tonometer. The patient is placed in the supine position and topical anesthetic applied. The examiner holds the lids open with the free hand, being careful not to apply any pressure to the globe. The patient is instructed to look straight ahead or fixate on a point on the ceiling with the fellow eye. Holding the instrument by the handles with the other hand, it is gently applied perpendicularly to the cornea until the foot plate rests on the cornea. Usually, when the instrument is properly positioned, there will be a gentle pulsation of the pointer, corresponding to the ocular pulse. The plunger, with the attached load weight, pushes down on the cornea and indents it to the amount allowed by the resistance of the intraocular pressure. This causes the jewel-mounted plunger to push back on the convex hammer, causing the pointer to deflect off zero on the inclined scale. Since the lever ratio is 1:20, the reading corresponds to the amount of corneal indentation × 0.05 mm. Once the scale reading has been determined, the intraocular pressure is read from the calibration chart.

corneal thickness less than 555 μm had a 36% chance. Similarly, many eyes with 'normal tension glaucoma' have been shown to have thinner than average corneas, and eyes with thinner than average corneas have also been show to be at higher risk for glaucoma progression. Clinically, it is essential to put intraocular pressure measurements within the context of central corneal thickness measurements in order to properly assess a patient's risk for developing glaucoma or of it progressing. Although the exact relationship between true intraocular pressure, central corneal thickness, and intraocular

pressure as measured by the Goldmann applanation tonometer is not known, it has been estimated that the pressure varies by 1 mmHg for each 20 μm of thickness above or below 540 μm. This is summarized in Table 4.2. It is possible that in the near future we will have new tonometers available that will better approximate true intraocular pressure, either by incorporating central corneal thickness into their measurements, or by applying new measuring principles. One such tonometer under investigation as of this writing is the dynamic contour tonometer.

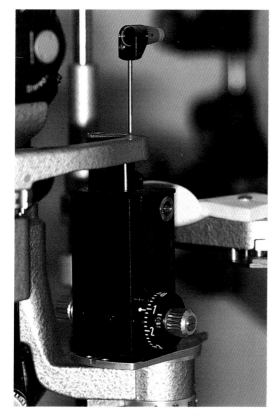

Figure 4.7 The Goldmann tonometer. Mounted on a slit lamp, the Goldmann tonometer consists of a tip attached by a rod to a coiled spring contained within the instrument housing. The tension on the spring, determined by the position of the calibrated knob, supplies the force used to flatten 3.06 mm of the central cornea. The tip contains a prism which splits the circular image of the flattened corneal surface into two semicircles, one above the other.

In using the Goldmann applanation tonometer, the flattening force to the cornea is supplied by a coiled spring contained in the housing of the instrument, controlled by a rotating knob at the base, and is applied to the anesthetized eye by the tip of a split prism device through which the cornea may be viewed with the slit lamp. The area of cornea flattened is 3.06 mm in diameter. Topical anesthetic and fluorescein are applied to the eye, and the tear film illuminated using the cobalt blue filter of the slit lamp. As the instrument is applied to the eye (Figure 4.8), the applanating head creates a circular tear film meniscus which may be viewed through the slit lamp. The prism in the applanating head splits the circular image into two semicircles, and the end point of the measurement is determined by adjusting the knob until the inside edges of the semicircles are just touching (Figure 4.9). The intraocular pressure is then determined by multiplying the reading on the scale on the knob by ten.

HAND-HELD TONOMETERS

The Perkins tonometer

The Perkins tonometer (Figure 4.10) is a battery-powered hand-held applanation tonometer which functions identically to the Goldmann tonometer. The mires are viewed directly through the instrument so a slit lamp is not necessary. It may be used in situations where the patient cannot sit at the slit lamp. The instrument is counterbalanced to allow it to be used in a variety of positions.

Table 4.2 Relationship between central corneal thickness and intraocular pressure	
Central corneal thickness (μm)	**'Correcting factor' (mmHg)**
405	7
425	6
445	5
465	4
485	3
505	2
525	1
545	0
565	−1
585	−2
605	−3
625	−4
645	−5
665	−6
685	−7
705	−8

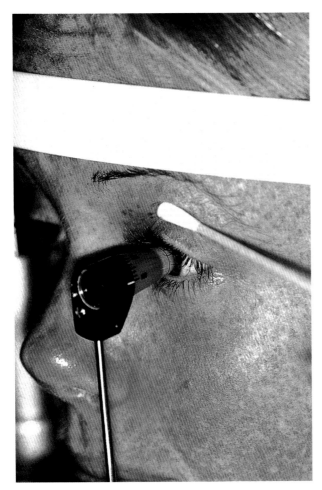

Figure 4.8   Measuring intraocular pressure with the Goldmann tonometer. The eye is anesthetized and the tear film stained with fluorescein. The instrument is then brought into the appropriate position on the slit lamp and the cobalt blue filter placed in the light path. The slit aperture should be opened widely. The tip of the instrument is gently placed against the cornea, and the image of the tear film is viewed through the biomicroscope. The knob is turned until the inner edges of the semicircles are just touching, indicating that 3.06 mm of corneal flattening has been attained, corresponding to the intraocular pressure. The reading on the knob is multiplied by ten to obtain the pressure reading.

The Mackay–Marg tonometer

The Mackay–Marg tonometer (Figure 4.11) was designed to measure intraocular pressure in eyes with scarred, irregular, or edematous corneas using a tip that is approximately half the diameter of that of the Goldmann tonometer. The movable tip protrudes from a surrounding foot plate and is supported by a spring connected to a transducer. The transducer senses the tension on the spring and translates that tension into a pressure reading. Basically, by advancing the tip on to the cornea, the bending pressure of the cornea (opposed by the intraocular pressure) is measured. Pressure readings are recorded on a moving paper strip.

(a)

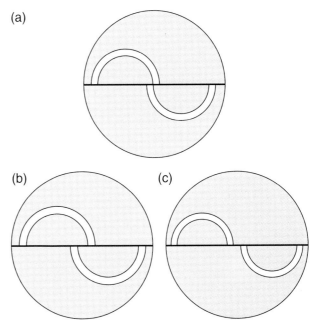

(b)   (c)

Figure 4.9   Tear film meniscus.   Appearance of tear film meniscus as viewed through the Goldmann tonometer during applanation tonometry. (a) Correct appearance of the mires when the applied force to the cornea is equal to the intraocular pressure. (b) Appearance of the mires when the applied force is greater than the intraocular pressure or the instrument is pushed too far into the eye, indicating that the cornea has been overflattened. (c) Appearance of the mires when the applied force is less than the intraocular pressure, indicating that the cornea has been underflattened.

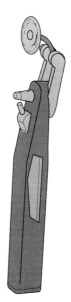

Figure 4.10 The Perkins tonometer. This tonometer employs the same principles as the Goldmann tonometer. The prism is mounted on a counterbalanced arm and the change in force obtained by rotation of a spiral spring. The disc at the top of the instrument is placed against the patient's forehead as a brace. The instrument can be used in any position and does not need to be held vertically.

The pneumatic tonometer

Another device useful for measuring pressure in eyes with scarred, irregular, and/or edematous corneas is the pneumatic tonometer (Figure 4.12). Measurements can also be made over bandaged contact lenses.

The Tonopen™

Advances in electronics and miniaturization have led to the development of a self-contained, compact, hand-held applanation tonometer that works on the same principle as the Mackay–Marg tonometer.

This has been marketed as the Tonopen (Figure 4.13). The device is gently applied to the anesthetized cornea (Figure 4.14) and intraocular pressure is displayed on a digital readout after five readings have been obtained. The spread of the measurements is also displayed as a percentage (Figure 4.15).

NON-CONTACT TONOMETRY

The non-contact (or air-puff) tonometer (Figure 4.16) was originally developed to allow the measurement

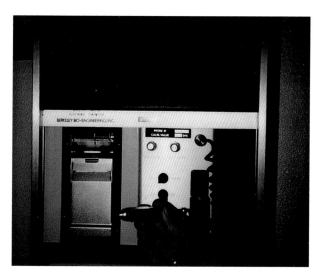

Figure 4.11 The Mackay–Marg Tonometer. This is another applanation-type device in which the movement of the tip is sensed by a transducer contained in the hand piece. The bending pressure of the cornea, opposed by the intraocular pressure, is determined. The instrument is useful for measuring the intraocular pressure in scarred, irregular, and/or edematous corneas.

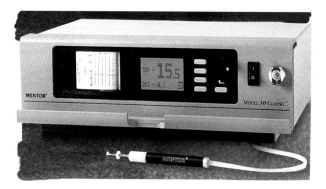

Figure 4.12 The pneumatic tonometer. The measuring device consists of a gas-filled chamber with a transducer capable of sensing the pressure in the chamber. As the device is applied to the eye, the counterpressure in the eye pushes back on the tip, raising the pressure on the gas until the end point is reached and recorded, either on a moving paper strip or displayed on a digital readout. This device may also be used for tonography.

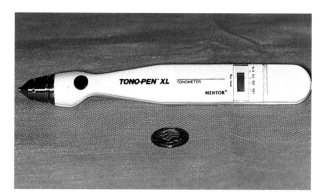

Figure 4.13 The Tonopen™. This miniaturized electronic applanation tonometer is battery powered and can be used in any position. It is very useful for measuring intraocular pressure in patients who cannot sit at a slit lamp. It is also useful for measuring pressures in patients with irregular corneas, since the applanation area is much smaller than that of the Goldmann instrument.

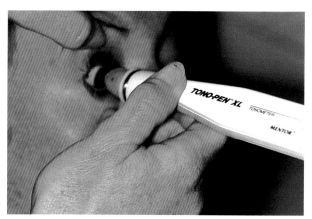

Figure 4.14 Measurement of intraocular pressure with the Tonopen™. The eye is anesthetized and the instrument tip is covered with a latex sleeve. The examiner holds the upper lid open, rests the hand holding the instrument on the patient's cheek, and gently and quickly touches the central cornea with the tip, moving the instrument rapidly on to and off the eye. A short beep will be emitted by the instrument when a measurement has been recorded, and the reading displayed when five successive measurements are obtained.

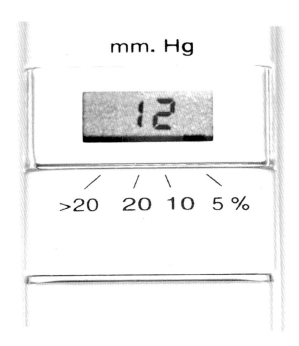

Figure 4.15 Intraocular pressure reading displayed on the Tonopen. The number indicates the average of the five readings in mmHg. A solid line will appear at the bottom of the printout corresponding to the percentage spread of the five readings (5%, 10%, 20%, or >20%).

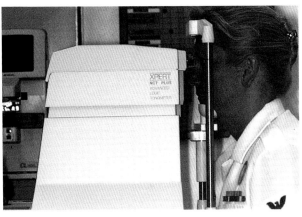

Figure 4.16 The non-contact tonometer. A patient is properly positioned for measurement of intraocular pressure with this instrument. The operator is seated to the left. No anesthetic is used. The eye to be measured is viewed on a CRT monitor, and, when the eye is properly aligned, the operator pushes a button which releases the air jet. Light sensors positioned on either side of the jet determine the degree of corneal flattening and when the end point has been reached. The patients usually react to the air jet with a slight startled response, but the measurement is not uncomfortable.

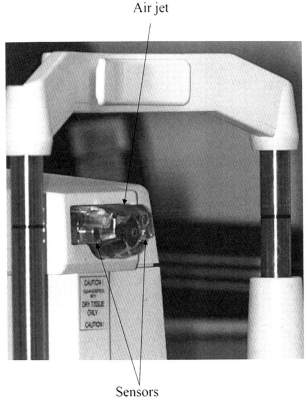

Figure 4.17 The 'business' end of a non-contact tonometer. The air jet is in the middle, with the two sensors on either side. As the air jet increases in force, the sensors determine when the end point of corneal flattening has been reached. The time required to reach this end point is directly related to the force opposing the flattening, i.e. the intraocular pressure.

of intraocular pressure by non-medical personnel since measurements may be obtained without the use of topical anesthetics. No part of the device touches the eye. The device uses a jet of air to applanate the cornea. Figure 4.17 shows the air jet and the sensors detect corneal flattening by means of reflected light. When activated, an air jet is blown at the cornea with increasing force over time. The cornea is illuminated with a collimated light beam which is reflected back to a detector, which determines when the reflected light reaches a maximum, corresponding to flattening of a corneal area 3.06 mm in diameter. The time required to reach this maximum reflection is directly related to the force of the air jet, counterbalanced by the intraocular pressure, and is translated into the intraocular pressure reading (Figure 4.18).

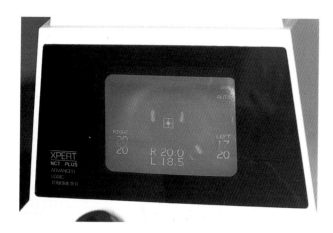

Figure 4.18 The display of a non-contact tonometer. The eye can be seen faintly in the center of the CRT. The pressure readings obtained for each eye are displayed, with the average in the middle.

Further reading

Brubaker RF. Tonometry. In: Duane's Clinical Ophthalmology, Vol 3. Philadelphia, PA: JB Lippincott, 1994

Ehlers N, Bramen T, Sperling S. Applanation tonometry and central corneal thickness. Acta Ophthalmol 1975; 53: 34–43

Gordon MO, Beiser JA, Brandt JD, et al., for the Ocular Hypertension Treatment Study Group. The Ocular Hypertension Treatment Study: baseline factors that predict the onset of primary open angle glaucoma. Arch Ophthalmol 2002; 120: 714–20

Herndon LW. Rethinking pachymetry and intraocular pressure. Rev Ophthalmol 2002; 9

Hitchings RA. Primary glaucoma. In: Slide Atlas of Ophthalmology, Vol 7. London: Gower Medical, 1984

Hoskins HD Jr, Kass M, eds. Becker–Shaffer's Diagnosis and Therapy of the Glaucomas, 6th edn. St Louis, MO: Mosby, 1989: 67–88

Mosaed S, Liu JH, Weinreb RN. Correlation between office and peak nocturnal intraocular pressures in healthy subjects and glaucoma patients. Am J Ophthalmol 2005; 139: 320–4

5 Gonioscopy

Ronald Fellman

INTRODUCTION

Collectively, primary angle closure and open angle glaucoma continue to be the leading causes of irreversible blindness afflicting at least 60 million people worldwide with over 7 million legally blind. Gonioscopy, the evaluation of the angle of the anterior chamber of the eye, is the only method to consistently diagnose and accurately differentiate these glaucomas. The long-term goal of gonioscopy is to reduce visual disability through the systematic evaluation and management of the chamber angle.

Gonioscopy is an essential component of vision care but continues to be underutilized. Recent studies of initial office visits for glaucoma in the United States found gonioscopy documented in less than half of all cases while evaluation of the disc was noted in 94%. Gonioscopy at an early stage of glaucomatous disease separates narrow from open angles with the resultant appropriate laser therapy and prevention of visual disability.

WHY PERFORM GONIOSCOPY?

Gonioscopy is underutilized because the function and appearance of the angle is typically inferred from the view of the anterior chamber as seen at the slit lamp. In addition, the reserve of the chamber angle is immense and may hide disease for years. Thus, even though the anterior chamber is always evaluated during routine slit lamp biomicroscopy, the chamber angle, with its vital outflow system and diagnostic clues, is hidden from ordinary view due to total internal reflection of light rays. Many examiners use the van Herick test to estimate depth of the peripheral anterior chamber. It is a screening tool designed to estimate depth of the iridocorneal angle but not a substitute for gonioscopy.

The intraocular pressure (IOP) is normal, and the chamber looks quiet. Why perform gonioscopy? (Table 5.1). It is good medical care to initially document the appearance of the chamber angle, just as it is to record the baseline appearance of the optic nerve for future reference.

The insurmountable problem of total internal reflection of light at the air–cornea–aqueous boundary is overcome with gonioscopy. With appropriate training, gonioscopy is easily integrated into a busy office schedule with minimal effort. This facilitates the differentiation of normal from abnormal angle structures and allows the early detection of ophthalmic disease. One gonioprism will not suffice for all occasions; the best gonioprism to rapidly screen the chamber angle in the clinic is not the best for laser therapy of the chamber angle or the best for an examination under anesthesia (Figure 5.1). This is due to the variable size, contour, contact area, mirror size and handle of the multitude of goniolenses and gonioprisms introduced in the next section.

PRINCIPLES OF GONIOSCOPY

The most important gonioscopic principle is to understand why total internal reflection of light occurs in the anterior compartment of the eye. Conquering this optical problem allows a more thorough appreciation of angle optics. Light rays emanating from the iris undergo four possible optical properties as they emerge from the cornea: (1) emerge bent; (2) emerge unbent or parallel; (3) follow the boundary; or (4) reflect internally. The observer does not see light rays from the chamber angle because of the last property, total internal reflection. A basic understanding of geometric optics is useful. Figure 5.2 is a good example of a patient with iris defects that involve angle structures that are clearly appreciated only through gonioscopy.

Table 5.1   Minimum indications for gonioscopy

Patient history reveals

Family member with angle closure or open angle disease

Symptoms compatible with angle closure disease

High-risk angle closure heritage (Asian, Alaskan, Indian heritage)

History of any type of glaucoma, field loss or disc damage

Ocular blunt trauma or history of foreign body

Diabetes mellitus or proliferative retinopathy

Ocular tumor

Failing vision

Topamax usage

Prior ocular surgery especially scleral buckle, penetrating keratoplasty, laser therapy, glaucoma surgery and cataract surgery

New patient examination or absence of gonioscopy for 2–4 years

Chart review reveals the absence of baseline gonioscopy

Patient examination reveals

Any sign of angle closure disease (glaucomflecken, iritis, iris atrophy)

Any iris lesion, vessel, coloboma, or cyst deserving gonioscopy

Positive van Herick or 'shallow chamber'

Elevated IOP, especially a significant change from baseline

Hyperopia

History of nanophthalmos

Pigment dispersion syndrome

Pseudoexfoliation syndrome

Anticipated trabeculoplasty

Retinal vascular occlusion

Hyphema

Posterior embryotoxon (prominent Schwalbe's line)

Inflammation with flare and cell

Miscellaneous

Preoperative cataract or glaucoma surgery to look for PAS

Following laser peripheral iridotomy or iridoplasty

After addition of pilocarpine

Post-trabeculectomy or non-penetrating glaucoma surgery

IOP rise post-dilatation with IOP greater than 6 mmHg

Without gonioscopy it is impossible to know how serious the angle pathology is.

The two most common clinical methods of viewing the chamber angle include direct and indirect gonioscopy (Figure 5.3). A Koeppe goniolens represents the prototype direct view of the angle and is most commonly used in the operating room. This is an excellent method to view the angle during an examination under anesthesia. A hand held slit lamp magnifies the view, creating a beautiful stereoscopic view of angle structures. The angle structures are viewed directly through the goniolens as seen in Figure 5.2c. Indirect gonioscopy is a rapid and efficient office-based approach to indirectly view the chamber angle as seen in Figure 5.2e. The light is reflected to the examiner from angle structures 180° away from the mirror. This is an important distinction because angle structures are directly viewed through a goniolens and indirectly seen through a gonioprism.

THE NORMAL ANGLE

An understanding of the immense variability of the normal angle is imperative in order to recognize the abnormal angle. Each angle is unique and changes as the patient ages, further complicating

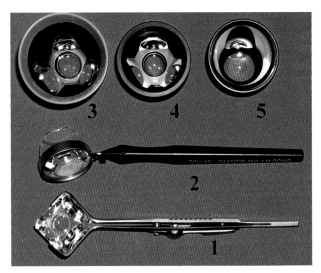

Figure 5.1 Office-based gonioscopy. A variety of gonio-prisms are necessary to accomplish a thorough examination and treatment of the chamber angle. Gonioprism number 1 is the Zeiss prism attached to an Unger handle. It is easily cleaned with alcohol because it is durable and made of glass. However, the silver coating may peel after extended use. The small 9-mm contact area of the Zeiss allows the patient's own tear film to act as a capillary bridge and a viscous gel is unnecessary. The same applies to prism 2, the Gaasterland prism (Ocular Instruments, Bellevue, Washington). Its small 9-mm contact area allows efficient compression gonioscopy, which is essential to differentiate appositional from synechial closure. The Gaasterland lens is a new generation lens that does not require a coating, making it easier to clean and maintain. Prisms 1 and 2 are excellent clinic gonioprisms because they are easily cleaned and disinfected and allow a rapid, efficient method to visualize the angle without patients complaining of discomfort from a larger more cumbersome prism. Gonioprism number 3 is the classic three-mirror Goldmann lens. This versatile lens is helpful when looking for peripheral retinal tears or ciliary body pathology. These lenses are bonded with a broad band antireflective coating to minimize reflections. The Goldmann-type prisms have a variable number of reflective mirrors and contact areas. The contact areas range from 13 to 20 mm. Patients with small palpebral fissures require the smaller Goldmann prisms ranging from 13 to 15 mm. Gonioprism 4 represents a smaller contact area and is useful for laser trabeculoplasty in patients with small palpebral fissures. Gonioprism 5 is the Magnaview lens made by Ocular Instruments. It provides additional magnification for trabeculoplasty.

our understanding of lifetime angle anatomy. Serious students of gonioscopy describe their angle findings and accurately record them, usually with a classification system.

There are six key anatomic landmarks to differentiate during gonioscopy (Figure 5.4):

1. Pupil border. Start the scan of the iridocorneal angle with the pupillary border, looking for blood vessels, iris cysts, ectropion uveae, and dandruff-like particles. At this point, examine the posterior chamber for diagnostic clues of misdirection, tumors, cyclitic membranes, cysts, and intraocular lens position. You may also view the fundus through the contact lens.

2. Peripheral iris. Identify the apparent site of iris insertion onto the inner wall of the eye, describe the peripheral configuration of the iris (flat, bows, concave, plateau), and characterize the angular approach of the iris to the cornea, 0° to 40°.

3. Ciliary body band. The ciliary body band is that portion of the ciliary body muscle seen on gonioscopy. The band has an average width of 0.75 mm and is usually tan, gray, or dark brown, and typically narrower in hyperopes and wider in myopes. The root of the iris usually inserts at the ciliary body band directly posterior to the scleral spur. If the iris inserts directly onto the scleral spur, the ciliary body band is difficult to see. A higher insertion of the iris may be normal in individuals of Asian or African descent. Ethnicity may reveal clues as to normal variation of the angle. If the iris inserts well posterior to the scleral spur, a wide ciliary body band is seen. The scleral spur is difficult to see in infants, but as the angle matures, the finer detail of the outflow system emerges.

4. Scleral spur. The scleral spur is the most notable landmark in the chamber angle. This white band represents the attachment of the ciliary body to the sclera and, if found, the trabecular meshwork is directly anterior and uveoscleral outflow posterior. The scleral spur separates conventional trabecular outflow from uveoscleral outflow and cyclodialysis clefts appear posterior to the spur and trabeculoplasty is carried out anterior to the spur. This is a critical structure in the delineation of iridocorneal anatomy.

5. Trabecular meshwork. The trabecular meshwork extends from the scleral spur to Schwalbe's line and initially has a ground-glass appearance. The average anterior-to-posterior measurement of the meshwork is 0.8 mm. Pigment in the meshwork usually accumulates in the posterior division and facilitates identification. However, any angle structure may accumulate pigment. The junction of the middle and posterior meshwork is the favored location for trabeculoplasty. When there is no pigment in the meshwork, the characteristic ground-glass appearance can be best seen with sclerotic scatter or by identification of the corneal optical wedge.

6. Schwalbe's line. Schwalbe's line represents the termination of Descemet's membrane and is the most visible anterior angle structure. Schwalbe's line marks the forward limit of the trabecular meshwork and is best appreciated through a Goldmann lens where the anterior and posterior reflections of the corneal optical wedge meet.

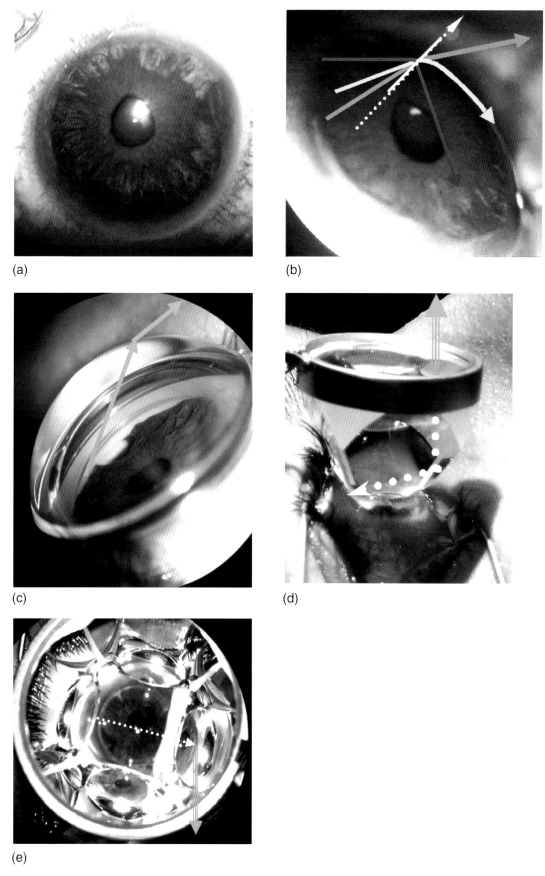

(a)

(b)

(c)

(d)

(e)

Figure 5.2   The natural inability to see the chamber angle.   (a) Iris atrophy. Routine biomicroscopy reveals iris atrophy but nothing definitive about the chamber angle. Clearly, any patient with iris anomalies requires gonioscopy. This patient has mesodermal dysgenesis. (b) Light rays. No matter how hard one tries, it is impossible to see into the chamber angle due to the physical interaction of light rays as they cross the aqueous–cornea–air interface. The construct of a light ray is grounded on establishing a perpendicular line at the air–cornea–aqueous boundary, called the normal (white line).

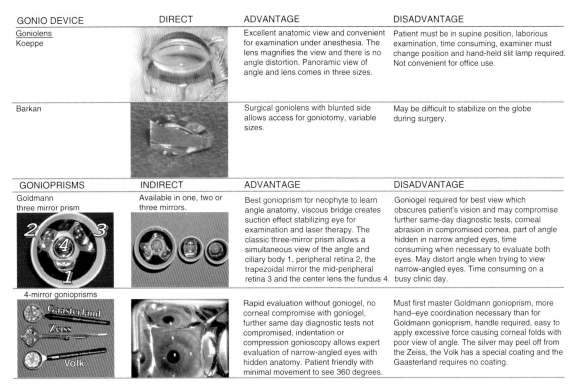

GONIO DEVICE	DIRECT	ADVANTAGE	DISADVANTAGE
Goniolens Koeppe		Excellent anatomic view and convenient for examination under anesthesia. The lens magnifies the view and there is no angle distortion. Panoramic view of angle and lens comes in three sizes.	Patient must be in supine position, laborious examination, time consuming, examiner must change position and hand-held slit lamp required. Not convenient for office use.
Barkan		Surgical goniolens with blunted side allows access for goniotomy, variable sizes.	May be difficult to stabilize on the globe during surgery.

GONIOPRISMS	INDIRECT	ADVANTAGE	DISADVANTAGE
Goldmann three mirror prism	Available in one, two or three mirrors.	Best gonioprism for neophyte to learn angle anatomy, viscous bridge creates suction effect stabilizing eye for examination and laser therapy. The classic three-mirror prism allows a simultaneous view of the angle and ciliary body 1, peripheral retina 2, the trapezoidal mirror the mid-peripheral retina 3 and the center lens the fundus 4.	Goniogel required for best view which obscures patient's vision and may compromise further same-day diagnostic tests, corneal abrasion in compromised cornea, part of angle hidden in narrow angled eyes, time consuming when necessary to evaluate both eyes. May distort angle when trying to view narrow-angled eyes. Time consuming on a busy clinic day.
4-mirror gonioprisms Gaasterland Zeiss Volk		Rapid evaluation without goniogel, no corneal compromise with goniogel, further same day diagnostic tests not compromised, indentation or compression gonioscopy allows expert evaluation of narrow-angled eyes with hidden anatomy. Patient friendly with minimal movement to see 360 degrees.	Must first master Goldmann gonioprism, more hand–eye coordination necessary than for Goldmann gonioprism, handle required, easy to apply excessive force causing corneal folds with poor view of angle. The silver may peel off from the Zeiss, the Volk has a special coating and the Gaasterland requires no coating.

Figure 5.3 Advantages and disadvantages of direct and indirect gonioscopy. Direct and indirect gonioscopic techniques constitute the two major methods of overcoming total internal reflection of light rays and visualizing the angle. The comprehensive ophthalmologist must be proficient with both techniques in order to diagnose and treat glaucoma.

NORMAL ANGLE VARIABILITY

Routine gonioscopy reveals wide variations in chamber depth, iris processes, ciliary body band width, angular approach, trabecular pigment and vessels (Figure 5.5). An appreciation of this immense variability facilitates early identification of angle pathology. This variability is rarely seen, because gonioscopy is not routinely performed unless ocular pathology, such as rubeosis iridis, prompts the examiner to look further. The depth and peripheral configuration of the anterior chamber are the most important factors that lead to visual disability. If the central anterior chamber depth is very shallow, the patient is more likely to have an occludable angle. An anterior chamber depth less than 2.22 mm measured by optical pachymetry is significant. The depth of the anterior chamber is highly variable

Light rays emerging from the iris either are bent (refracted), exit parallel (unbent) to the normal of the cornea, follow the critical angle or reflect internally. The dotted white arrow represents a light ray emerging unbent from the cornea because it emerges parallel to the normal. When an incident light ray (green arrow) approaches the normal obliquely, then the ray will emerge bent according to Snell's Law. (n_1 * sine i = n_2 * sine r) with n_1 = index of refraction of medium (aqueous), sine i = the sine of the angle of incidence, n_2 = index of refraction of medium (air), sine r = the sine of the angle of refraction. The ray is bent away from the normal as it emerges because the index of refraction of the aqueous humor is greater than that of air. Similarly, when you try to look into the angle, light rays are bent away from the angle towards the pupil because the index of refraction of aqueous is greater than that of air (1.38 vs. 1.0). Light emanating from the peripheral iris creates an even larger oblique incident ray and, according to Snell's Law, a critical angle occurs when the ray is bent 90° from the normal (yellow arrow). The critical angle does not emerge from the cornea and is unseen by the examiner. The critical angle is 46.5° for the anterior chamber. Any ray of light that exceeds 46.5° will be reflected back into the anterior chamber (red arrow). This represents total internal reflection of light and is the reason the angle cannot be visualized without a gonioprism. (c) Direct gonioscopy with a Koeppe lens. The Koeppe lens eliminates total internal reflection of light rays by two methods. First, the index of refraction of the lens is 1.4, very close to that of aqueous. This practically eliminates any significant bending of light at the cornea–air interface and the light passes through. The curvature of the Koeppe is steeper than the cornea, further allowing the light ray to pass to the examiner. Indirect gonioscopy with a gonioprism, lateral view (d) and frontal view (e). This gonioprism also eliminates the problem of total internal reflection of light rays through an indirect view of the angle. The Gaasterland lens (Ocular Instruments) is constructed of glass. The index of refraction of glass approximates that of the aqueous, thereby allowing light to pass through the cornea into the lens (white dotted line). Either a mirror or in this case the high index refraction of the glass acts as a mirror and reflects the light to the observer (green arrow).

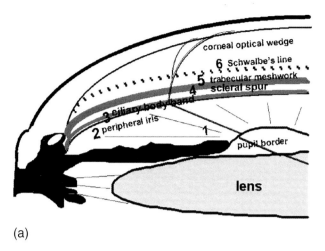

(a)

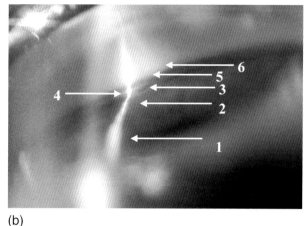

(b)

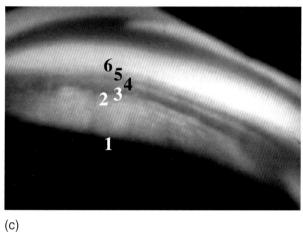

(c)

Figure 5.4 Six key anatomic landmarks of the normal chamber angle. The typical 140° panoramic view of the angle as seen through a gonioprism can be overwhelming unless the observer purposely seeks to find the six key structures in every patient. The scleral spur (4) is the most reliable gonioscopic landmark. This circular white roll bar is the scleral anchor for the ciliary body, which separates trabecular from uveoscleral outflow. It consistently is the least variable of the angle structures. View the diagram, identify the six key structures and refer to the six-point gonioscopy checklist. Correlate the drawing with the slit beam and the overview goniophotographs.

and dependent on multiple factors including genetics, refractive error, age, sex, size of the lens and even diurnal factors.

Gonioscopy is important for family members of angle closure glaucoma patients, for they are more likely to have occludable angles especially noted by a marked anterior convexity that is five times greater than that of controls. In addition, patients with angle closure disease have a higher insertion of the iris, shallower recess and greater iris convexity than controls. The iris is more likely to insert anteriorly in Eskimos–Inuit > Asians > Blacks > Whites. An understanding of the ethnic traits of the iridocorneal angle facilitates the early diagnosis of glaucoma.

Figure 5.5 Normal variability of the chamber angle.   (a) Serpentine angle vessel. Blood vessels are normally visible in the angle in 62% of individuals with blue eyes and 9% with brown eyes. These circular vessels are nestled in the face of the ciliary body and do not cross the scleral spur. As seen during gonioscopy, any vessel that crosses the scleral spur (green arrow) is considered abnormal. (b) Blood in Schlemm's canal. Blood may reflux into Schlemm's canal during gonioscopy and appear as a red band. It is not unusual to have a segmental appearance as the canal has many branches. Blood is more likely to reflux into the canal associated with hypotony or elevated episcleral venous pressure. (c) Iris processes. Iris processes are present in approximately 35% of normal eyes. They are pigmented in brown eyes and gray in blue eyes. Iris processes (green arrow) are typically finer than PAS, most common nasally and allow some view of posterior angle structures. The white arrow points to the scleral spur. (d) Absence of trabecular pigment. Lack of trabecular pigment further blurs outflow boundaries as seen gonioscopically. This juvenile angle reveals the ciliary body band (green arrow) but the scleral spur is not distinct (white arrow), and there is no pigment in the trabecular meshwork (red arrow). (e) Mild trabecular pigment. This goniophotograph of a 5-diopter myope reveals a variable insertion of the iris onto the ciliary body band (green arrows). The scleral spur is seen (white arrow), and trabecular pigment (red arrow) is minimal. It is common to see some pigment dusting the angle, especially in individuals over age 50. Excessive trabecular pigment at the 12 o'clock position occurs in only 2.5% of individuals and is usually pathological. (f) Deep anterior chamber. The insertion of the iris into the ciliary body band along with its curvature is partly genetically determined. This goniophotograph of a deep anterior chamber makes it easy to see the scleral spur and trabecular meshwork. (g) Shallow anterior chamber. A shallow anterior chamber greatly increases the likelihood of angle closure disease. The best method to detect a shallow chamber is with gonioscopy, because the chamber depth may appear deep at the slit lamp, but the angle may already demonstrate peripheral anterior synechiae.

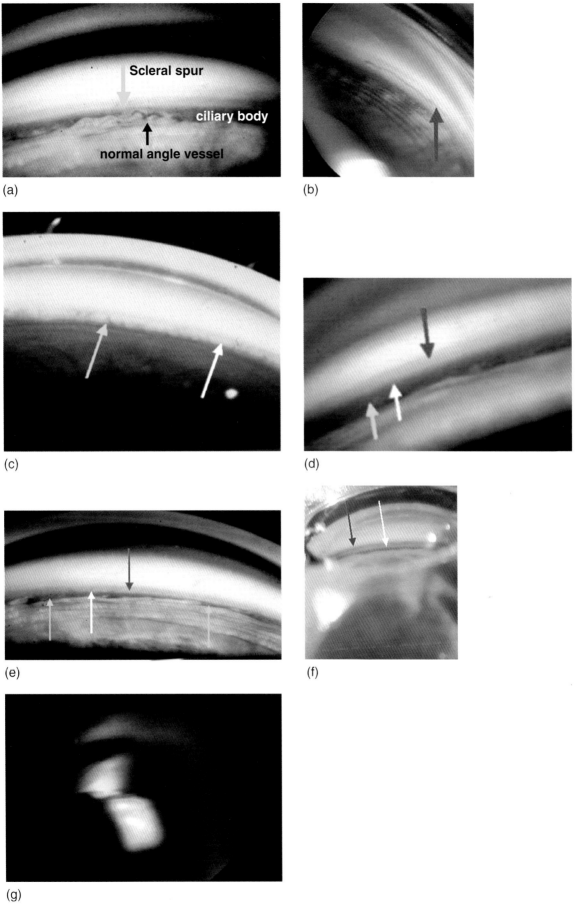

(a)

(b)

(c)

(d)

(e)

(f)

(g)

This marked variability of the configuration of the angle has stimulated an evolution of classification systems.

ANGLE CLASSIFICATION SYSTEMS

One of the stumbling blocks related to gonioscopy is the concise documentation of angle findings. A reliable system is crucial to document and understand how the chamber angle changes (Figure 5.6). Chart documentation should accurately reflect angle findings. The chamber angle is a very complex structure. For example, during a new patient examination it is not enough to say the angle is 'open' or 'narrow.' This is tantamount to saying the optic nerve is 'normal.' Even if the nerve looks normal, its appearance is documented with a picture, drawing, or description in order to establish a baseline for future reference. The chamber angle is no different – it can change yearly, or daily, especially if pharmacologically provoked. The standard of care is to document findings according to one of the angle classification systems or to completely annotate descriptive initial findings. Future reference may indicate that the angle has not changed and is 'open', but initially a full angle description is required. For example, a more appropriate angle description is 'wide open for 360°, ciliary body band easily seen and moderate trabecular pigmentation.' This angle can be dilated safely. In addition to classification systems, additional findings such as pigmentation, synechiae, iris processes, clefts, recession, vessels, precipitates, cysts, etc. are noted with their clock hour location. The Schaefer and Scheie systems are well known and have significantly improved angle grading. However, in the 21st century, thorough descriptions of angle anatomy are now driven by age, gender, and population.

The Spaeth Gonioscopy System evaluates three angle variables and continues to gain global momentum. The reason is that it enhances the description of the angle because the iris may insert onto the inner wall of the eye differently in an Asian compared to a Caucasian and this is easy to communicate with the system. It adds validity to any examiner's description of the angle by forcing them to describe in alphanumeric form what they see. The mandatory decisiveness of the system is its key to success. After learning the system, a three-dimensional view of the angle is communicated in alphanumeric form (Figure 5.7) compared to a simple 'angle is open'.

INDENTATION GONIOSCOPY AND THE NARROW-ANGLED EYE

Additional skills are required to view the crowded or narrow-angled eye (Figure 5.8). To diagnose and treat the narrow angle adequately, the gonioscopist must understand the relationship between the

SYSTEM	SYSTEM BASIS	ANGLE STRUCTURES	CLASSIFICATION	
Scheie 1957	Extent of angle structures visualized	all structures seen iris root not seen ciliary body band not seen posterior trabeculum obscured only Schwalbe's line visible	Wide open Grade I narrow Grade II narrow Grade III narrow Grade IV narrow	
Shaffer 1960	Angular width of the recess	wide open (30°–45°) moderately narrow (20°) extremely narrow (10°) partly or totally closed	Grade 3–4, closure improbable Grade 2 closure possible Grade 1 closure probable Grade 0 closure present	
Spaeth 1971	Three variables: 1. Angular approach to the recess 2. Configuration of peripheral iris 3. Insertion of iris root	**1. Level of iris insertion** Anterior to Schwalbe's line Behind (posterior) to Schwalbe's sCleral spur Deep into ciliary body band Extremely deep **2. Angular approach to recess** **3. Peripheral iris configuration** flat approach bowing (forward bow, 1 to 4 plus) concave (post. bow, 1 to 4 plus) p = plateau	A B C D E 0°–40° f b c p	

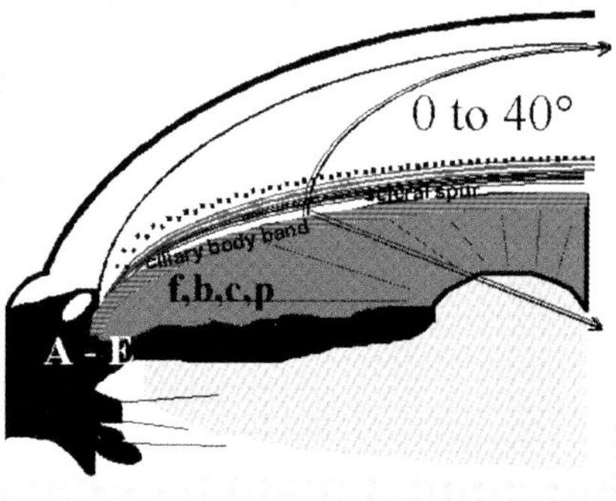

Figure 5.6 Angle classification systems. Classification systems of the angle vary widely. These systems continue to evolve. The author uses the Spaeth system, which forces the examiner to grade three critical areas of the outflow system.

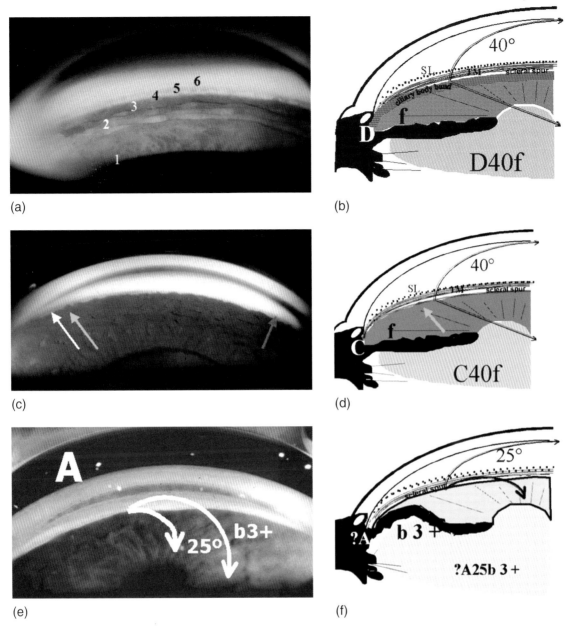

(a)

(b)

(c)

(d)

(e)

(f)

Figure 5.7 Gonioscopic classification systems. Scheie designed the first system around visible posterior angle structures and the amount of pigmentation in the posterior trabecular meshwork. The Shaffer system, still popular today, revolves around the width of the recess. Spaeth thought the chamber angle too complex to describe with one variable. The Spaeth system requires the observer to evaluate not only the angular approach as in the Shaffer system but, in addition, the site of insertion of the iris onto the inner wall of the eye and the peripheral configuration of the iris. Indentation gonioscopy is an integral part of the Spaeth classification system and is explained in the next section. (a) Deep angle goniophotograph. This is an obviously deep angled goniophotograph. Classify the angle according to the three systems. Scheie = wide open; Shaffer = 4; Spaeth = D40f. Note the wide ciliary body band (3) and the scleral spur (4). (b) Spaeth D40f. The Spaeth system requires identifying where the iris inserts onto the inner wall of the eye, the peripheral shape of the iris, and the angular approach. This is a common angle configuration for individuals of European ancestry. This is the Spaeth classification of the goniophotograph from (a). (c) Deep angle goniophotograph. This is another deep angled goniophotograph; however, note the difference in classification systems and to what they relate. Scheie = grade I, Shaffer = 4; Spaeth C40f. (d) Spaeth C40f. Even though the angle is 'wide open', creeping angle closure is more likely in this individual of African-American descent, because the iris inserts much higher onto the inner wall of the eye, closer to the meshwork. The Spaeth system denotes this through the C nomenclature; the other classification systems do not differentiate this insertion point. The green arrow points to the variable high insertion; this is not a peripheral anterior synechia. (e) Narrow angle goniophotograph. This angle is clearly narrow (Scheie = III, Shaffer = Grade 2 and Spaeth ?A25b3+); however, there is more to the Spaeth grading as divulged in the next section. (f) Spaeth ?A25b3+. This system dictates that the iris appears to insert high, but is it possible the iris inserts further into the angle and the true insertion site is hidden by the iris? The angular approach is worrisome and designated by 3+.

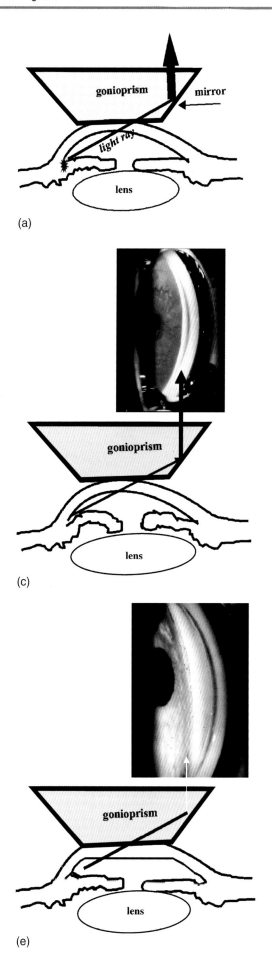

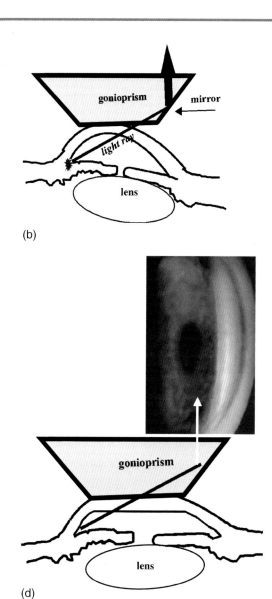

Figure 5.8 Additional methods of viewing the narrow-angled eye. (a) Angle–mirror alignment. In the narrow-angled eye, the last roll of the iris may block the view of the peripheral angle. In this drawing, it is difficult to see far into the angle recess. (b) Angle–mirror alignment improved with gaze. Instruct the patient to look towards the mirror of regard. This will further rotate angle structures into the plane of the mirror, allowing visualization of the angle. (c) View through Zeiss gonioprism without indentation. The iris hides the outflow structures. (d) View through Zeiss gonioprism with indentation, appositional closure. Compression gonioscopy forces the iris backwards, opening the angle. The scleral spur is seen along with the trabecular meshwork. This angle is optically or appositionally closed. (e) View through Zeiss gonioprism with indentation, synechial closure. With indentation, there are broad PAS. This angle is severely compromised by angle closure disease.

anterior chamber angle, the viewing mirror, and dynamic or indentation gonioscopy. Gonioprisms with a large cornea-contact area are not well suited for dynamic gonioscopy because they distort the iridocorneal angle. Indentation or dynamic gonioscopy facilitates the differentiation between appositional and synechial angle closure. Indentation gonioscopy is best performed with a small contact surface diameter of 9 mm, as seen with a Zeiss-type gonioprism. Dynamic or indentation gonioscopy consists of a firm forward motion of the gonioprism against the central portion of the cornea. This forces the aqueous posteriorly, pushing the iris backwards, opening the peripheral angle to reveal either appositional or synechial closure (Figure 5.9).

ANGLE PATHOLOGY

Angle pathology may be subtle, especially during the nascent stage of a disease, or the presentation may be dramatic depending on a congenital or traumatic structural abnormality. Gonioscopy may help clinch the diagnosis in many cases – a simple elegant method of augmenting one's diagnostic skills.

One area of confusion centers on the differential between mesodermal dysgenesis, iridocorneal endothelial syndrome (ICE), and posterior polymorphous dystrophy (Figure 5.10).

The angle in aniridia is another very confusing picture (Figure 5.11). There may be a small stump of iris remaining, and outflow structures are obscured. It is imperative to differentiate between sporadic and autosomal dominant forms of aniridia in order to determine the risk for Wilms' tumor. Angle surgery in aniridia may be impossible due to the lack of development of Schlemm's canal.

Angle findings post-intraocular surgery may enhance diagnosis or at least help explain visual symptoms (Figure 5.12). Any surgeon who performs intraocular surgery should be aware of epithelial implantation cysts, which may become apparent years after surgery. Many patients respond to alcohol injection into the cyst. This patient has undergone penetrating keratoplasty.

Any patient with a pigmented iris lesion deserves gonioscopy (Figure 5.13). This patient harbored significant angle pathology and, when discovered, required complex iridocyclectomy to remove a malignant melanoma of the ciliary body. The patient had no visual complaints.

Ocular trauma causes a myriad of anterior segment findings. One of the most difficult to appreciate is a cyclodialysis cleft, especially if small. All patients with a significant cleft demonstrate hypotony with poor vision (Figure 5.14). Another consequence of trauma is angle recession (Figure 5.15). The discovery of angle recession may help prompt the patient to remember a traumatic ocular event that occurred decades earlier. These patients should be followed for life for the development of secondary glaucoma.

A gonioprism is also useful to magnify structures in the posterior chamber and lens area in children during an examination under anesthesia. The Koeppe lens facilitates evaluation of the anterior segment by revealing dragged ciliary body processes on the posterior lens capsule (Figure 5.16). This was easily seen with a hand-held slit lamp with the Koeppe lens.

Peripheral anterior synechiae may be subtle or dramatic and may be confused with iris processes. Review the differences between PAS and iris processes (Figure 5.17). In early neovascularization of the angle, vessels grow over the scleral spur into the trabecular meshwork area and then arborize laterally; compare to normal vessels (Figure 5.5a). The angle is laced with vessels and, when the associated fibrovascular membrane contracts, it closes the angle (Figure 5.17d).

Gonioscopy is an immensely useful adjunctive tool to diagnose and treat eye disease. A thorough understanding of normal is a prerequisite to appreciate early angle pathology. The ability to scan the angle rapidly, indent when necessary, record findings and compare this to future and past examinations will reduce blindness due to a number of eye diseases. There are a plethora of books and chapters on gonioscopy and the reader is encouraged to review these valuable sources.

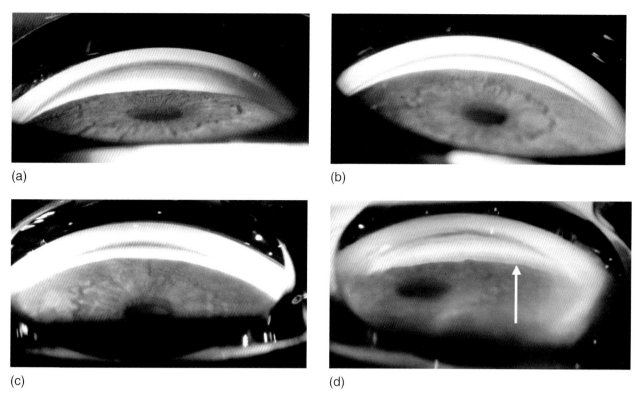

(a)

(b)

(c)

(d)

Figure 5.9 Indentation gonioscopy. The goniophotograph of the narrow angle in Figure 5.7f demands further evaluation. The observer does not know whether the closure is appositional (optical) or synechial (PAS) in nature. (a) Goldmann view of narrow angle. Indentation gonioscopy is not possible with this size lens; it is impossible to see any angle detail without distorting the angle. (b) Goldmann view of narrow angle with gaze shifted into the mirror. Even when the patient shifts their gaze further into the mirror, the details of the angle are not evident. (c) Zeiss view without indentation. It is still impossible to see any angle detail with the Zeiss prism Spaeth A25b3+. (d) Zeiss view with indentation. Finally, with compression or indentation gonioscopy, the iris is easily displaced posteriorly, demonstrating the scleral spur and trabecular meshwork. This angle is appositionally or optically closed. The angle as seen prior to indentation is noted in parenthesis. Following indentation, the insertion site is recorded as seen: (A)C25 b3plus,1+PTM, no PAS. (e) Zeiss view post-iridotomy. The angle deepens considerably following laser iridotomy. Pigment dusts the angle liberated from the iridotomy. Spaeth C40f. The classification system facilitates the recording of how the angle changes following intervention. (f) Zeiss view of narrow-angled eye. It is impossible to see into the peripheral angle. This is an apparent A insertion with a 30° approach and marked bowing of the iris, A30b3+. (g) Zeiss view with indentation of (f). Indentation gonioscopy reveals significant angle pathology. The dark area that the iris inserts into is actually the pigmented trabecular meshwork, not the ciliary body. The white area above that is the anterior trabecular meshwork and the pigment above that is dusting Schwalbe's line. (A)B30b3+. This alphanumeric explanation of the angle informs the examiner that the iris appears to insert into the cornea, but with compression inserts into the trabecular meshwork and the angle bows significantly. Clearly, this patient needs a peripheral iridotomy. Without indentation gonioscopy, it is impossible to see into the depths of the angles in this narrow-angled eye. This amount of detail would be impossible to obtain accurately with a standard Goldmann-type gonioprism.

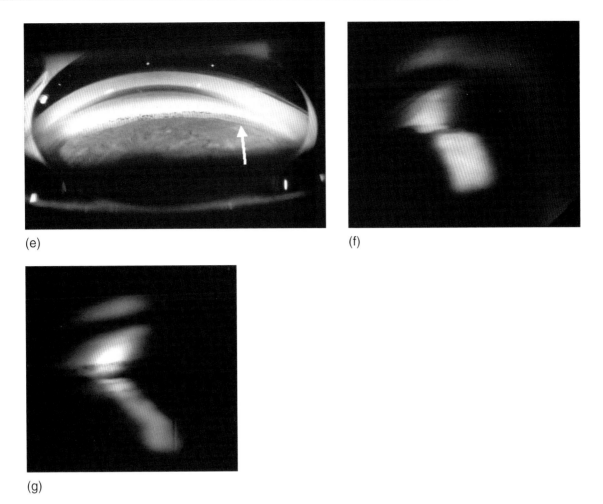

(e)

(f)

(g)

Figure 5.9 *Continued.*

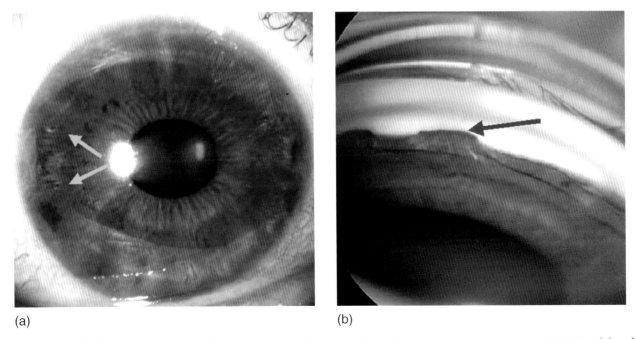

(a)

(b)

Figure 5.10 **Angle pathology. Differentiating mesodermal dysgenesis from iridocorneal endothelial syndromes (ICE).** (a) and (b) Iris atrophy with ICE syndrome. Note the iris atrophy (green arrow). Iris anomalies should always prompt an angle examination. The iris is dragged far onto the cornea. The goniophotograph (b) reveals very high PAS. Only a few diseases cause very high anterior PAS, such as ICE, posterior polymorphous dystrophy, rubeosis iridis, and mesodermal dysgenesis.

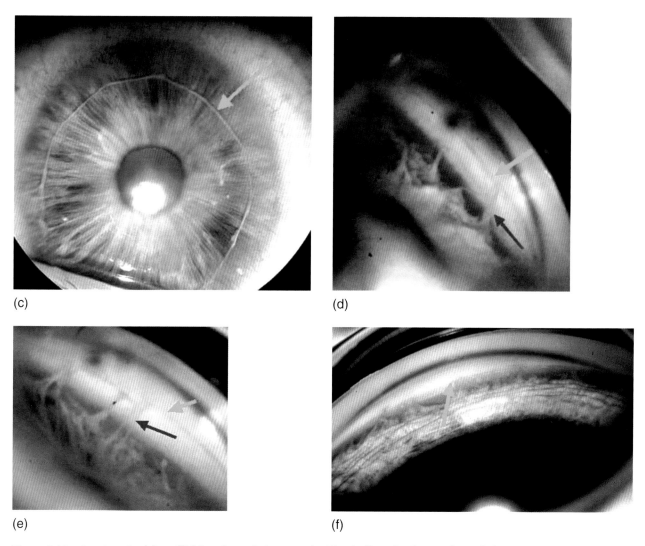

(c)

(d)

(e)

(f)

Figure 5.10 *Continued.* (c) to (f) Mesodermal dysgenesis. The hallmark of mesodermal dysgenesis is a prominent anteriorly displaced Schwalbe's line, or posterior embryotoxon. Posterior embryotoxon is an isolated finding in 15% of the population but may be seen only on gonioscopy. The slit lamp photograph (c) demonstrates posterior embryotoxon (green arrow), which is on the endothelial side of the cornea. This line should always prompt an angle examination. The goniophotographs (d) and (e) reveal the posterior embryotoxon (green arrow), with fine iris strands bridging the angle (red arrow). This is a case of Axenfeld's anomaly, with bilateral involvement, currently normal IOP, and no extraocular findings to consider Axenfeld–Reiger syndrome. (f) From another patient with Axenfeld's anomaly with broader iris strands and optic nerve damage with developmental glaucoma. Angle findings vary considerably with mesodermal dysgenesis and 50% develop glaucoma, which may be very refractory to conventional medical and surgical therapy. Patients with secondary glaucoma at birth with cloudy corneas have the most guarded prognosis. Review Figure 5.2c, a patient with broad synechiae due to autosomal dominant Axenfeld–Reiger syndrome. Approximately 10% of cases do not have a prominent Schwalbe's line, as seen in Figure 5.2c.

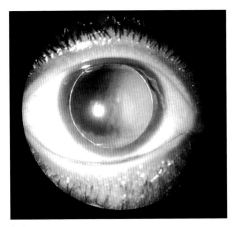

(a)

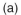

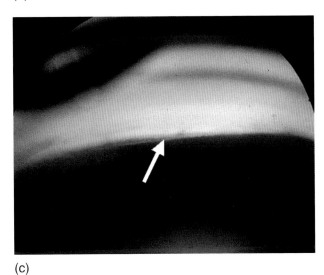

(b)

(c)

Figure 5.11   Aniridia.   This slit lamp photograph (a) reveals the typical appearance of the crystalline lens in the absence of the iris. A small stump of iris may remain as seen on gonioscopy. In the goniophotograph (b) the white arrow points to a portion of the ciliary body, which initially was thought to be a stump of iris. In this advanced case, there was no stump of iris, the ciliary body was nearly absent, the ciliary processes were seen (red arrow) and the glaucoma was severe. The aniridia was familial and no Wilms' tumor was found. A trabeculotomy was attempted with some of the angle responding to partial cleavage (c). The white arrow denotes the area of successful trabeculotomy with cleavage of Schlemm's canal.

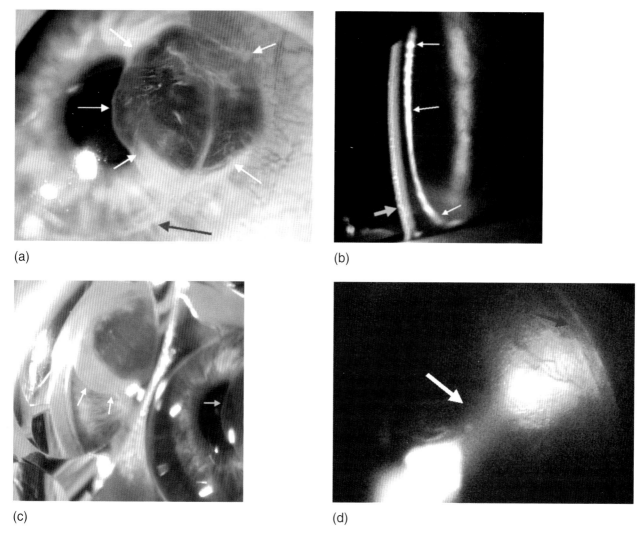

(a)

(b)

(c)

(d)

Figure 5.12 Implantation cyst post-penetrating keratoplasty.   This epithelial invasion took the form of a cyst and was discovered 1 year post-penetrating keratoplasty (PK). In (a) note the surgical wound site (red arrow), and the walls of the cyst (white arrows). The slit beam view is seen in (b). Clearly this is a large cyst. Green arrow shows the cornea, white arrow the anterior wall of the cyst. The goniophotograph (c) reveals the angle involvement. Gonioscopy is very helpful in the operating room to delineate the boundaries of the cyst and to help guide needle sclerosis of the cyst with alcohol. Implantation cysts usually accumulate turbid fluid (d), because the lining is stratified squamous epithelium often mixed with goblet cells. The red arrow denotes the back wall of the cyst and the white arrow the flare. Glaucoma surgery and anterior segment reconstruction related to this entity is extremely difficult. Surgical invasion or even laser shrinkage may convert the problem into sheets of epithelial ingrowth.

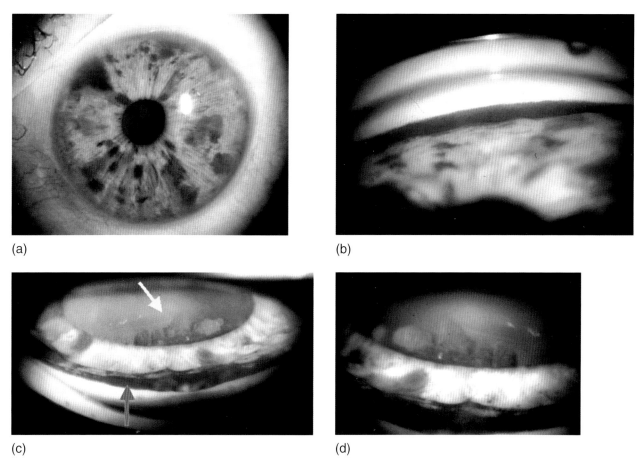

(a)

(b)

(c)

(d)

Figure 5.13 Pigmented iris lesion in asymptomatic patient. Pigmented iris lesions are common findings during slit lamp examination. They are usually benign but not in this case of ciliary body melanoma with seeding of the angle and iris. *Pigmented iris lesions, even in asymptomatic patients, should always prompt an angle examination.* This iris demonstrates multiple areas of excessive pigment (a). The gonioscopy view is striking. This goniophotograph of the inferior angle (b) reveals heavy pigmentation and the same was seen for 360°. In this situation it is mandatory to dilate the pupil to search for the site of origin of the pigment, especially the ciliary body (c). A large ciliary body tumor (yellow arrow) is easily seen with pupil dilatation and gonioscopy. The red arrow reveals the excessive pigment in the superior angle. A higher magnification of the tumor is seen in (d). Even after enucleation, this aggressive tumor spread to the liver, claiming the life of this patient.

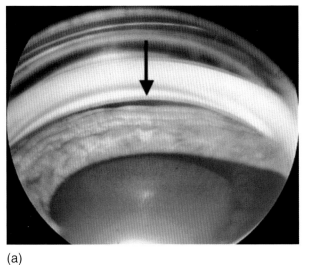

(a)

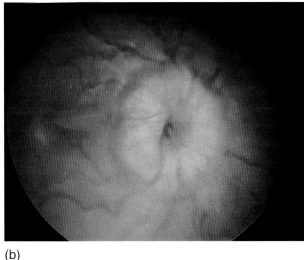

(b)

Figure 5.14 Traumatic cyclodialysis cleft causing hypotony maculopathy. Skilled gonioscopists are definitely rewarded when seeking a cyclodialysis cleft associated with low intraocular pressure. The IOP was zero; the hypotony maculopathy was severe, resulting in hand motions vision. A cyclodialysis cleft is a separation of the ciliary body from the scleral spur (black arrow; (a)). This separation results in a significant increase in uveoscleral outflow and decrease in IOP, leading to disc and macular edema (b). Cyclodialysis cleft repair involves either laser therapy to close the cleft or a direct suture cyclopexy.

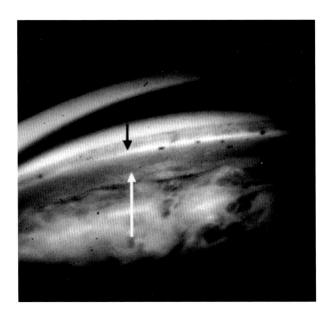

Figure 5.15 Traumatic angle recession. Angle recession is due to blunt trauma to the face of the ciliary body, shearing the muscle fibers. The quickest way to diagnose angle recession is to compare angles between right and left eyes. The unaffected eye will have the more normal appearance of iris insertion. In the affected eye, the iris insertion (yellow arrow) may vary as one scans the angle. An associated iridodialysis may be found.

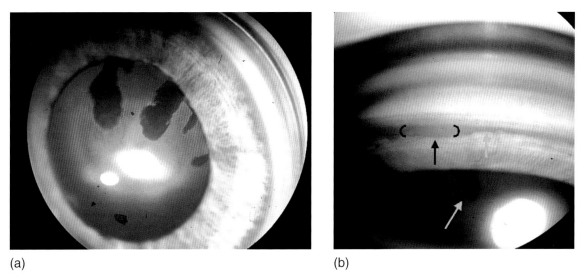

(a)   (b)

Figure 5.16 Persistent hyperplastic primary vitreous (persistent fetal vascular syndrome). This child had a decreased red reflex found during routine examination with decreased visual acuity. The referring physician was worried about an ocular tumor. At examination under anesthesia, the abnormality was easier to discern with a Koeppe lens viewed through a hand-held slit lamp (a). The overview as seen through the Koeppe localized the problem to the ciliary body processes. They were dragged onto the posterior surface of the lens and this appeared to be a developmental problem, not a tumor. Even the angle (b) had a variable insertion of the iris onto the inner wall of the eye (black arrow, deep insertion; green arrow, closer insertion; and yellow arrow, dragged ciliary body process). The differential diagnosis is limited with this finding and it was thought to be a forme fruste of persistent fetal vascular syndrome.

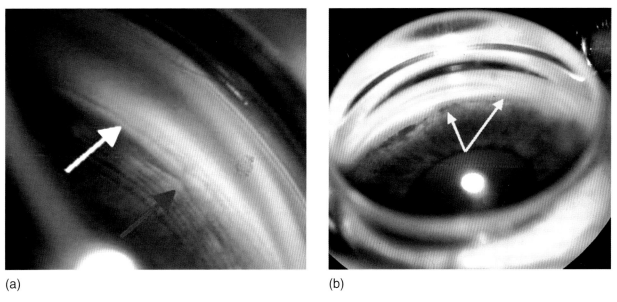

(a)   (b)

Figure 5.17 Peripheral anterior synechiae (PAS). The development of PAS always indicates eye disease. These adhesions may be very subtle in their nascent stages and only adhere to the ciliary body (red arrow). Synechiae do not have to cross the scleral spur (white arrow) to be considered pathological. In early angle closure, this may be the very first manifestation of disease, often nestled in the superior angle. Larger synechiae are more obvious and cross the spur into the trabecular meshwork as seen in (b) (yellow arrows). Iris processes (c) may be confused with PAS. With iris processes the examiner is still able to appreciate angle structures through the iris tissue and this is not possible with PAS. Neovascularization of the anterior segment is an increasing health problem leading to angle closure (d). If retinal ablation is performed in time, these vessels that lace the angle will regress, sparing outflow structures. Early recognition of rubeosis may often spare the patient considerable visual loss.

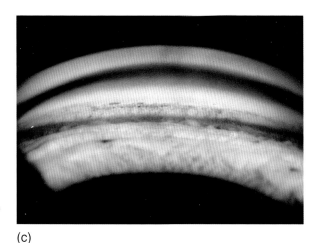

(c)

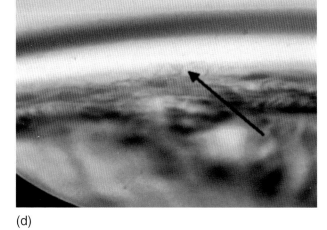

(d)

Figure 5.17 *Continued.*

Further reading

Campbell DG. A comparison of diagnostic techniques in angle-closure glaucoma. Am J Ophthalmol 1979; 88: 197–204

Chandler PA, Grant WM. Lectures on glaucoma Philadelphia, PA: Lea & Febiger, 1954

Fellman RL, Spaeth GL, Starita RJ. Gonioscopy: key to successful management of glaucoma. In: Focal points: clinical modules for ophthamologists. San Francisco, CA: American Academy of Ophthalmology, 1984

Fellman RL, Starita RJ, Spaeth GL. Reopening cyclodialysis cleft with Nd:YAG laser following trabeculectomy. Ophthalmic Surg 1984; 15: 285–8

Fellman RL, Spaeth GL. Gonioscopy. In: Tasman, Jaeger, eds. Duane's Clinical Ophthamology vol 3, revised edition. Philadelphia: Lippincott, Williams and Wilkins, 2005

Forbes M. Gonioscopy with corneal indentation. A method for distinguishing between appositional closure and synechial closure. Arch Ophthalmol 1966; 76: 488–92

Henkind P. Angle vessels in normal eyes. A gonioscopic evaluation and anatomic correlation. Br J Ophthalmol 1964; 48: 551–7

Lichter PR. Iris processes in 340 eyes, Am J Ophthalmol 1969; 68: 872–8

Lynn JR, Fellman RL, Starita RJ. Full circumference trabeculotomy: an improved procedure for primary congenital glaucoma. Ophthalmology 1988; 95(suppl): 168

Palmberg P. Gonioscopy. In: Ritch R, Shields MB, Krupin T, eds. The glaucomas, 2nd edn. St Louis, MO: Mosby, 1996

Scheie H. Width and pigmentation of the angle of the anterior chamber: A system of grading by gonioscopy. Arch Ophthalmol 1957; 58: 510–12

Shaffer RN. Gonioscopy, ophthalmoscopy and perimetry. Trans Am Acad Ophthalmol Otolaryngol 1960; 64: 112–25

Shields MB. Axenfeld-Rieger syndrome. A theory of mechanism and distinctions from the iridocorneal endothelial syndrome. Trans Am Ophthal Soc 1983; 81: 736

Shields MB. Aqueous humor dynamics. II. Techniques for evaluating. In: Textbook of glaucoma, 3rd edn. Baltimore, MD: Williams & Wilkins, 1992, 38–40

Spaeth GL. The normal development of the human anterior chamber angle: a new system of descriptive grading. Trans Ophthalmol Soc UK 1971; 91: 709–39

Starita RJ, Rodrigues MM, Fellman RL, Spaeth GL. Histopathologic verification of position of laser burns in argon laser trabeculopathy. Ophthalmic Surg 1984; 15: 854–8

Sugar HS. Concerning the chamber angle. Am J Ophthalmol 1940; 23: 853–66

6 The optic nerve in glaucoma

Gustavo E Gamero, Robert D Fechtner

INTRODUCTION

The glaucomas are characterized by optic nerve (ON) and retinal nerve fiber layer (rNFL) damage and corresponding changes in visual function often revealed through visual field testing. An appreciation of the anatomy of the normal ON and the pathological changes that occur in glaucomatous optic neuropathy (GON) is essential for the early detection and monitoring of these diseases.

ANATOMY OF THE OPTIC NERVE

Normal nerve

Structure

The optic nerve (cranial nerve II) originates in the ganglion cells of the retina. The ganglion cell axons (also known as nerve fibers) converge in the posterior pole of the eye and exit through the scleral canal constituting most of the ON tissue. In a healthy

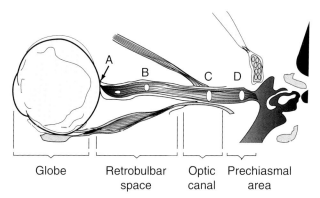

Globe   Retrobulbar   Optic   Prechiasmal
           space   canal   area

Figure 6.1   Division of the optic nerve.   Topographic division of the optic nerve from its origin in the globe to the optic chiasm. (A) Intraocular; (B) intraorbital; (C) intracanalicular; and (D) intracranial. (Drawing adapted from: Hogan MJ, Zimmerman LE. Ophthalmic Pathology. An Atlas and Textbook. Philadelphia: Saunders, 1962: 57.)

middle-aged adult the ON is composed of approximately 0.8–1.2 million axons. This number is higher in the newborn and diminishes gradually throughout life as a result of an estimated loss of 5000 nerve fibers per year, although these figures have been challenged. From its origin in the eye until it reaches the optic chiasm in the anterior cerebral fossa the ON can be divided into four segments as illustrated in Figure 6.1: intraocular (1 mm) which in turn consists of the nerve fiber layer (NFL), prelaminar, laminar and retrolaminar portions; intraorbital (20–25 mm), intracanalicular (4–10 mm) and intracranial (10 mm).

The intraocular portion of the ON is also referred to as the optic nerve head (ONH). The visible most anterior part of the ONH is known as the optic disc. The average optic disc is slightly more elongated vertically (1.9 mm) than horizontally (1.7 mm). There is significant variation in the size, shape, and topography of normal optic discs. Histologically its most anterior portion, the NFL, is composed mainly of non-myelinated axons with some astroglial tissue in between. After traveling on the surface of the retina, these axons turn 90° away from the retinal surface at the scleral canal to exit the eye arranged in approximately 1000 bundles or fascicles. The more peripheral (superficial) nerve fibers turn into the ON closer to the scleral rim, therefore occupying the periphery of the ON. The more central (axial) fibers exit the eye closer to the center of the scleral canal and thus travel more centrally within the ON, as seen in Figure 6.2.

As the ganglion cell axons pass through the prelaminar portion of the optic nerve (at the level of the retina and peripapillary choroid), they are still surrounded by astroglia and exit the eye through a modified region of the sclera known as the lamina cribrosa. Despite being surrounded by scleral tissue the lamina cribrosa has a distinctive histological structure. Its extracellular matrix consists of collagen and non-collagen components such as fibronectin and elastin. Studies have shown that aging results

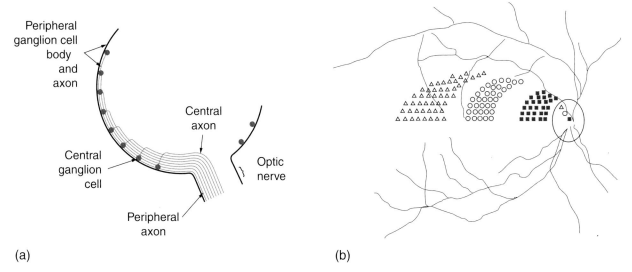

(a)

(b)

Figure 6.2 Retinotopic organization of the ganglion cell axons in the retina and optic nerve. (a) Axons from peripheral retinal ganglion cells occupy a more superficial position in the optic nerve. Axons from retinal areas closer to the disc are located more centrally in the nerve. (b) Frontal view of the distribution pattern of axons as shown in (a). The retina–optic nerve correspondence of fibers is again represented. (From Minckler DS. Arch Ophthalmol 1980; 98: 1630.)

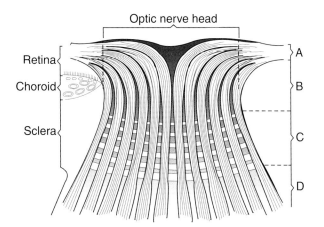

Figure 6.3 Schematic division of the optic nerve head. (A) Nerve fiber layer; (B) prelaminar; (C) laminar, and (D) retro-laminar. (Reproduced with permission from Shields MB. A Study Guide for Glaucoma. Baltimore: Williams & Wilkins, 1982: 79.)

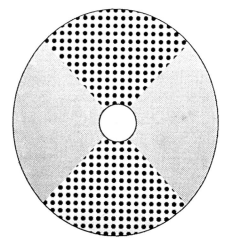

Figure 6.4 Lamina cribrosa. Diagram shows the regional variation of the laminar orifices or pores. The larger orifices are located in an hour-glass configuration, corresponding to the most frequently damaged areas of the ONH in glaucoma.

in a decrease of fibronectin and an increase of elastin. The lamina cribrosa is composed of 8–12 roughly parallel layers of connective and elastic tissue with 500 to 600 orifices or pores of variable diameter which convey the nerve fascicles. This specialized tissue provides mechanical and nutritional support to the axons. The lamina cribrosa, nerve bundles, capillaries and astroglia constitute the laminar portion of the ONH (Figure 6.3). The superior and inferior pores of the lamina cribrosa are larger than the nasal and temporal pores. The larger pores accommodate thicker nerve fascicles and fibers. It is interesting

that glaucomatous damage is often first observed at the superior and inferior poles. This could be the result of relatively less mechanical and nutritional support as less connective and elastic tissue exists in between the larger pores. Therefore, superior and inferior fibers may be more susceptible to damage by various factors, including intraocular pressure (IOP). This may have clinical implications in the pattern of development of glaucomatous ON damage (Figure 6.4). The central retinal artery and vein emerge from the nerve near the center of the optic cup in most eyes.

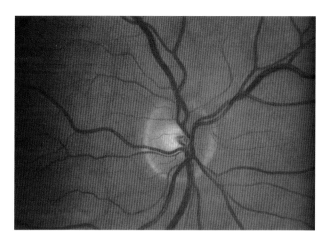

Figure 6.5 Appearance of an average normal optic disc. Note its sharp margins and the orange area (neural rim), composed of the ganglion cell axons and capillaries. The retinal vessels exit near the center of an average-size 0.3 cup. The inferior neural rim is the thickest, followed by the superior, nasal and temporal (the ISNT rule, see text).

Upon clinical examination the optic disc is generally described as consisting of the neural rim (the nerve axons) and the optic cup (the central area of the disc, surrounded by the neural rim). The optic cup is relatively devoid of nerve fascicles and normally appears as a round to oval depression of variable size, usually of a lighter color; the laminar orifices may be noticeable (Figure 6.5). The cup represents a topographic change in the surface of the disc, independent of the color of the tissue. Therefore, the visible area of the laminar orifices should not be used to gauge the size of the cup, which could be significantly larger. The diameter of the optic cup divided by the diameter of the optic disc is known as the cup/disc ratio (C/D ratio) and is expressed in decimal notation (0.1, 0.2, etc.). When recording C/D ratio both vertical and horizontal C/D ratios should be measured and documented. Ninety per cent of normal individuals have an average C/D ratio of less than 0.5 measured by direct ophthalmoscopy. However, data obtained by stereoscopic examination and topographic analysis have revealed slightly larger C/D ratios. The size of the optic cup tends to be proportional to the size of the optic disc; a larger disc has a larger cup. Assuming discs of equal size, both optic cups usually appear fairly symmetric in normal individuals. Only 1–2% have more than a 0.2 difference between the cups. The area occupied by the neural rim is normally pink–orange and ranges from 1.4 to 2.0 mm^2 in normal subjects. It probably diminishes somewhat with age but does not correlate well with the size of the optic disc or the cup.

The cup is not central but is typically displaced superiorly and temporally. As a result the neural rim is thickest inferiorly, then superiorly, nasally, and is thinnest temporally. This is known as the ISNT rule (inferior, superior, nasal, temporal). This is a fairly consistent rule and any optic nerve that does not follow it should raise the suspicion of GON.

The retrolaminar portion of the optic nerve is short and corresponds to the area where myelin produced by oligodendroglia begins to 'wrap' the nerve, nearly doubling its diameter to 3–4 mm. The intraorbital, intracanalicular and intracranial portions of the ON, like the brain, are surrounded by pia mater, arachnoid and dura mater.

Vasculature

Glaucomatous optic neuropathy was once believed to represent a purely mechanical injury of the ganglion cell axons at the level of the lamina cribrosa induced by elevated IOP. In recent years it has been appreciated that GON is probably a multifactorial entity. There has been great interest in the role of microvasculature in the etiology of GON. Emerging technologies are providing new information about blood flow characteristics in glaucoma. While this information has not yet had an impact on the office management of glaucoma, it may in the future. A thorough knowledge of the blood supply to the ON and its regulatory mechanisms in health and disease may better allow us to understand and treat the causes of some types of glaucoma.

The blood supply of the ONH derives entirely from the ophthalmic artery, mainly through the short posterior ciliary arteries (SPCAs), as seen in Figures 6.6 and 6.7. Some reports have drawn conflicting conclusions regarding the blood supply to the various portions of the ONH. Current evidence shows that the rNFL is supplied mainly by branches of the central retinal artery. The prelaminar portion of the ONH is supplied by direct branches of the SPCAs and the circle of Zinn–Haller (an intrascleral vascular structure around the ONH, not always continuous, and originating from branches of the SPCAs). Direct choroidal contribution to the blood supply of the prelaminar region is minimal. The laminar portion is mainly supplied by the SPCAs, with lesser contribution of the circle of Zinn–Haller and occasionally of the peripapillary choroid. The contribution of the choroid to the ONH circulation may have clinical significance. The choroid is a relatively high-flow, low-pressure system with less capacity for autoregulation than the retinal circulation. Consequently, the choroidal circulation may be more susceptible to local or systemic factors. The retrolaminar region is supplied by the SPCAs, some intraneural branches of the central retinal artery and perforating pial branches.

Despite regional differences in the architecture of the various capillary plexuses of the ONH they are interconnected. The endothelial cells of these non-fenestrated capillaries exhibit tight junctions constituting the blood–nerve barrier. The venous

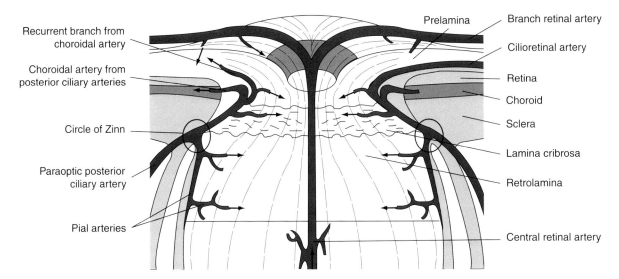

Figure 6.6   The arterial vasculature of the ONH.   Note the extensive contribution of the short posterior ciliary arteries as well as the intraneural branches from the central retinal artery in the retrolaminar region. (Reproduced with permission from Varma R, Minckler DS. Anatomy and pathophysiology of the retina and optic nerve. In: Ritch R, Shields MB, Krupin T, eds. The Glaucomas, 2nd edn. St Louis, MO: Mosby-Year Book, 1996: 153.)

drainage of the ONH occurs mainly via the central retinal vein.

Variations

The appearance of the ONH depends on various anatomical factors. These include: size and shape of the scleral canal, size and shape of the disc, angle at which the nerve exits the globe, and number and configuration of axons and vessels passing through this canal. Despite the large variability in the relative sizes of optic discs and C/D ratios in normal subjects, the nerve rim area tends to remain fairly constant, as it correlates with the total number of axons.

There are other factors that affect the appearance of a normal ONH:

- *Age*   New studies using recent imaging technology (scanning laser tomography) have confirmed that optic cup size and C/D ratio tend to increase with age. In addition, total retinal thickness and rNFL thickness significantly decrease with age, as shown in studies using optical coherence tomography.
- *Race*   Blacks and Asians have larger discs, cups and C/D ratios than Whites, with Latinos having intermediate sizes.
- *Sex*   Men tend to have slightly larger optic nerves and cups than women.
- *Refractive error*   Hyperopic individuals have smaller globes, discs and cups than emmetropes. High myopes have larger globes, discs and cups, but no direct relationship between disc size and axial length (or refractive error) has been found in lower degrees of myopia. Myopic cups are more difficult to assess due to their shallowness

and indistinct margins. Furthermore, these discs tend to appear tilted due to an oblique insertion of the ON. This is illustrated in Figure 6.8. There is evidence that suggests that, for a given level of IOP, ON damage may be more pronounced in highly myopic persons with large discs.

GLAUCOMATOUS OPTIC NEUROPATHY

The changes in the morphology of the ONH in glaucoma have been characterized extensively in several reviews. The inferior and superior poles of the ONH tend to be affected earlier, causing characteristic arcuate visual field defects. The inferotemporal rim is the most commonly damaged early in the course of the disease.

Even though different patterns of GON have been described, many of the following signs are common to many types of glaucoma and should guide the clinician in the early diagnosis and detection of progressive ON damage.

Specific signs

A number of findings are highly suggestive of GON and are important in the diagnosis and follow-up of glaucoma patients.

Progressive enlargement and/or deepening of the cup ('cupping'), when documented, is the hallmark of GON (Figures 6.9 and 6.10). This appearance is the direct result of axonal loss and backward bowing of the lamina cribrosa. Some enlarged cups can remain shallow despite extensive axonal loss, but usually advanced cupping produces undermining of the rim, creating what has been called a 'bean pot' appearance.

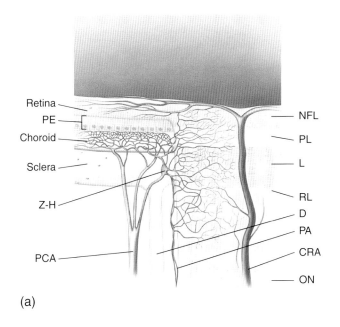

(a)

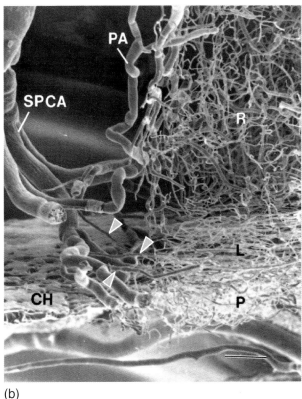

(b)

Figure 6.7 The arterial circulation of the ONH. (a) Diagram of the arterial circulation of the ONH. Note major direct contributions from the posterior ciliary arteries (PCA) and from the circle of Zinn–Haller (Z-H), which originates from the SPCA. Additional blood supply derives from pial arteries (PA) and the central retinal artery (CRA). A few choroidal branches contribute to the arterial supply of the ONH. PE, retinal pigment epithelium; NFL, nerve fiber layer; PL, prelaminar region; L, lamina cribrosa; RL, retrolaminar region; D, dura mater. (b) Microvascular corrosion casting of the human anterior optic nerve. Short posterior ciliary arteries (SPCA) are the main contributors. Some connections (arrowheads) to the pial system (PA) can be seen. CH, choroid; P, prelaminar region; L, lamina cribrosa; R, retrolaminar region. (c) Microvascular corrosion casting of the human anterior optic nerve head (ON). The circle of Zinn–Haller (arrowheads) can be seen originating from the posterior ciliary arteries (red arrows). In this specimen choroidal contributory branches (asterisks) can be seen. CH, choroid. (Reproduced with permission from Cioffi GA, Van Buskirk EM. Vasculature of the anterior optic nerve and peripapillary choroid. In: Ritch R, Shields MB, Krupin T, eds. The Glaucomas 2nd edn. St Louis, MO: Mosby-Year Book, 1996: 179.)

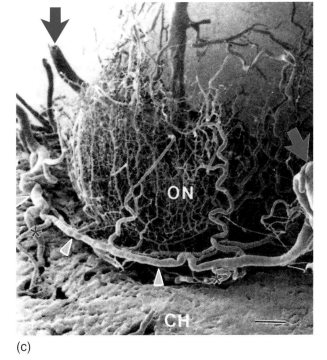

(c)

Vertical elongation of the cup (Figure 6.9) results from preferential loss of the superior and inferior nerve fibers, perhaps due to histological laminar features previously discussed. When present, it represents a highly specific sign of glaucoma, or disease progression in established cases.

Localized nerve rim thinning ('notching,' Figure 6.11) occurs. A notch of variable magnitude results from focal ON rim damage and usually corresponds with visual field changes and NFL loss. Whether this is caused by pressure or focal ischemia (or both) is still controversial. An acquired notch should be differentiated from a congenital disc pit.

Neural rim hemorrhages (Figure 6.12) ('disc hemorrhages') are usually small and splinter or flame-shaped and occur at the level of the rNFL. They tend to be located on the temporal rim, where they are more common inferiorly than superiorly.

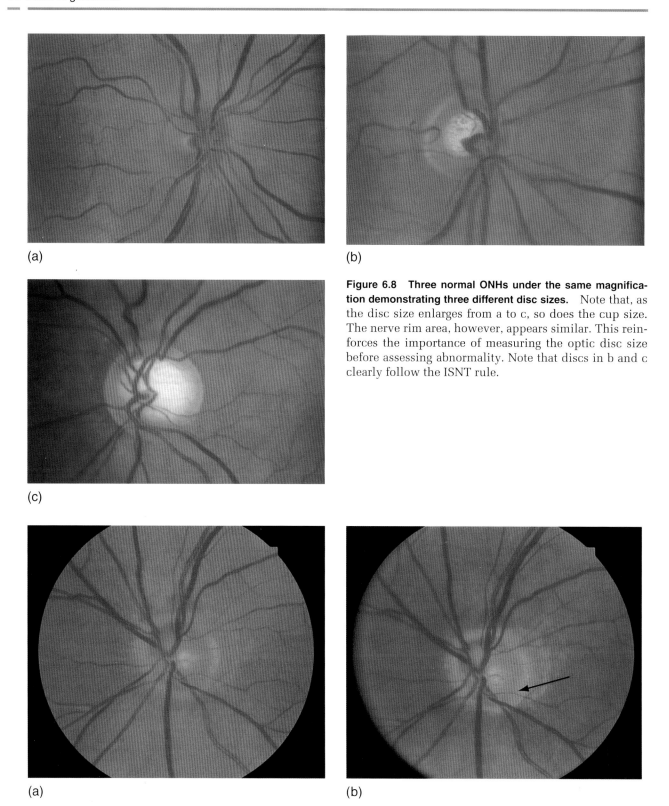

(a)

(b)

Figure 6.8 Three normal ONHs under the same magnification demonstrating three different disc sizes. Note that, as the disc size enlarges from a to c, so does the cup size. The nerve rim area, however, appears similar. This reinforces the importance of measuring the optic disc size before assessing abnormality. Note that discs in b and c clearly follow the ISNT rule.

(c)

(a)

(b)

Figure 6.9 Enlargement of the optic nerve excavation. Sequential photographs ((a) and (b)) showing subtle but definite enlargement of the size of the optic nerve excavation with vertical extension of the cup and a change in the position of a vessel (arrow). This patient showed a new, corresponding new visual field defect.

Rarely they can occur nasally. They eventually resolve often leaving a focal rNFL loss and, depending on the severity, a corresponding visual field defect. These hemorrhages are more common in eyes with normal-tension glaucoma and have prognostic significance, usually indicating progression of disease.

Since they often precede the occurrence of a focal notch on the ONH, it is possible that both findings originate through the same mechanism.

Nerve fiber layer defects (Figure 6.13) can be highly specific for the diagnosis of glaucoma. They occur as a result of axonal loss at the ONH and can

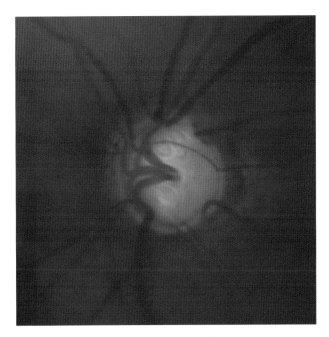

Figure 6.10 'Bean-pot' appearance. Extensive cupping as a result of advanced axonal loss, giving the ONH a 'bean-pot' appearance.

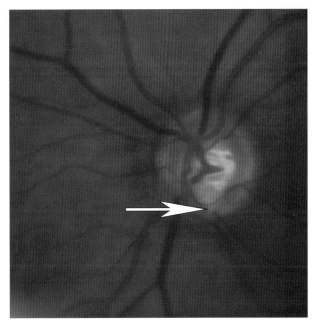

Figure 6.11 Moderately advanced cupping and 'notch'. Moderately advanced cupping in addition to a localized nerve rim loss ('notch') in the inferior region of the ONH (arrow).

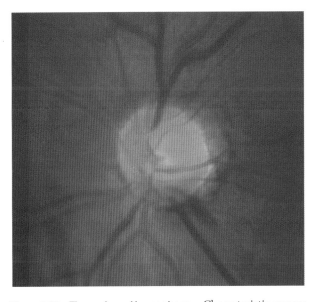

Figure 6.12 Flame-shaped hemorrhage. Characteristic appearance and location of a flame-shaped hemorrhage in the inferotemporal portion of the nerve rim.

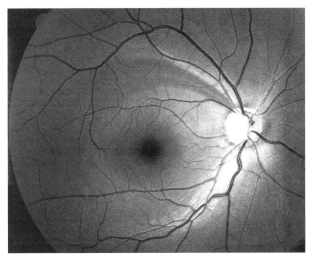

Figure 6.13 Nerve fiber layer defects. Black-and-white nerve fiber layer photograph showing a typical defect compatible with glaucomatous optic nerve damage. (Courtesy of Frederick Mikelberg, MD.)

Non-specific signs

Less specific but still significant signs in patients suspected of having glaucoma are as follows.

A large C/D ratio (greater than 0.5) in Caucasian individuals is a suspicious finding. Keeping in mind age- and race-related differences in cup size, a given C/D ratio bears limited clinical significance unless additional signs of ONH damage described here are present. The ISNT rule can be helpful when evaluating an ON with a large C/D ratio.

Nasal displacement of central vessels can occur in glaucoma. This change is not early, can also occur in large physiological or myopic cups in the absence

precede the appearance of ONH changes or visual field defects. The morphology of these defects follows the normal architectural pattern of the rNFL in the retina and will be discussed later. Their recognition requires a methodical, purposeful examination of the fundi.

Asymmetric cups (Figure 6.14) are sometimes the first objective sign of glaucoma. As mentioned earlier it is unusual for normal individuals to have a cup asymmetry greater than 0.2. Comparing two stereo color disc photographs is the most effective way of detecting subtle differences between cups.

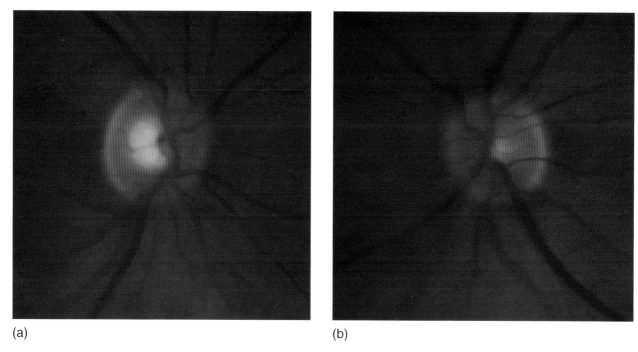

(a)   (b)

Figure 6.14 Asymmetric cups in slighty asymmetric discs. The right cup measures 0.4 and the left cup measures 0.2. Neither eye had detectable evidence of glaucomatous damage but long-term follow-up is indicated.

of glaucoma, and is usually seen in many eyes with advanced disease.

Segmental ('sloping') or generalized ('saucerization') depression of the ONH surface results from partial nerve tissue loss. This topographic change can best be recognized by stereoscopic examination under appropriate dilatation, magnification and illumination.

An increased space between a vessel and the underlying nerve surface ('overpass sign') can result from localized loss of supporting nerve tissue, although an increased transparency without actual surface change has been suggested as an explanation.

Peripapillary atrophy of the choroid and retinal pigment epithelium (Figure 6.15) has been frequently associated with glaucoma. When atrophy involves the choroid alone it appears as a whitish discoloration of the peripapillary tissue known as zone beta. It often corresponds to areas with greater nerve tissue loss and visual field defects. A retinal pigment epithelium crescent surrounding zone beta may also be present. This is known as zone alpha, and lacks the specificity of zone beta.

Baring of the lamina cribrosa with prominent laminar pores can result from significant loss of nerve fibers. However, it can also be seen in large nerves with deep, large cups in the absence of glaucoma.

Optic disc pallor can occur in GON. Typically the degree of cupping will exceed the degree of pallor. When pallor exceeds cupping, other ON diseases must be suspected and ruled out. In glaucomatous nerves pallor can sometimes affect the neural rim in a localized manner. This change is believed to result from thinning of the nerve tissue and capillary

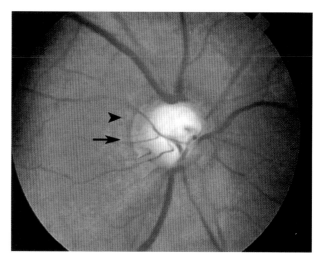

Figure 6.15 Peripapillary changes in glaucoma. Note the whitish area of choroidal sclerosis surrounding the nerve (zone beta, arrow). A pigment epithelium crescent is also present (zone alpha, arrowhead).

dropout. In addition, mild to moderate diffuse disc pallor can result after an attack of acute angle-closure glaucoma.

The presence of a circumlinear vessel was once thought to be a sign of glaucoma. This vessel characteristically follows the margin of the cup and is present in many normal nerves. A recession of the cup margin resulting from glaucomatous tissue loss may create a space between the vessel and the cup margin known as baring of a circumlinear vessel. This finding is more specific but can also occur in the absence of glaucoma.

Differential diagnosis

Careful evaluation of the ONH characteristics and associated clinical findings will in most cases allow one to differentiate GON from non-glaucomatous optic neuropathy. Nonetheless, a number of clinical conditions may mimic GON and must be considered and excluded (see Figures 6.16a–e). These include:

- A physiological or congenitally large optic cup (Figure 6.8c). Examination of close relatives may reveal a similar configuration and will help in the differential diagnosis. A large disc with a normal number of nerve fibers is likely to have a large cup.
- Congenital anomalies of the optic nerve, such as congenital pits, colobomas (Figure 6.16a), the morning glory syndrome, and the tilted disc syndrome can occasionally mimic the appearance of a glaucomatous nerve.
- Pale, cupped nerves can sometimes result from other entities. Arteritic ischemic optic neuropathy can result in an enlarged cup, but in this case peripapillary atrophy is lacking. Demyelinating disease, central retinal artery occlusion, toxic optic neuropathy, traumatic optic atrophy and compressive lesions can also result in glaucoma-like cupping. Age-related macular degeneration has been shown to produce enlarged cups. A thorough history and physical examination will often guide the clinician in the appropriate direction and reveal the underlying condition.
- Tilted normal nerves in myopic patients (Figure 6.16b) can simulate glaucomatous cupping and require careful differentiation. Examination of the visual fields and rNFL can be very useful in these cases.

Theories of etiology of glaucomatous optic neuropathy

Glaucomatous optic neuropathy probably represents the final common pathway for various mechanisms of injury. It is generally appreciated that IOP alone cannot explain the occurrence of GON in every patient. As understanding of the pathophysiology of GON expands, so too will diagnostic and therapeutic approaches to these diseases. Outlined briefly below are several of the current theories regarding the mechanisms of damage in GON.

Mechanical

This theory supports the opinion that elevated IOP is the primary mechanism responsible for the damage to neural cells through biomechanical or structural factors. It is commonly recognized that IOP is probably the single most important identifiable risk factor in the development of GON and the only one currently treatable. Levels of IOP appear to correlate with degrees of ONH damage in many patients.

Disturbances in one or more components of axoplasmic flow at the level of the lamina cribrosa can result in axonal injury and subsequent cell death as a result of increased IOP. The precise mechanisms by which this occurs are not known, but it is thought that backward bowing of the lamina from elevated IOP causes 'kinking' of the axons within the pores, resulting in a disruption of axoplasmic flow. Left untreated, the nerve fiber eventually dies. Another proposed mechanism is the obstruction of the retrograde axoplasmic flow, which may alter the normal delivery of neurotrophic factors at the lamina cribrosa, resulting in ganglion cell death.

Vascular

This theory proposes that the basic pathogenic mechanism responsible for the death of ganglion cells in glaucoma is an insufficient blood supply to the ONH. Despite extensive investigation, the precise level at which this abnormality occurs is at this time unknown. It is therefore not clear at what location an ischemic injury must occur to produce the characteristic findings of GON. This mechanism has been postulated as being responsible for the optic neuropathy seen in many patients with GON and normal IOP (normal-tension glaucoma). Several non-invasive methods to measure the circulation of the posterior pole of the eye and the orbit have recently been developed. For example, color Doppler ultrasonographic analysis has allowed estimates of blood supply through the ophthalmic artery, nasal and temporal short posterior ciliary arteries and central retinal artery. Posterior ciliary, retinal and choroidal circulation differences between normals and glaucoma patients have been reported, but the precise significance of these findings is at this time of uncertain clinical significance. It is difficult to estimate the degree to which these or other mechanisms play a role in a particular patient, since these theories are not exclusive. Decreased circulation and a tendency to an elevated IOP are two known occurrences in elderly individuals in the Western world. There is evidence that significant nocturnal systemic arterial hypotension can occur in some individuals, theoretically compromising the blood supply to the optic nerves. In addition, some data suggest that, in some elderly patients with glaucoma, the damage to the optic nerve may result from a chronic vascular occlusive process, at least partly independent of the level of IOP. It is therefore difficult to separate the mechanical and vascular mechanisms as isolated causes of GON in a given patient.

Biochemical

Multiple alterations have been found at the cellular and molecular levels in optic nerves with glaucoma. These include abnormal astrocyte deposition of collagen IV in the lamina cribrosa and changes

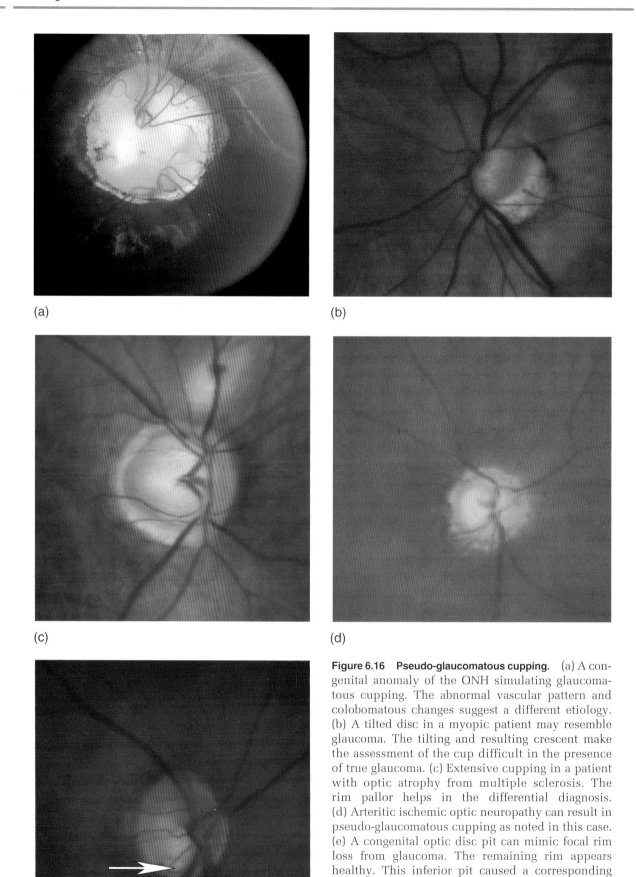

(a)

(b)

(c)

(d)

(e)

Figure 6.16 Pseudo-glaucomatous cupping. (a) A congenital anomaly of the ONH simulating glaucomatous cupping. The abnormal vascular pattern and colobomatous changes suggest a different etiology. (b) A tilted disc in a myopic patient may resemble glaucoma. The tilting and resulting crescent make the assessment of the cup difficult in the presence of true glaucoma. (c) Extensive cupping in a patient with optic atrophy from multiple sclerosis. The rim pallor helps in the differential diagnosis. (d) Arteritic ischemic optic neuropathy can result in pseudo-glaucomatous cupping as noted in this case. (e) A congenital optic disc pit can mimic focal rim loss from glaucoma. The remaining rim appears healthy. This inferior pit caused a corresponding superior nerve fiber bundle visual field defect.

in the composition of the extracellular matrix. Alterations in elastin, tropoelastine, fibronectin, glial fibrillary acidic protein and hyaluronic acid have been demonstrated. It must be noted that some of these biochemical changes have been found in normal, aging optic nerves without evidence of glaucoma.

Neurochemical

It is well known that typical glaucomatous ONH changes occur in eyes without documented elevated IOP or demonstrable circulatory ('vascular') insufficiency. A third proposed mechanism of neuronal injury is one of a neurochemical nature. A number of substances have been shown to have a damaging effect on neural cells and deserve mention.

The excitotoxins (excitatory neurotransmitters) are found in normal neural tissue and, in high concentrations, have been shown to be toxic to neurons. One of these compounds, glutamate, was found in high amounts in glaucomatous eyes. Later studies have failed to confirm this finding.

An uncontrolled accumulation of intracellular calcium can cause neuronal damage and subsequent cell death. Calcium channel blockers have shown not only a vasodilating action in cases of normal tension glaucoma attributed to vasospasm, but also a decrease in the intracellular concentration of calcium.

Astrocytes have been shown to increase the expression of certain molecules (e.g. nitric oxide synthase) under hyperbaric conditions. Nitric oxide can act as a neurotransmitter and has vasodilating effects. It has also shown toxic effects (probably glutamate-mediated) on neurons. A group of substances produced by the vascular endothelium called endothelins have shown a marked vasoconstrictive effect on the ONH, and their role in the pathogenesis of GON is being investigated. An increase in oxygen free radicals has been found in certain neurological diseases, and a role in ganglion cell damage appears possible.

The future importance of these alternative mechanisms in the pathogenesis of glaucoma lies in the possibility of pharmacological intervention. This may allow us to 'protect' the cells and in some cases halt or even reverse the alleged chemically mediated neuronal damage.

Apoptosis

It has been shown that ganglion cell loss occurs in the optic nerves of normal individuals throughout life at a fairly steady rate. Much attention has been given recently to a specific and distinct process of cellular death called apoptosis that occurs in many cells, including neurons. Each cell carries a predetermined ('programmed') intrinsic self-destruction mechanism that ultimately results in its death. There is evidence that apoptosis occurs in eyes with experimental glaucoma. Glaucoma could theoretically result from accelerated or premature apoptosis due to defective

control mechanisms, possibly genetic in origin. Further research will define the possible role of this mechanism in the pathogenesis of glaucoma.

CLINICAL EXAMINATION TECHNIQUES

Optic nerve damage and rNFL damage are the hallmarks of glaucoma. Careful clinical examination is the key to detection of glaucoma. While obvious GON is not difficult to identify, the subtle early changes may escape detection unless the clinician is systematic about optic nerve examination. Each examination of the optic nerve should include evaluation of the optic nerve size, neuroretinal rim (ISNT rule), region of peripapillary atrophy, retinal nerve fiber layer, and disc hemorrhage documentation. Systematic examination will allow detection of the early changes of GON.

Glaucomatous optic neuropathy is at this time considered an irreversible process. Its detection at the earliest stages becomes of the utmost importance in order to prevent or ameliorate functional loss. Several subjective, qualitative methods of examination have traditionally been used to evaluate glaucomatous damage. Newer objective methods have been developed to evaluate the ONH and rNFL. Comparisons between these methods have been conducted, showing that at present no single method is clearly the best in detecting early glaucomatous damage. Like any diagnostic process in most areas of medicine, these techniques appear to complement each other. Evidence has suggested that up to 40% of the nerve fibers may have been destroyed before a diagnostic visual field defect is shown by standard automated perimetry. Therefore, some clinical techniques have detected the presence of ONH and NFL abnormalities prior to the occurrence of typical glaucomatous visual field defects. Still, careful examination by an experienced observer remains one of the best tools to detect glaucomatous damage.

Although a careful observer can obtain excellent reproducibility, the variability between observers using subjective techniques and the lack of standardized terminology to describe various clinical observations have created the need for more objective techniques to record the appearance of the ONH. Examination techniques currently in use by clinicians in the assessment of the ONH include the following.

Direct ophthalmoscopy

Direct ophthalmoscopy has been used for many years to examine the posterior pole of the eye. A direct ophthalmoscope yields a virtual, upright image with a 15× magnification, with good illumination but a limited field of view. The major drawback of this monocular technique is the lack of a three-dimensional view. Subtle yet important topographic changes in the

ONH may be overlooked. A rough idea of the topography of the optic nerve can be obtained by direct ophthalmoscopy. It can be quite useful for detecting optic nerve hemorrhages and for estimating disc size but it remains a suboptimal method for thorough evaluation of the optic nerve. It is nonetheless a useful tool for non-ophthalmologist physicians, for screening purposes, and whenever a small pupil precludes other types of ophthalmoscopy.

Standard binocular indirect ophthalmoscopy

In this technique peripheral light rays from the patient's retina are 'captured' by aspheric condensing lenses and projected into the examiner's retina allowing a much wider field of view. A real and inverted image is formed between the lens and the examiner. The power of the lenses used for indirect ophthalmoscopy varies from 15 to 30 diopters, yielding a lateral magnification that ranges from 2× to 4×. Although a stereoscopic view is obtained, these levels of magnification are inadequate for the evaluation of fine details. Under these conditions the assessment of subtle variations in ONH color and surface is difficult to make. An increase in axial magnification adds to this inconvenience. It is not recommended that one rely on standard indirect ophthalmoscopy when examining glaucoma patients.

Slit lamp biomicroscopy

The excellent illumination, high magnification and stereoscopic view obtainable through a slit lamp biomicroscope with a supplemental lens makes this type of examination highly desirable for the clinical evaluation of the ONH.

The Hruby lens (adapted to the slit lamp) is a plano-concave lens of −55 D of power. It provides an upright virtual image with good magnification. Unfortunately, the small field of view makes this technique challenging and may preclude good stereopsis. It is a non-contact technique that has largely been replaced by more convenient lenses.

The Goldmann fundus contact lens, like the Hruby lens, creates an upright virtual image. Its use requires a coupling material between the lens and the cornea. This allows some control of the globe during the examination. Adequate magnification can be obtained from the optical system of the slit lamp (up to 16× and higher), since the lens itself provides little magnification. With a fully dilated pupil and good illumination, this technique provides the best view available for the clinical assessment of the ONH. Unfortunately, the use of coupling material can affect the view during subsequent examination or fundus photography.

Condensing bi-convex aspheric lenses of high power allows the use of the slit lamp for binocular indirect ophthalmoscopy. The availability of high magnification makes this an effective technique ('biomicroscope indirect ophthalmoscopy'). A real, inverted image is created between the examiner and the lens. Lenses of 78 D and 90 D of power are most commonly used today although a wide range of powers are available. As a non-contact technique, it is comfortable for the patient and does not interfere with further eye examination since no coupling material is needed. Good illumination and magnification can be obtained from the slit lamp. The 78 D lens gives better magnification while the 90 D lens allows examination through smaller pupils. There are 54 D and 60 D lenses available that give image magnification close to 1×. With increasing power, a reduced depth perception results from the inherent optics of these lenses, which can result in an underestimation of cupping and other topographic changes. A lower power lens should be used for better depth perception.

Nerve fiber layer examination

The fundamental pathological process occurring in the glaucomatous optic nerve is a loss of retinal ganglion cells and their axons. This loss of nerve fibers follows the pattern of their structural arrangement in the retina and defines the sequence of the natural course of the disease. A normal NFL has a striated appearance radiating from the optic disc and is more prominent in the superior and inferior poles of the nerve, where the nerve bundles have a larger diameter. Temporal and nasal fibers are thinner and tightly arranged, giving the peripapillary retina a more uniform appearance. Thus, focal NFL loss will show a radiating wedge-shaped defect of variable width on the surface of the retina. Diffuse NFL loss will show a uniform decrease in the NFL pattern, being more difficult to identify in its early stages or when both types of defect coexist.

Biomicroscopy

Even though large NFL defects can often be seen with white light, more subtle defects require special variations in technique and instrumentation. A better view is obtained at the slit lamp after pupillary dilatation using a red-free (green) filter and good illumination. As this is a subjective examination, the potential for interobserver variability is always present.

Photography

Different photographic techniques have been described and attempts have been made to enhance visibility of the NFL. It appears that the use of blue or green filters with proper focusing gives the best results. A high-contrast, fine-grain black-and-white film is currently recommended. Even though NFL photographic analysis has been greatly improved, it remains a technically challenging (subjective and qualitative) examination with variable results depending on the experience of the examiner (Figure 6.13). False-positive results can be obtained since localized defects can occur in normal patients.

Recording the optic nerve examination

Drawings

Careful, standardized drawing of the optic disc appearance is a useful clinical endeavor that requires the clinician to be meticulous and pay attention to small but important details. While several systems have been proposed, no uniform drawing system has been widely accepted. Detailed, written descriptions of the observed changes complement a drawing and provide valuable additional information. Interobserver variation, different drawing styles, and the general availability of fundus photography make this a less-than-ideal method to document and follow the progression of the disease. This becomes critical when multiple observers are providing care. When no other method of recording the appearance of the discs is available, detailed and descriptive drawings are necessary.

Photography

Color fundus photography is widely available and as of today represents the standard to document and follow ONH morphology. While monoscopic color disc photographs examined by a meticulous clinician can yield useful and reliable information, it is most desirable to obtain a stereo pair of photographs. High magnification can be achieved and three-dimensional analysis of subtle features such as color, surface, and vascular patterns can be performed with appropriate techniques. A standard fundus camera can be used to obtain sequential optic nerve images from two different angles by varying the position of the camera. A similar result can be obtained by using the Allen Stereo Separator, a glass plate that pivots right-to-left around its vertical axis. Photographs are taken in two positions to obtain dissimilar images and create a stereoscopic effect. Images obtained by these two methods are then simultaneously viewed and a near-stereoscopic view is obtained.

Simultaneous stereo-photography requires a special camera with beam-splitting prisms to image the ONH. Stereo fundus cameras are specifically designed for this purpose and resulting images produce the most consistent three-dimensional view of the fundus. Currently available cameras place two images in a single frame (Figure 6.17), resulting in less magnification than the sequential stereo techniques. Stereo photography is the ideal photographic technique to document the appearance of the ONH in patients with glaucoma. These models include the traditional 35 mm camera and the digital variety

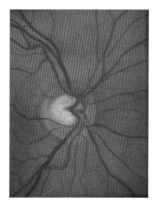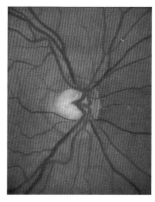

Figure 6.17 Simultaneous stereoscopic color disc photographs taken with a Nidek camera. Digital and 35 mm photography are now available. This technique gives the best stereoscopic view of the ONH currently available.

which adds convenience, allows immediate reading and appears to be fairly equivalent in terms of diagnostic accuracy. The subjective component of this technique is determined by the experience and expertise of the observer, resulting in variable outcomes in some cases. Careful review of high-quality photographs may reveal subtle findings not appreciated during clinical examination.

The techniques recently described tend to be affected by a large subjective component. There is substantial intra- and interobserver variability. Despite this, studies have shown that there is acceptable consistency when well-trained and experienced observers try to determine the degree of suspicion of glaucoma when examining an optic nerve.

SUMMARY

Most if not all clinical signs and symptoms seen in the most common types of glaucoma appear to result from an injury to the ganglion cells that constitute the optic nerve head. The precise pathophysiological mechanisms and anatomic substrate of this injury are not completely understood. Intraocular pressure remains as the single most widely recognized risk factor linked to the development of GON. Additional proposed factors include genetic, circulatory, neurochemical and other mechanisms of disease. Early diagnosis of ONH damage and prompt detection of disease progression remain as critical goals. Towards these objectives, multiple diagnostic techniques can assist but not take the place of a careful clinical examination. To date, no single technique has proved to be clearly superior to others; rather, they complement each other. The clinical examination of the fundus remains the cornerstone of the diagnostic process in glaucoma, and can be supplemented by a number of newer techniques covered in another section of this Atlas. These techniques can add meaningful information but do not replace the careful, thoughtful examination by the ophthalmologist. New therapeutic approaches other than lowering of IOP are being considered, as diverse pathogenic mechanisms are investigated. Assessing the status of the ONH remains a crucial tool in the diagnosis, therapy and follow-up of patients with glaucoma.

Further reading

Airaksinen PJ, Nieminen H. Retinal nerve fiber layer photography in glaucoma. Ophthalmology 1985; 92: 877–9

Airaksinen PJ, Drance SM, Douglas GR, et al. Diffuse and localized nerve fiber loss in glaucoma. Am J Ophthalmol 1984; 98: 566–71

Airaksinen PJ, Tuulonen A, Werner EB. Clinical evaluation of the optic disc and retinal nerve fiber layer. In: Ritch R, Shields MB, Krupin T, eds. The Glaucomas, 2nd edn. St Louis, MO: Mosby-Year Book, 1996: 617–57

Alamouti B, Funk J. Retinal thickness decreases with age: an OCT study. Br J Ophthalmol 2003; 87: 899–901

Albon J, Karwatowski WS, Easty DL, et al. Age related changes in the non-collagenous components of the extracellular matrix of the lamina cribrosa. Br J Ophthalmol 2000; 84: 311–17

Anderson DR. Ultrastructure of human and monkey lamina cribrosa and optic nerve head. Arch Ophthalmol 1969; 82: 800–14

Armaly MF. Genetic determination of cup/disc ratio of the optic nerve. Arch Ophthalmol 1967; 78: 35–43

Bishop KI, Werner EB, Krupin T, et al. Variability and reproducibility of optic disc topographic measurements with the Rodenstock optic nerve head analyzer. Am J Ophthalmol 1988; 29: 1294–8

Bohem AG, Koeller AU, Pillunat LE. The effect of age on optic nerve head blood flow. Invest Ophthalmol Vis Sci 2005; 46: 1291–5

Brown GC. Differential diagnosis of the glaucomatous optic disc. In: Varma R, Spaeth GL, eds. The Optic Nerve in Glaucoma. Philadelphia: JB Lippincott, 1993: 99–112

Burgoyne CF, Morrison JC. The anatomy and pathophysiology of the optic nerve head in glaucoma. J Glaucoma 2001; 10 (Suppl 1): S16–S18

Burgoyne CF, Downs JC, Bellezza AJ, et al. The optic nerve head as a biomechanical structure: a new paradigm for understanding the role of IOP-related stress and strain in the pathophysiology of glaucomatous optic nerve head damage. Prog Retin Eye Res 2005; 24: 39–73

Caprioli J, Prum B, Zeyen T. Comparison of methods to evaluate the optic nerve head and nerve fiber layer for glaucomatous change. Am J Ophthalmol 1996; 121: 659–67

Carpel EF, Engstrom PF. The normal cup–disc ratio. Am J Ophthalmol 1981; 91: 588–97

Chauhan BC, Le Blanc RP, McCormick TA, Rogers JB. Re-test variability of topographic measurements with confocal scanning laser tomography in patients with glaucoma and control subjects. Am J Ophthalmol 1994; 118: 9–15

Chi T, Ritch R, Stickler D, et al. Racial differences in optic nerve head parameters. Arch Ophthalmol 1989; 107: 836–9

Ciarelli L, Falconieri G, Cameron D, et al. Schnabel cavernous degeneration: a vascular change of the aging eye. Arch Pathol Lab Med 2003; 127: 1314–19

Cioffi GA, Van Buskirk EM. Anatomy of the ocular microvasculature. Surv Ophthalmol 1994; 38: S107–16

Cioffi GA, Van Buskirk EM. Vasculature of the anterior optic nerve and peripapillary choroid. In: Ritch R, Shields MB, Krupin T, eds. The Glaucomas, 2nd edn. St Louis, MO: Mosby-Year Book, 1996: 177–88.

Cioffi GA, Robin AL, Eastman RD, et al. Confocal laser scanning ophthalmoscope: reproducibility of optic nerve head topographic measurements with the confocal scanning laser ophthalmoscope. Ophthalmology 1993; 100: 57–62

Colenbrander A. Principles of ophthalmoscopy. In: Tasman W, Jaeger EA, eds. Duane's Clinical Ophthalmology, Revised Edition. Philadelphia: Lippincott-Raven, 1995; 1: 1–21

Dandona L, Quigley HA, Jampel HD. Reliability of optic nerve head topographic measurements with computerized image analysis. Am J Ophthalmol 1989; 108: 414–21

Drance SM, Fairclough M, Butler DM, Kottler MS. The importance of disc hemorrhage in the prognosis of chronic open angle glaucoma. Arch Ophthalmol 1977; 95: 226–8

Dreher AW, Reiter K. Scanning laser polarimetry of the retinal nerve fiber layer. Proc SPIE Int Soc Opt Eng 1992: 1746: 34–8

Dreher AW, Reiter KR. Retinal laser ellipsometry: a new method for measuring the retinal nerve fiber layer thickness distribution. Clin Vision Sci 1992: 7481–8

Dreher AW, Tso PC, Weinreb RN. Reproducibility of topographic measurements of the normal and glaucomatous optic nerve head with the laser tomographic scanner. Am J Ophthalmol 1991; 32: 2992–6

Dreyer EB, Zurakowski D, Schumer RA, et al. Elevated glutamate in the vitreous body of humans and monkeys with glaucoma. Arch Ophthalmol 1996; 114: 299–305

Emdadi A, Kono Y, Sample PA, et al. Parapapillary atrophy in patients with focal visual field loss. Am J Ophthalmol 1999; 128: 595–600

Fechtner RD. Reproducibility of topographic measurements of the normal and glaucomatous optic nerve head with a new confocal laser scanning system. Proceedings of the American Academy of Ophthalmology 1992. Annual Meeting. Dallas, 1992

Fechtner RD, Weinreb RN. Examining and recording the appearance of the optic nerve head. In: Starita RJ, ed. Clinical Signs in Ophthalmology: Glaucoma Series, Vol XII, No. 5. St Louis, MO: Mosby-Year Book, 1991: 2–15

Fechtner RD, Weinreb RB. Mechanisms of optic nerve damage in primary open angle glaucoma. Surv Ophthalmol 1994; 39: 23–42

Fechtner RD, Ikram F, Essock EA. Advances in quantitative optic nerve analysis. In: Burde R, Slamovitz TL, eds. Advances in Clinical Ophthalmology, Vol 3. St Louis, MO: Mosby-Year Book, 1996: 203–24

Harris A. Non-invasive assessment of ocular hemodynamics in glaucoma: a review of the literature. In: Medical Educational Resources Program of Indiana University. 1995: 1–16

Harris A, Rechtman E, Siesky B, et al. The role of optic nerve blood flow in the pathogenesis of glaucoma. Ophthalmol Clin North Am 2005; 18: 345–53

Hayreh SS. Blood supply of the optic nerve head and its role in optic atrophy, glaucoma, and oedema of the optic disc. Br J Ophthalmol 1969; 53: 721–48

Hayreh SS, Jonas JB. Optic disc morphology after arteritic anterior ischemic optic neuropathy. Ophthalmology 2001; 108: 1586–94

Herschler J, Osher RH. Baring of the circumlinear vessel: an early sign of optic nerve damage. Arch Ophthalmol 1980; 98: 865–9

Hitchings RA, Spaeth GL. The optic disc in glaucoma. I: Classification. Br J Ophthalmol 1976; 60: 778–85

Johnson BM, Miao M, Sadun AA. Age-related decline of human optic nerve axon populations. Age 1987; 10: 5–9

Jonas FB, Dichtl A. Evaluation of the retinal nerve fiber layer. Surv Ophthalmol 1996; 40: 369–78

Jonas JB, Budde WM. Optic nerve damage in highly myopic eyes with chronic open-angle glaucoma. Eur J Ophthalmol 2005; 15: 41–7

Jonas JB, Zach F, Gusek GC, Naumann GOH. Pseudoglaucomatous physiologic large cups. Am J Ophthalmol 1989; 107: 137–44

Jonas JB, Fernandez MC, Naumann GOH. Glaucomatous parapapillary atrophy. Occurrence and correlations. Arch Ophthalmol 1992; 110: 214–22

Katz LJ. Optic disc drawings. In: Varma R, Spaeth GL, eds. The Optic Nerve in Glaucoma. Philadelphia: JB Lippincott, 1993: 147–58

Kruse FE, Burk ROW, Volcker GE, et al. Reproducibility of topographic measurements of the optic nerve head with laser tomographic scanning. Ophthalmology 1989; 96: 1320–4

Law FU. The origin of the ophthalmoscope. Ophthalmology 1986; 93: 140–1

Law SK, Sohn YH, Hoffman D, et al. Macular degeneration and glaucoma-like optic nerve head cupping. Am J Ophthalmol 2004; 138: 38–45

Levin LA, Louhab A. Apoptosis of retinal ganglion cells and anterior ischemic optic neuropathy. Arch Ophthalmol 1996; 114: 488–91

Lichter PR. Variability of expert observers in evaluating the optic disc. Trans Am Ophthalmol Soc 1976; 74: 532–72

Maumenee AE. Causes of optic nerve damage in glaucoma. Ophthalmology 1983; 90: 741–52

Mikelberg FS, Drance SM, Schulzer M, et al. The normal human optic nerve. Ophthalmology 1989; 96: 1325–8

Mikelberg FS, Wijsman K, Schulzer M. Reproducibility of topographic parameters obtained with the Heidelberg retina tomograph. J Glaucoma 1991; 2: 101–3

Mikelberg FS, Parfitt CM, Swindale NV, et al. Ability of the Heildelberg retina tomograph to detect early glaucomatous visual field loss. J Glaucoma 1995; 4: 242–7

Miller NR, ed. Anatomy and physiology of the optic nerve. In: Walsh & Hoyt's Clinical Neuro-Ophthalmology, 4th edn. Baltimore, MD: Williams & Wilkins, 1982; 1: 41–59

Minckler DS. Optic nerve damage in glaucoma: 1. Obstruction to axoplasmic flow. Surv Ophthalmol 1981; 26: 128–36

Motolko M, Drance SJ. Features of the optic disc in preglaucomatous eyes. Arch Ophthalmol 1981; 99: 1992–4

Netland PA, Chaturvedi N, Dreyer EB. Calcium channel blockers in the management of low tension and open-angle glaucoma. Am J Ophthalmol 1993; 115: 60–8

Nicolela MT, Drance SM. Various glaucomatous optic nerve appearances. Clinical correlations. Ophthalmology 1996; 103: 640–9

O'Connor DJ, Zeyen T, Caprioli J. Comparison of methods to detect glaucomatous optic nerve damage. Ophthalmology 1993; 100: 1498–503

Orgul S, Meyer P, Cioffi A. Physiology of blood flow regulation and mechanisms involved in optic nerve perfusion. J Glaucoma 1995; 4: 427–43

Orgul S, Cioffi GA, Bacon DR, Van Buskirk EM. Sources of variability of topometric data with a scanning laser ophthalmoscope. Arch Ophthalmol 1996; 113: 161–4

Orgul S, Cioffi GA, Wilson DJ, et al. An endothelin-1 induced model of optic nerve ischemia in the rabbit. Invest Ophthalmol Vis Sci 1996; 37: 1860–9

Osher RH, Herschler J. The significance of baring of the circumlinear vessel: a prospective study. Arch Ophthalmol 1981; 99: 817–18

Pederson JE, Anderson DR. The mode of progressive disc cupping in ocular hypertension and glaucoma. Arch Ophthalmol 1980; 98: 490–5

Peli E, Hedges TR, Schwartz B. Computerized enhancement of retinal nerve fiber layer. Acta Ophthalmol 1986; 64: 113–22

Pendergast SD, Shields MB. Reproducibility of optic nerve head topographic measurements with the glaucoma-scope. J Glaucoma 1994; 4: 170–6

Pickard R. A method of recording disc alterations and a study of the growth of normal and abnormal disc cups. Br J Ophthalmol 1923; 80: 81–90

Quigley HA, Addicks EM. Regional differences in the structure of the lamina cribrosa and their relation to glaucomatous optic nerve damage. Arch Ophthalmol 1981; 99: 137–43

Quigley HA, Miller NR, George T. Clinical evaluation of nerve fiber layer atrophy as an indicator of glaucomatous optic nerve damage. Arch Ophthalmol 1980; 98: 1564–71

Quigley HA, Addicks EM, Green WR. Optic nerve damage in human glaucoma. III. Quantitative correlation of nerve fiber loss and visual field defect in glaucoma, ischemic neuropathy, papilledema and toxic neuropathy. Arch Ophthalmol 1982; 100: 135–46

Quigley HA, Dunkelberger GR, Green WR. Retinal ganglion cell atrophy correlated with automated perimetry in human eyes with glaucoma. Am J Ophthalmol 1989; 107: 453–64

Quigley HA, Katz J, Derick R, et al. An evaluation of optic disc and nerve fiber layer examinations in monitoring progression of early glaucoma damage. Ophthalmology 1992; 99: 19–28

Quigley HA, Nickells RW, Kerrigan LA, et al. Retinal ganglion cells death in experimental glaucoma and after axotomy occurs by apoptosis. Invest Ophthalmol Vis Sci 1995; 36: 774–86

Rankin SJA, Drance SM, Buckley AR, Walman BE. Visual field correlations with color Doppler studies in open angle glaucoma. J Glaucoma 1996; 5: 15–21

Repka MX, Quigley HA. The effect of age on normal human optic nerve fiber and diameter. Ophthalmology 1989; 96: 26–32

Saheb NE, Drance SM, Nelson A. The use of photogrammetry in evaluating the cup of the optic nerve head for a study in chronic simple glaucoma. Can J Ophthalmol 1972; 7: 466–71

Schumer RA, Podos SM. The nerve of glaucoma! Arch Ophthalmol 1994; 112: 37–44

Schwartz JT, Reuling FH, Garrison RJ. Acquired cupping of the optic nerve head in normotensive eyes. Br J Ophthalmol 1975; 59: 216–22

Shaffer RN, Ridgway WL, Brown R, Kramer SG. The use of diagrams to record changes in glaucomatous discs. Am J Ophthalmol 1975; 80: 460–4

Sharma NK, Hitchings RA. A comparison of monocular and 'stereoscopic' photographs of the optic disc in the identification of glaucomatous visual field defects. Br J Ophthalmol 1983; 67: 677–80

Snead MP, Rubinstein MP, Jacobs PM. The optics of fundus examination. Surv Ophthalmol 1992; 36: 439–45

Sommer A. Intraocular pressure and glaucoma. Am J Ophthalmol 1994; 118: 1–8

Sommer A, Miller NR, Pollack I, et al. The nerve fiber layer in the diagnosis of glaucoma. Arch Ophthalmol 1977; 95: 2149–56

Sommer A, D'Anna SA, Kues HA, George T. High-resolution photography of the retinal fiber layer. Am J Ophthalmol 1983; 96: 535–9

Sommer A, Quigley HA, Robin AL, et al. Evaluation of nerve fiber layer assessment. Arch Ophthalmol 1984; 102: 1766–71

Sommer AS, Katz J, Quigley HA, et al. Clinically detectable nerve fiber atrophy precedes the onset of glaucomatous field loss. Arch Ophthalmol 1991; 109: 77–83

Spaeth GL. Optic nerve damage in glaucoma: 2. Insufficiency of blood flow. Surv Ophthalmol 1981; 26: 128–48

Spaeth GL. Development of glaucomatous changes of the optic nerve. In: Varma R, Spaeth GL, eds. The Optic Nerve in Glaucoma. Philadelphia: JB Lippincott, 1993: 63–81

Spaeth GL, Hitchings RA. The optic disc in glaucoma: pathogenic correlation of five patterns of cupping in chronic open angle glaucoma. Trans Am Acad Ophthalmol Otolaryngol 1976; 81: 217–23

Tielsch JM, Katz J, Quigley HA, et al. Intraobserver and interobserver agreement in measurement of optic disc characteristics. Ophthalmology 1988; 95: 350–6

Trobe JD, Glaser JS, Cassady JC. Optic atrophy. Differential diagnosis by fundus observation alone. Arch Ophthalmol 1980; 98: 1040–5

Trobe FD, Glaser JS, Cassady J, et al. Nonglaucomatous excavation of the optic disc. Arch Ophthalmol 1980; 98: 1046–50

Van Buskirk EM, Cioffi GA. Glaucomatous optic neuropathy. Am J Ophthalmol 1992; 113: 447–52

Varma R, Minckler DS. Anatomy and Pathophysiology of the Retina and Optic Nerve. In: Ritch R, Shields MB, Krupin T, eds.

The Glaucomas, 2nd edn. St Louis, MO: Mosby-Year Book, 1996: 139–75

Varma R, Steinmann WC, Scott IU. Expert agreement in evaluating the optic disc for glaucoma. Ophthalmology 1992; 99: 215–21

Varma R, Tielsch JM, Quigley HA, et al. Race-, age-, gender-, and refractive error. Related differences in the normal optic disc. Arch Ophthalmol 1994; 112: 1068–76

Wang L, Cioffi GA, Van Buskirk EM. The vascular pattern of the optic nerve and its potential relevance in glaucoma. Curr Opin Ophthalmol 1998; 9: 24–9

Weinreb RB. Why study the ocular microcirculation in glaucoma? J Glaucoma 1992; 1: 145–7

Weinreb RN. Diagnosing and monitoring glaucoma with confocal scanning laser ophthalmoscopy. J Glaucoma 1995; 4: 225–7

Weinreb RN, Lusky M, Bartsch DU, Morsman D. Effect of repetitive imaging on topographic measurements of the optic nerve head. Arch Ophthalmol 1993; 111: 636–8

Weinreb RN, Shakiba S, Zangwill L. Scanning laser polarimetry to measure the nerve fiber layer of normal and glaucomatous eyes. Am J Ophthalmol 1994; 119: 627–36

Wiegner SW, Netland PA. Optic disc hemorrhages and progression of glaucoma. Ophthalmology 1996; 103: 1014–24

Wilensky JT, Kolker AE. Peripapillary changes in glaucoma. Am J Ophthalmol 1976; 81: 341–5

Wisman RL, Asseff DF, Phelps CD, et al. Vertical elongation of the optic cup in glaucoma. Trans Am Acad Ophthalmol Otolaryngol 1973; 77: 157–61

Zeyen TG, Caprioli J. Progression of disc and field damage in early glaucoma. Arch Ophthalmol 1993; 111: 62–5

7 Scanning laser imaging

Christopher Bowd, Linda M Zangwill, Rupert RA Bourne, Robert N Weinreb

OPTIC DISC AND RETINAL NERVE FIBER LAYER TOPOGRAPHY IN GLAUCOMA

As described in previous chapters, glaucoma is a progressive optic neuropathy that causes a slow degeneration of retinal ganglion cells resulting in characteristic defects of the optic nerve and retinal nerve fiber layer (RNFL). These defects generally manifest anatomically as diffuse or focal thinning of the neuroretinal rim and/or RNFL. Evidence suggests that rim thinning is most pronounced inferiorly and superiorly in early glaucoma, and that RNFL defects are first detectable in the inferior and superior parapapillary areas (Figure 7.1).

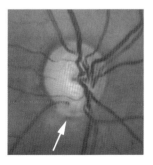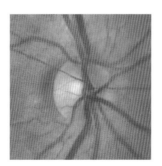

Figure 7.1 A glaucomatous eye. A glaucomatous eye (left) with focal neuroretinal rim thinning in the inferior quadrant (arrow). An associated RNFL defect also is present. Patient is a 59-year-old male with a repeatable superior arcuate defect measured using standard automated perimetry (SAP). SAP mean deviation at the time of imaging was –2.79 ($p < 2\%$), pattern standard deviation was 2.93 ($p < 2\%$) and Glaucoma Hemifield Test result was outside of normal limits. A healthy eye (right), with healthy neuroretinal rim and RNFL, is shown for comparison. The healthy eye shows a characteristic rim thickness pattern, with the inferior and superior quadrants thickest, followed by nasal and temporal quadrants. This pattern often is violated in glaucoma, providing evidence of glaucomatous damage.

RATIONALE FOR COMPUTER-BASED LASER IMAGING FOR DETECTING AND MONITORING GLAUCOMA

Detecting optic disc and RNFL damage and change is critical for glaucoma management. Currently, many ophthalmologists do not objectively document the condition of the optic disc and parapapillary retina during examination. Frequently the disc size, cup/disc ratio and characteristics of the RNFL are subjectively documented by drawing. This technique is unlikely to be sensitive to detection of change on follow-up. Stereophotography of the optic disc provides objective documentation but, like drawings, requires subjective assessment. Furthermore, in the case of analog photographs, processing is required, making photographs unavailable for assessment or comparison to previous photographs at the time of a patient's visit.

Computer-based optic disc and RNFL imaging, introduced over the past 15 years, provides objective documentation, allows objective assessment and provides immediate, automated feedback. In addition, the need for ocular dilatation and clear ocular media are reduced, compared to photography. Current imaging techniques require little expertise for operation.

THE NEED FOR A NORMATIVE DATABASE

The number of retinal ganglion cell axons in a healthy eye can range from approximately 750 000 to 1 500 000. This can limit the ability of any structural measure to perfectly discriminate between healthy and glaucomatous eyes. It is, therefore, often difficult to detect ganglion cell loss manifested in neuroretinal rim and RNFL thickness based on measurements alone, without knowing the range of these measurements in a sample of healthy eyes. To facilitate the detection of abnormalities, most imaging software compares parameter measurements to a normative database. These comparisons frequently provide probabilities of abnormality for each parameter based on measurements from healthy eyes included in the normative database. Examples of normative database comparisons, for each imaging instrument, are shown below in several figures.

IMAGING TECHNOLOGIES CURRENTLY AVAILABLE

Four laser imaging techniques currently are in clinical use for detecting and monitoring glaucoma. Each technique uses different optical principles and relies on different properties of the measured tissue. In addition, available techniques measure different characteristics of the eye. All techniques provide numerous measurements and summary parameters designed for clinical use.

Confocal scanning laser ophthalmoscopy

The most recent commercially available confocal scanning laser ophthalmoscope is the HRT II (available since 1999) (Heidelberg Engineering, Dossenheim, Germany), which is designed to measure optic disc topography (Figure 7.2). In common with its predecessor the HRT, the HRT II uses confocal technology in which multiple shallow-depth-of-field images are combined to provide a three-dimensional topographic image of the retinal surface, specifically the 15 × 15° field centered on the optic disc. A variable number of confocal images (determined by the desired depth of the scan, e.g. from retinal surface to lamina cribrosa) are obtained at 16 images per millimeter.

Most HRT II optic disc topography measurements are defined relative to a user-defined contour line placed along the optic disc margin and a reference

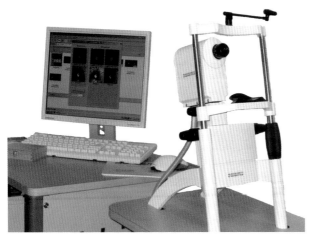

Figure 7.2 The Heidelberg Retina Tomograph (HRT) II.

plane placed 50 μm below the contour line in the temporal 5° sector (the papillomacular bundle which is assumed to change only late in the course of progressive glaucoma) (Figure 7.3).

Optical coherence tomography

The most recent commercially available optical coherence tomograph is the StratusOCT (available since 2002) (Carl Zeiss Meditec, Dublin, CA), which is designed to measure RNFL thickness, optic disc topography and macular thickness (Figure 7.4). To measure tissue thickness, OCT technology relies on interferometry in which a near-infrared light beam (low coherence light source) is split into two beams: a measurement beam and a reference beam. The measurement beam is projected onto, and reflected from, the retina while the reference beam is projected onto, and reflected from, a reference mirror (at a known distance). The pattern of interference of the reflected measurement beam on the reflected reference beam provides information regarding thickness of tissue. The resulting image is a color-coded reflectivity-based map.

To automatically obtain circumpapillary RNFL thickness measurements, a circular scan is centered on the optic disc. OCT software first determines the retinal boundaries (i.e. retinal thickness) defined by the vitreoretinal interface and the retinal pigment epithelium. These boundaries are relatively easy to define because they are sites of abrupt changes in reflectivity. Next, the RNFL itself is defined by the vitreoretinal interface, anteriorly, and the retinal pigment epithelium and an area of predefined threshold reflectance adjacent to the neurosensory retina, posteriorly.

Optic disc topography is measured based on retinal thickness measurements from six radial scans centered on the optic disc. The disc margin is defined as the ends of the retinal pigment epithelium/choricapillaris in each scan and is interpolated between scans. A straight line connects the edges of the retinal pigment epithelium/choriocapillaris of each radial scan, and a reference plane placed 150 μm above this line delineates the neuroretinal rim from the optic cup.

Macular thickness is measured on the basis of retinal thickness measurements from six radial scans centered on the fovea and is interpolated between scans, similar to optic disc topography measurement (Figure 7.5).

Scanning laser polarimetry

The most recent commercially available scanning laser polarimeter (SLP) is the GDx VCC (available since 2002) (Carl Zeiss Meditec, Dublin, CA), which is designed to measure RNFL thickness (Figure 7.6). SLP technology measures RNFL based on the change

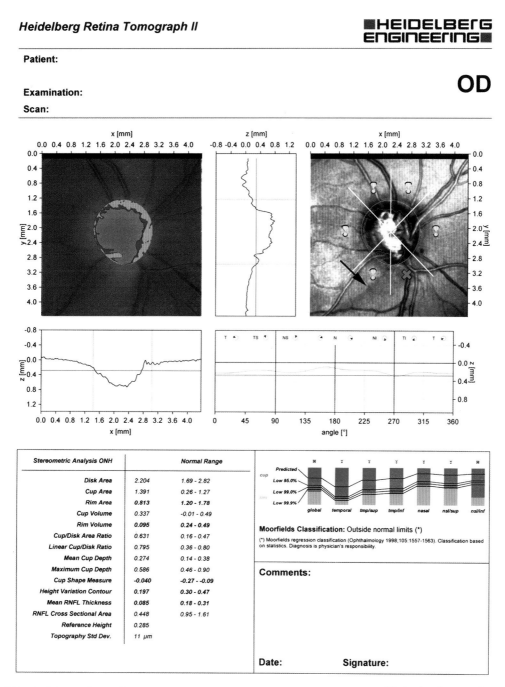

Figure 7.3 HRT II clinical printout from the glaucomatous eye pictured in Figure 7.1. Clinical printouts from the HRT II ('Standard Report' and 'Moorfields Report') contain a topography image (left), reflectance image (right), one vertical and one horizontal cross-section through the topography, the stereometric parameters (e.g. rim area and volume, cup area and volume, mean and maximum cup depth, cup shape, with associated normal ranges derived from the internal normative database), a color-coded optic disc assessment in which the disc is divided into rim (green), 'sloping rim' (blue) and cup (red), a graphical representation of the mean height of the contour line along the optic disc margin, and a bar graph representation of the Moorfields Regression Analysis results (analysis in which measured rim area, relative to disc area, is compared to an age-adjusted expected value based on normative data).

For the glaucomatous eye, an inferior RNFL defect is visible on the reflectance image (arrow) and a corresponding 'notch' (focal thinning) is visible on the topography (color-coded) image, corresponding to the Moorfields Regression Analysis classification of 'outside normal limits' in the inferior nasal sector. The other Moorfields Regression Analysis sectors indicate that rim thickness is 'borderline' and the overall Moorfields Regression Analysis result is 'outside normal limits'. Several stereometric parameters also are outside normal limits (indicated by bold type), including rim area, rim volume, cup shape, variation in the height of the contour line, and mean RNFL thickness.

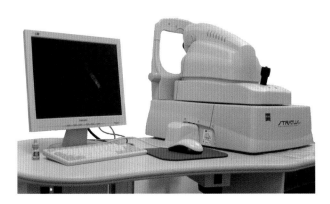

Figure 7.4 The StratusOCT.

in polarization (i.e. retardation) that occurs when light illuminates birefringent tissues, such as the RNFL. Thickness can be estimated from retardation

measurements according to the known linear relationship between the two. Because the cornea and lens also are birefringent structures, and their birefringence is not similar across all eyes, the GDx VCC incorporates a 'variable corneal compensator' that allows non-RNFL-related retardation to be subtracted from thickness measurements, for each eye individually (Figure 7.7).

Retinal thickness analysis

The retinal thickness analyzer (RTA, Talia Technology, Neve Ilan, Israel) was initially designed to measure retinal thickness of the posterior pole (Figure 7.8). An optic disc module has been available since 2003. To measure tissue thickness, a slit of laser light is scanned, in steps, across the retina and the retinal thickness is defined as the separation between

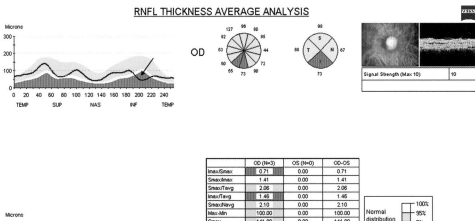

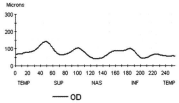

(a)

Figure 7.5 StratusOCT clinical printouts. (a) RNFL analysis; (b) optic disc analysis; (c) macular analysis from the glaucomatous eye pictured in Figure 7.1. (a) The StratusOCT 'RNFL Thickness Average Analysis' includes a graphical depiction of the RNFL thickness profile with comparison to normative values, RNFL thickness measurements by quadrant and 30° sector with normative comparisons, and several summary parameters with normative comparisons. A fundus image and false-colored reflectance image also are shown. For the glaucomatous eye, RNFL thinning outside normal limits is shown in the inferior temporal region on the RNFL thickness profile (arrow) and the 30° sector plot (as red). The inferior quadrant also is outside normal limits, as are several of the summary parameters including inferior maximum thickness/superior maximum thickness, inferior maximum thickness/temporal maximum thickness, inferior maximum thickness and inferior average thickness. (b) The StratusOCT 'Optic Nerve Head Analysis' includes a false-colored cross-sectional image of the optic nerve head obtained along one of the six radial scans. Images derived from the other radial scans are viewable with interactive software. A polar image of the optic nerve head and several summary parameters also are shown, without comparison to normative data. For the glaucomatous eye, neuroretinal rim thinning is apparent inferiorly (arrow) and measured cup/disc ratios (area, horizontal, vertical) range from 0.625 (area) to 0.829 (vertical). (c) The StratusOCT 'Retinal Thickness/Volume Tabular Output' analysis of the macula includes a polar color-coded continuous thickness map, a regional thickness map with normative comparisons, and multiple summary parameters with normative comparisons. For the glaucomatous eye, the inferior outer macular thickness is outside normal limits (yellow, $p \leq 5\%$) (polar plot, summary parameters) and the temporal-to-nasal outer macular thickness ratio is outside normal limits (red, $p \leq 1\%$).

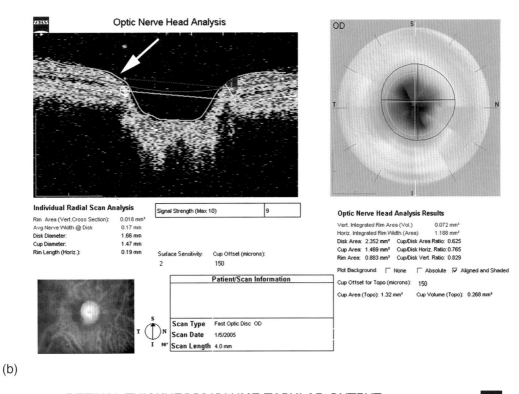

(b)

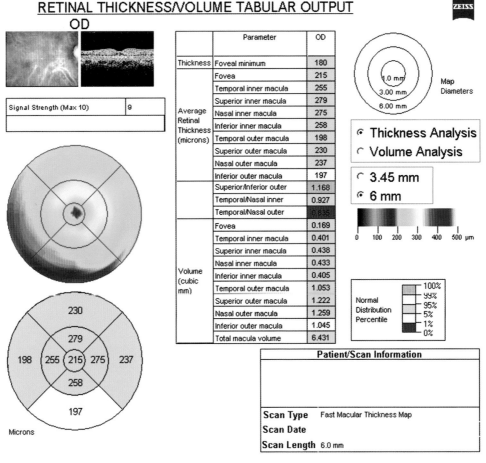

(c)

Figure 7.5 *Continued.*

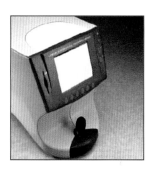

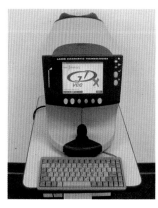

Figure 7.6   The GDx VCC.

the vitreoretinal interface and the chorioretinal interface (two reflective peaks that result from the oblique beam projection and the transparency of the retina). Each of several 3-mm^2 scans is composed of 16 optical sections. Interpolation is used to depict a continuous surface, and changes in fixation are used to place each scan over the area of interest.

Optic disc topography measurements are defined relative to a user-defined contour line placed along the optic disc margin and a reference plane placed 50 μm below the contour line in the temporal 5° sector, similar to HRT II. The RTA provides measurements for the same optic disc parameters provided by HRT II (Figure 7.9).

Nerve Fiber Analysis
With Variable Corneal Compensation

OD Right	Q: 9 Operator: lpw H: 1489 μm V: 1861 μm Date: 2/12/03 08:26

Right Fundus Image

TSNIT Parameters	OD Actual Val.	
TSNIT Average	37.6	
Superior Average	55.6	
Inferior Average	32.5	
TSNIT Std. Dev.	18.5	
NFI	52	

p>=5%	p<5%		p<1%	p<0.5%

Thickness Map Legend (microns)

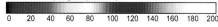

0   20   40   60   80   100   120   140   160   180   200

Right Nerve Fiber Thickness Map

Impression / Plan:
right (OD) Cornea: 37nm, -6.2deg; Res: 2nm, 19.7deg;

Right Deviation Map (from Normal)

Right Side Info: Mean Image Std Dev = 5.64

Signature:_____   Date:_____

p<5%		p<1%	p<0.5%

Right Nerve Fiber Layer

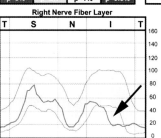

Figure 7.7   GDx VCC clinical printouts from the glaucomatous eye pictured in Figure 7.1. Clinical printouts from the GDx VCC contain the fundus image, nerve fiber layer thickness map (showing color-coded RNFL thickness where brighter colors represent increased thickness), deviation (from normal values) map, 'TSNIT' (temporal, superior, nasal, inferior, temporal RNFL thickness measured under an ellipse in the peripapillary region), plot (with normal range shaded in green), TSNIT parameters (e.g. TSNIT average, superior average, inferior average), and NFI (Nerve Fiber Indicator, based on machine-learning classification of multiple measurements where low values indicate a low likelihood of glaucoma and high values indicate a high likelihood of glaucoma on a scale of 1 to 100). For the glaucomatous eye, an inferior RNFL defect, relative to normative values (deviation map), is visible with thickness in the < 5% of normal to < 0.05% of normal range. This defect is evident on the TSNIT plot (arrow) and is reflected in 'outside normal limits' TSNIT average and inferior average results. The NFI result is 52.

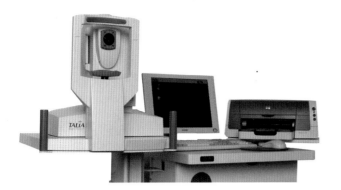

Figure 7.8 The retinal thickness analyzer (RTA).

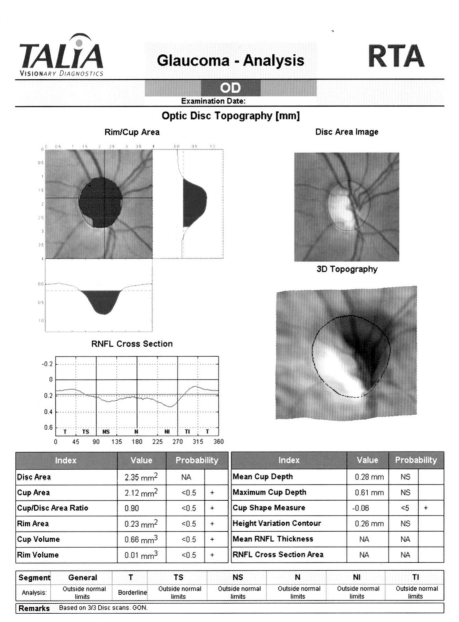

Index	Value	Probability		Index	Value	Probability	
Disc Area	2.35 mm²	NA		Mean Cup Depth	0.28 mm	NS	
Cup Area	2.12 mm²	<0.5	+	Maximum Cup Depth	0.61 mm	NS	
Cup/Disc Area Ratio	0.90	<0.5	+	Cup Shape Measure	-0.06	<5	+
Rim Area	0.23 mm²	<0.5	+	Height Variation Contour	0.26 mm	NS	
Cup Volume	0.66 mm³	<0.5	+	Mean RNFL Thickness	NA	NA	
Rim Volume	0.01 mm³	<0.5	+	RNFL Cross Section Area	NA	NA	

Segment	General	T	TS	NS	N	NI	TI
Analysis:	Outside normal limits	Borderline	Outside normal limits	Outside normal limits	Outside normal limits	Outside normal limits	Outside normal limits
Remarks	Based on 3/3 Disc scans. GON.						

Figure 7.9 RTA clinical printout ('Glaucoma Analysis') from the glaucomatous eye pictured in Figure 7.1. Clinical printouts from the RTA contain a color-coded Rim/Cup Area in which the disc is divided into rim (green) and cup (red), one vertical and one horizontal cross-section through the topography, a graphical representation of the RNFL cross-section, a fundus image (Disc Area Image), a three-dimensional topography measurement (3D Topography), stereometric parameters (including comparisons that provide probabilities relevant to a normative database), and the results from an analysis in which measured rim area, relative to disc area, is compared to an age-adjusted expected value based on normative data (similar to that available for HRT II). For the glaucomatous eye, the Rim/Disc Area map indicates an almost complete loss of neuroretinal rim, the RNFL cross-section graph shows a lack of RNFL nasally and especially inferonasally, and the 3D Topography shows an obvious inferior notch. Most stereometric parameters are outside normal limits and most regression analysis results are outside normal limits.

SUMMARY OF RESULTS FOR GLAUCOMA DETECTION

Historically, few studies have compared the performance of multiple laser imaging techniques for identifying glaucoma in a single population. Comparisons within the same population are more meaningful than comparisons across populations (i.e. across studies) because the demographic characteristics, including glaucoma severity, of single-population studies are controlled. Table 7.1 shows results from the only currently available study comparing new-generation CSLO (HRT II), OCT (StratusOCT) and SLP (GDx VCC) in one population. No other published studies have compared two or more of these techniques, at the time of writing.

Several studies investigating new-generation CSLO, OCT, SLP and RTA individually have shown that all techniques can discriminate between glaucomatous eyes (defined by abnormal standard automated perimetry) and healthy eyes. In addition, studies investigating previous-generation techniques showed similar results for CSLO and OCT. GDx VCC has been shown to discriminate better between glaucomatous and healthy eyes and to be better correlated with visual function measured with standard automated perimetry compared to the previous-generation SLP (GDx with fixed corneal birefringence compensator). Significantly fewer studies have investigated glaucoma detection using RTA, compared to CSLO, OCT and SLP.

TECHNIQUES FOR DETECTING CHANGE OVER TIME

An advantage of these imaging instruments is the plethora of quantitative and reproducible data that can be obtained. Given the large interindividual variability in the characteristics of the optic nerve head and RNFL which renders cross-sectional diagnosis of glaucoma problematic, these instruments offer the opportunity to objectively compare measurements longitudinally in a given individual and thereby establish the progressive nature of the disease. The high spatial resolution of these devices may allow structural changes to be measured over time that are too subtle to be detected by more conventional means such as photography. However, for a true change to be detected, the change needs to exceed the variability of the measurement. Measurement variability can be calculated by obtaining multiple scans at an imaging session. Change that exceeds this measurement variability can then be automatically measured and assessed for repeatability over successive imaging sessions in order to confirm that a change has truly occurred. Less sophisticated change analyses simply document the amount of change from baseline measurements by subtraction.

Confocal scanning laser ophthalmoscopy

The HRT II offers two methods of measuring change over time: Topographic Change Analysis and stereometric parameter change.

Topographic Change Analysis

This analysis is performed automatically once sufficient examinations have been acquired (at least three consecutive examinations are recommended). The baseline and follow-up topographies are normalized to each other by correcting for magnification, displacement, rotation, and tilt between images. This process is independent of a reference plane or contour line. Clusters of 4 × 4 adjacent pixels are combined to create super-pixels, which are colored if there is a significant local height change. The result is the change probability map, with red colors indicating significantly more depression in the follow-up examination – or glaucomatous progression (green colors indicate a significant elevation or improvement). A cluster of at least 20 connected super-pixels occurring in at least two or three (three is

---

Table 7.1 ROC curve areas and sensitivities at fixed specificities for discriminating between glaucomatous and healthy eyes using the 'best' (largest ROC curve area) HRT II, StratusOCT and GDx VCC parameter. Population included 75 glaucoma eyes with average standard perimetry MD = −4.87 dB (SD = 3.9 dB) and 66 healthy eyes

Parameter	Area under ROC curve	Sensitivity/specificity (%)
HRT II Vertical cup/disc ratio*	0.83	59/95, 69/80
StratusOCT inferior RNFL thickness	0.92	64/95, 89/80
GDx VCC Nerve Fiber Indicator	0.91	61/97, 87/80

*HRT Moorfields Regression Analysis results performed similarly to vertical cup/disc ratio, but results are not reported because ROC curve areas and sensitivities at fixed specificities cannot be calculated for categorical variables.

suggested) consecutive follow-up topographies indicates significant change (an error probability of < 5% compared to variability in the baseline topography) (Figure 7.10).

Stereometric parameter change

The stereometric parameter values can be examined for change over time. This requires a contour line to be placed around the optic nerve head on the baseline examination (see above). The parameter values inside that contour are then computed and the contour line automatically transferred to follow-up examinations that are normalized to the baseline. Stereometric parameter values are re-computed for follow-up examinations and compared to the baseline values. The result is the amount of change for each parameter. The significance of a detected change can be estimated from the typical variability of the parameter values of about 5%. The parameter values can be displayed in a diagram along the time axis (a trend analysis) (Figure 7.11).

Optical coherence tomography

For assessing RNFL thickness change, the StratusOCT incorporates both an 'RNFL Thickness Change Analysis' and an 'RNFL Thickness Serial Analysis'. The RNFL Thickness Change Analysis graphically presents the change in RNFL thickness (x-axis) around the optic disc (shown in TSNIT format along the y-axis) between two examinations. In addition, changes (in micrometers) for each quadrant and for 12, 30° sectors are shown as pie charts. The 'RNFL Thickness Serial Analysis' displays the RNFL thickness (x-axis) around the optic disc (y-axis) for up to four examinations on the same axes. Both reports can be used to compare RNFL thickness measurements between tests over time (Figure 7.12).

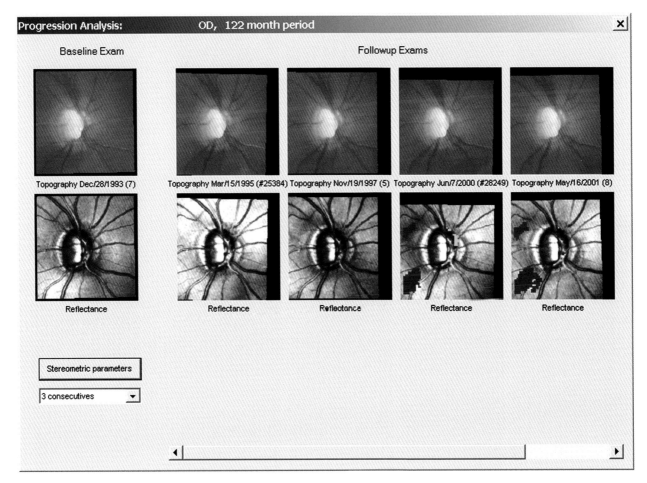

Figure 7.10 HRT II Topographic Change Analysis. HRT II Topographic Change Analysis of an optic disc of a glaucoma patient over a period of 8 years, using three consecutive follow-up topographies to confirm change. The topographical map on the left is the baseline topography, with the follow-up topographies arranged chronologically to the right. Areas of significant depression in local height measurements (colored red) denote areas of the neuroretinal rim and peripapillary retina that are progressively enlarging with time. A progressively enlarging area of depression of height is seen in the temporal-inferior peripapillary area.

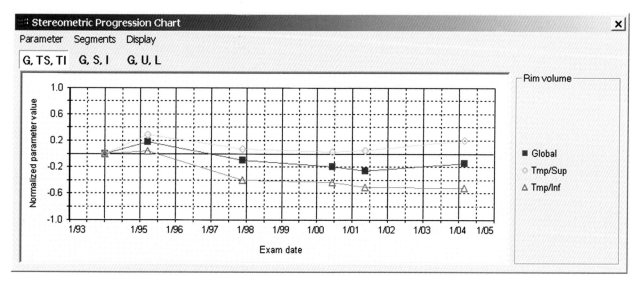

Figure 7.11 HRT II Trend Analysis. HRT II Trend Analysis report of the same patient illustrated in Figure 7.10. The global, temporal-inferior and temporal-superior regions are shown for neuroretinal rim volume. A progressive reduction of rim volume in the temporal-inferior region is evident and consistent with the temporal-inferior peripapillary depression shown in Figure 7.10.

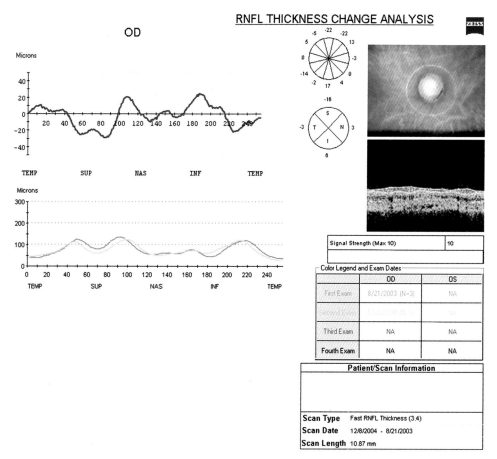

Figure 7.12 RNFL thickness change analysis. A composite figure illustrating available StratusOCT information for detecting RNFL thickness change over time. For the comparison graph, the purple curve is the first scan and the blue curve is the second. This glaucoma patient (different from that shown in Figures 7.10 and 7.11) shows some RNFL thinning superiorly, inferiorly and inferotemporally evident on the thickness change (top) and comparison thickness (bottom) graphs. The change is shown in micrometers by quadrant and 30° sector on the RNFL thickness charts. Some RNFL thickness improvement is also shown.

No change detection analyses currently are available for StratusOCT evaluation of optic disc topography or macular thickness.

Scanning laser polarimetry

The GDx VCC provides an 'Advanced Serial Analysis' report that displays a selection of up to four scans of the same eye chronologically, depicting the changes in RNFL with time (Figure 7.13). The report presents a Nerve Fiber Layer map, Deviation from Normal map, Difference from Baseline map, and TSNIT Parameter Table with trend analysis. The Deviation from Normal and Difference from Baseline maps are color coded to show probability of measurement compared to the normative database, and micrometer change from baseline, respectively. Additionally, a combination TSNIT graph shows the TSNIT RNFL thickness measurements at baseline and at each follow-up as a different-colored line, allowing comparison of the RNFL profile over time (Figure 7.13).

Retinal thickness analysis

The Retinal Thickness Analyzer (RTA) system allows the clinician to generate 'follow-up reports' for both retinal thickness and optic disc topography. These reports are produced when a patient is scanned at least twice using the same analysis type. For optic disc topography, a cup/disc area map is shown for each consecutive scan, a deviation map illustrates areas of thickness deviation compared to the baseline thickness map, and stereometric parameters, with deviation from baseline values, are shown for each follow-up examination. Regression analysis results also are shown for all images, and changes in these results may signal glaucomatous progression (Figure 7.14).

 Advanced Serial Analysis

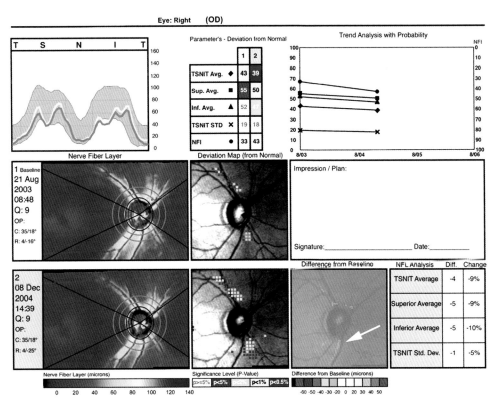

Figure 7.13 GDx VCC Scanning Laser Polarimeter. GDx VCC Scanning Laser Polarimeter 'Advanced Serial Analysis' report from the same patient illustrated in Figure 7.12. The examination at the top of the report is considered the reference (baseline) measurement for the selected serial analysis. Compared to baseline, the follow-up examination shows a slight decrease in RNFL thickness, based on the Nerve Fiber Layer map (left). This decrease is reflected as an increase in the area of the image that is outside normal limits based on the Deviation from Normal map, and a corresponding area of the image showing RNFL thinning compared to the reference image (arrow on Difference from Baseline map). In addition, one more TSNIT parameter is outside normal limits (inferior average RNFL thickness), the NFI has increased from 33 to 43, the Trend Analysis indicates a slight downward slope in all parameters, and the TSNIT graph shows a slight decrease in RNFL thickness superiorly and inferiorly.

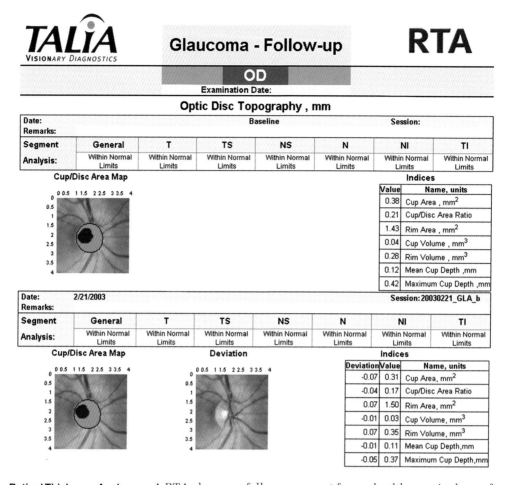

Figure 7.14   Retinal Thickness Analyzer.   A RTA glaucoma follow-up report from a healthy eye is shown for illustrative purposes. The upper figure includes the baseline disc area image, with overlying rim/cup area, and the lower figure includes the follow-up image. Potential changes in cup size would be shown on the deviation map. Deviation from baseline values for all parameters are shown in the lower right table.

SUMMARY OF RESULTS FOR CHANGE DETECTION

Because glaucoma is a slowly progressing disease, and because the newest-generation imaging technologies described in this chapter have been in use for only a few years, no studies have yet reported the ability of HRT II, StratusOCT, GDx VCC, and RTA optic disc topography measurement to detect change over time.

One relevant study showed change over time in retinal height measurements in glaucomatous eyes using a previous version of the currently available confocal scanning laser ophthalmoscopy topographic change analysis software for the HRT. This study showed significant change in retinal height (i.e. tissue thinning) in 69% of 77 eyes followed for approximately 5 years. Significant change in visual function accompanied 27% of these eyes and tissue thinning was corroborated by assessment of stereoscopic optic disc photographs in 80% of those eyes for which stereophotographs were available.

CONCLUSIONS

Computer-based imaging techniques show considerable promise for detecting abnormalities in eyes with glaucoma. The fact that they provide objective, reproducible, quantitative measurements on-demand makes them clinically attractive. While the new-generation instruments discussed in this chapter have not been well tested for glaucoma detection, they appear to perform as well as, or better than, their predecessors. Although it is not recommended that clinical diagnoses be made based solely on measurements from these instruments, it appears obvious that the measurements obtained can supplement other available clinical information. However, clinicians need to be aware of the strengths and limitations of these techniques, including understanding the importance of good image quality, before utilizing imaging data for clinical decision-making. Finally, although these instruments appear promising for the detection of glaucomatous change over time, available scientific data neither sufficiently support nor reject this claim. Further research is necessary to provide a strong, evidence-based recommendation for their use in the monitoring of this disease.

Further reading

Chauhan BC, McCormick TA, Nicolela MT, LeBlanc RP. Optic disc and visual field changes in a prospective longitudinal study of patients with glaucoma: comparison of scanning laser tomography with conventional perimetry and optic disc photography. Arch Ophthalmol 2001; 119: 1492–9

Greenfield DS. Optic nerve and retinal nerve fiber layer analyzers in glaucoma. Curr Opin Ophthalmol 2002; 13: 68–76

Medeiros FA, Zangwill LM, Bowd C, Weinreb RN. Comparison of the GDx VCC scanning laser polarimeter, HRT II confocal scanning laser ophthalmoscope, and stratus OCT optical coherence tomograph for the detection of glaucoma. Arch Ophthalmol 2004; 122: 827–37

Medeiros FA, Zangwill LM, Bowd C, et al. Evaluation of retinal nerve fiber layer, optic nerve head, and macular thickness measurements for glaucoma detection using optical coherence tomography. Am J Ophthalmol 2005; 139: 44–55

Reus NJ, Lemij HG. Diagnostic accuracy of the GDx VCC for glaucoma. Ophthalmology 2004; 111: 1860–5

Wollstein G, Garway-Heath DF, Hitchings RA. Identification of early glaucoma cases with the scanning laser ophthalmoscope. Ophthalmology 1998; 105: 1557–63

Zangwill LM, Medeiros FA, Bowd C, Weinreb RN. Optic nerve imaging: recent advances. In: Grehn F, Stamper R, eds. Glaucoma. Berlin: Springer-Verlag, 2004; 63–88

Zeimer R, Asrani S, Zou S, et al. Quantitative detection of glaucomatous damage at the posterior pole by retinal thickness mapping. A pilot study. Ophthalmology 1998; 105: 224–31

8 Psychophysical and electrophysiological testing in glaucoma: visual fields and other functional tests

Neil T Choplin

INTRODUCTION

The detection of nerve fiber loss and prevention of its development and progression is the ultimate goal of the ophthalmologist in the diagnosis and management of patients with glaucoma. At the present time, there is no proven reliable and consistent way to 'count' optic nerve fibers, compare the 'count' to known normals to determine the presence or absence of glaucomatous disease, and accurately determine whether the 'count' is changing over time. As axons are lost through the disease process, visual function declines in relation to the loss of fibers serving the region of the loss. Therefore, tests of optic nerve function are integral to the management of glaucoma patients as an indirect measure of the number of axons remaining.

Tests of optic nerve function can be objective or subjective. A variety of different test modalities have been investigated, looking for the ideal test that would be: (1) easy to administer; (2) mostly objective (requiring minimal decision-making or other efforts on the part of the patient); (3) highly sensitive to early loss or minimal change in the disease state; and (4) specific for glaucoma.

No objective test meeting these criteria has been found. Clinical functional testing for glaucoma consists mostly of 'psychophysical' tests, which by their very nature are highly subjective and susceptible to the shortcomings of human subjects. These tests require the patients to perceive something, intellectually interpret what was perceived, then

remember the instructions regarding what is supposed to be said or done if the correct 'something' was perceived, and effect some type of verbal or motor response. Perception, memory, interpretation and action thus characterize such psychophysical tests, and can all (individually, collectively or in some combination) lead to variability in the results. This can sometimes lead to false conclusions regarding the state of the disease process and inappropriate treatment.

FUNCTIONAL TESTS IN GLAUCOMA

There is good evidence that chronic glaucoma selectively damages large optic nerve fibers, although fibers of all sizes are damaged. Functional testing, therefore, should be directed at the visual tasks subserved by these axons in an attempt to identify early damage (Table 8.1). Some investigators have shown associated functional changes attributable to the loss of large optic nerve fibers, including declines in contrast sensitivity at high spatial frequencies, loss of pattern-evoked electroretinographic responses (PERG) after death of ganglion cells, and attenuation of PERG responses for high temporal frequencies of stimulation, supporting the idea that some part of glaucoma damage involves loss of the function of these large-diameter nerve fibers. Other investigators have suggested that the PERG may be helpful in identifying patients with ocular hypertension who will develop signs of glaucoma.

Table 8.1   Functional tests other than standard visual fields that have been used for glaucoma.   Many different electrophysiological and psychophysical tests have been investigated in glaucoma, particularly in an attempt to identify early damage or risk factors for development or progression of damage. This table lists the various modalities that have been investigated, how they are performed, what they measure and what the findings are in glaucoma patients

Test name	Objective or subjective	How performed	What it measures	Findings in glaucoma	Reference
Central contrast sensitivity	Subjective	Low-contrast flickering stimuli presented to the central four degrees	Minimum difference in luminance between stimulus and background of a flickering stimulus	Mean thresholds were lower than normal controls. Some ocular hypertensive patients also show reduction in threshold	Atkin et al., 1979; 1980
Temporal contrast sensitivity	Subjective	Stimulus of increasing frequency of flicker presented to the fovea	Intensity of stimulus required to perceive flicker at each presented flicker frequency	Frequency-specific loss at 15 Hz, non-frequency specific mean sensitivity loss greater in glaucoma patients than suspects	Breton et al., 1991
Pattern-evoked electro-retinographic responses (PERG)	Objective	Reversing checkerboard pattern presented on a television screen at varying contrast while standard ERG measurements are obtained	Waveform generated, latencies of responses and amplitudes for each wave component	Second negative wave selectively depressed in patients with glaucoma. Some ocular hypertensives showed similar responses	Trick, 1985; Weinstein et al., 1988
Contrast sensitivity	Subjective	Patient views figures of decreasing contrast at multiple spatial frequencies and identifies orientation of stripe pattern	Ability to detect correct orientation of stripe pattern as contrast decreases	Decreased contrast acuity in glaucoma patients, particularly at high spatial frequencies	Nadler et al., 1990
Color vision	Subjective	Farnsworth–Munsell 100 Hue Test, Farnsworth D-15 Test, Nagel or Pickford–Nicholson anomaloscope	Defects in color vision	Blue-yellow defects may occur early in glaucoma, red-green defects appear with advanced optic neuropathy	Sample et al., 1986
Color contrast sensitivity	Subjective	Computer-driven color television system	Color contrast threshold as a fraction of the maximum color available for color combinations on each color axis	Sensitivity to blue and red lights (relative to green) significantly less than controls	Gunduz et al., 1988

Test name	Objective or subjective	How performed	What it measures	Findings in glaucoma	Reference
Scotopic retinal sensitivity	Subjective	Patient dark adapted then presented with flickering stimulus increasing in luminance until seen	Sensitivity of dark-adapted retina to a flashing light	Reduction in absolute whole-field retinal sensitivity	Glovinsky et al., 1992
Flicker perimetry	Subjective	Static visual field testing performed with target flickering at 25 flashes/second	Threshold for target luminance against constant background	Flicker threshold elevated in glaucoma patients compared to normals but not compared to nonflickering stimulus	Feghali et al., 1991
Flicker visual-evoked potential	Objective	Standard VEP recording while viewing a flickering stimulus of varying frequency	Amplitude and phase responses of VEP	Glaucoma patients showed amplitude loss at high flicker frequencies, correlating with visual field damage	Schmeisser et al., 1992
Color pattern-reversal visual-evoked potential	Objective	Standard VEP recording while viewing a reversing checkerboard of black-white, black-red or black-blue	P1-wave peak time and amplitude for each pattern	Glaucoma and ocular hypertensives showed significant decreases in the measured parameters compared to normal, especially to the black-red and black-blue checkerboards	Shih et al., 1991
Visual-evoked potentials after photostress	Objective	Standard VEP measurement before and following 30 seconds of photostress	Time for VEP recording to return to prestress baseline	Longer VEP recovery time required for glaucoma patients with intermediate values in ocular hypertensives compared to normals	Parisi and Bucci, 1992
High-pass resolution perimetry	Subjective	Rings of varying size presented to peripheral retina, patient indicates seen or not seen	'Ring' threshold, peripheral visual acuity	Similar to standard perimetry except that target size, rather than luminance, is the variable	Sample et al., 1992
Blue-on-yellow perimetry (short-wavelength automated perimetry or SWAP)	Subjective	Modified automated static threshold perimeter with yellow background and blue projected stimuli	Visual field thresholds to blue stimuli on a yellow background	Abnormalities to blue-on-yellow may precede those to standard white-on-white and may predict which patients will develop loss or progress	Johnson et al., 1993a; 1993b
Multifocal visual-evoked potentials	Objective	Standard VEP recording while viewing a reversing white-black checkerboard which tests 60 locations simultaneously	P1-wave peak time and amplitude for each location	Decreased amplitude in a cluster of ≥ 3 test locations	Goldberg et al., 2002

Damage to the optic nerve is not limited only to loss of large-diameter axons. There is considerable evidence that axonal loss occurs in bundles which may be visible ophthalmoscopically. Typical glaucomatous loss favors the superior and inferior poles of the disc. Areas of retina which have lost bundles of nerve fibers will manifest a loss of sensitivity compared to surrounding areas. Such areas of decreased sensitivity are detectable on visual field testing; these scotomas and other defects in the mid-peripheral portion of the visual field begin to emerge as large numbers of axons are lost. Diffuse loss of axons may occur early in certain types of glaucoma or late in uncontrolled and progressive cases, resulting in generalized reduction in visual sensitivity. Other visual functions affected by loss of nerve fibers

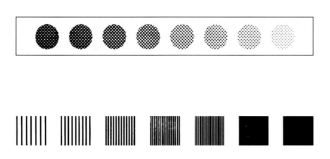

Figure 8.1 Testing contrast sensitivity. One method of testing contrast sensitivity requires the patient to discern the orientation of a pattern of stripes of increasing spatial frequency (more lines per unit area or degree of visual angle) and decreasing contrast. The top of the figure is an example of decreasing contrast between the test object and the background; the bottom of the figure illustrates a series of stimuli showing increasing spatial frequency, i.e. the pattern of stripes gets 'tighter' as the patient looks from left to right, making it harder to determine the orientation of the stripes. Tests involving these types of stimuli determine grating acuity.

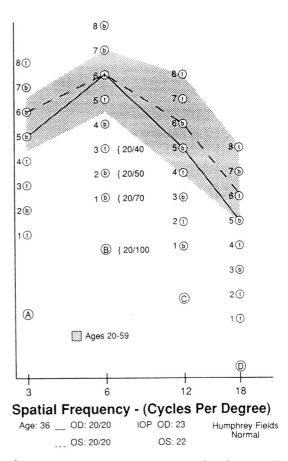

Figure 8.2 Decreased contrast sensitivity. Glaucoma may cause a decrease in contrast sensitivity in the absence of visual field defects or reduction in visual acuity. This figure is an example of decreased contrast sensitivity as determined by the Vectorvision system. The left side of the figure illustrates a reduction in sensitivity, particularly at the higher spatial frequencies (12 and 18 cycles per degree) in a patient with newly diagnosed open-angle glaucoma. The left eye, which has higher intraocular pressure, is worse. The gray area on the chart represents normal data. The right side of the figure illustrates normalization of the curves following institution of medical therapy and reduction in intraocular pressure.

include contrast sensitivity (Figures 8.1 and 8.2), temporal contrast sensitivity, multifocal visual-evoked potentials, color vision, scotopic retinal sensitivity, flicker perimetry, flicker visual-evoked potential, color pattern-reversal visual-evoked potentials, visual-evoked potentials following photostress, regional retinal visual acuity and foveal acuity. Loss of foveal acuity usually occurs late in the course of the disease but may occasionally occur early.

Purely objective tests of visual function, such as electro-oculography, electroretinography and visual-evoked potentials lack specificity for glaucoma. Other objective tests, such as multifocal visual-evoked potentials, flicker visual-evoked potential, color pattern-reversal visual-evoked potentials and pattern-evoked electroretinographic responses, have so far proved to have limited clinical applicability due to equipment requirements (e.g. cost, complex engineering, lack of commercial availability), lack of familiarity to clinicians, complexity of interpretation, and ease of performance.

VISUAL FIELDS IN GLAUCOMA

Of the subjective tests currently available, visual field testing remains the mainstay, and the use of automated perimetry has allowed the development of standardized tests for obtaining quantitative measurements (Figures 8.3–8.26). Such measurements can be compared to known normal values to determine the presence of abnormalities, and can easily be followed over time for change. Statistical packages have been developed to help in the interpretation of quantitative visual field data, both for determining abnormality in a single visual field examination and for determining the significance of observed changes in a series of visual fields measured over time. Newer testing algorithms such as the Swedish Interactive Thresholding Algorithm (SITA) can shorten test time by 50%, resulting in less patient fatigue while maintaining excellent sensitivity and specificity. Although the examples in this chapter were obtained with the full threshold algorithm (and illustrate the types of visual field defects that may be found in patients with glaucoma), SITA has become widely accepted as the 'standard' for computerized automated perimetry. Other researchers have investigated the combination of the known objective effects of optic nerve disease on color vision with the familiar types of subjective automated perimetry to determine if a blue stimulus on a yellow background will detect earlier defects than standard white-on-white perimetry. This has been named 'short-wavelength automated perimetry', or 'SWAP'. Although helpful in detecting early loss, SWAP may be affected by media opacities such as cataracts. Also, it is a somewhat more lengthy and tiring test for the patient. Use of the SITA testing algorithm for SWAP visual fields may address this issue. Visual field defects in glaucoma are summarized in Table 8.2.

Table 8.2 Visual field defects in glaucoma. Visual field defects in glaucoma are well known. None of the defects that can occur in glaucoma is 100% specific; any defect that respects the horizontal meridian may occur in any optic nerve disorder. The interpretation of any visual field defect with regards to a differential diagnosis of disorders that can produce it must be made with regard to the entire clinical picture of the patient – intraocular pressure level, optic nerve appearance, family history and other risk factors. This table lists the visual field defects that occur in glaucoma, and indicates the frequency with which those defects have been observed to be initial defects

Type of defect	Glaucoma patients manifesting this as their initial defect (%)
Increasing scatter (fluctuation)	Probably all
Diffuse depression, i.e. increased threshold	
Paracentral defects	41
Nasal steps	54
Arcuate enlargement of the blind spot	30
Arcuate scotomata not connected to the blind spot	90
Nerve fiber bundle defects	
Altitudinal defects	
Temporal wedge defects	3
Central and temporal islands	
End-stage (temporal island only)	

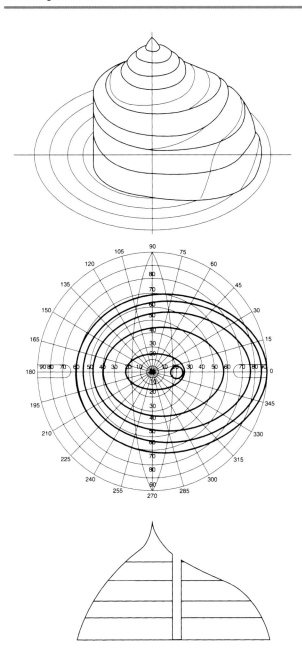

Figure 8.3 The normal visual field and methods to 'map' it. The visual field defines all that is visible to one eye at a given time. It has been likened to an 'island' or 'hill' of vision in a 'sea of blindness'. The job of visual field testing is to draw a map of the island of vision. The top of the figure represents the three-dimensional structure of a normal island of vision. The fovea is the 0,0 point on the x and y axes. The z axis represents the height of the island of vision at any point x,y above the 'sea', and is equivalent to the sensitivity of the retina at that point. Two different methods are available for drawing a map of the island. The middle of the figure represents the island as viewed from above as drawn by isopter perimetry, such as the tangent screen or Goldmann perimeter. An isopter may be thought of as the boundary of a retinal area within which all points have equal or greater sensitivity to those at the boundary. Each curved line, equivalent to the lines on the top figure, thus represents an isopter boundary. The lines are determined by moving test objects of fixed size and intensity from areas of non-seeing towards the center until the patient indicates it has been seen, thus giving this type of testing the name 'kinetic' perimetry. The smaller circles indicate areas determined by smaller and/or dimmer stimuli. By comparing the isopter locations and shapes to known normals, visual field defects can be determined. The bottom of the figure represents a 'slice', or profile of the island of vision through any meridian. It is determined by varying the intensity of a stimulus of fixed size at each point along the meridian until threshold has been determined. This type of testing has been termed 'static' perimetry, since the object does not move to determine threshold, and is typified by the Octopus perimeters and the Humphrey Field Analyzer (Zeiss-Humphrey Inc., San Leandro, CA). Testing multiple meridians and putting them together will give the three-dimensional picture of the island. Comparing the measured sensitivities to known normals allows for the detection of defects. Since quantitative information is generated (i.e. sensitivity values), statistical techniques can be applied for determining abnormalities and significant changes over time.

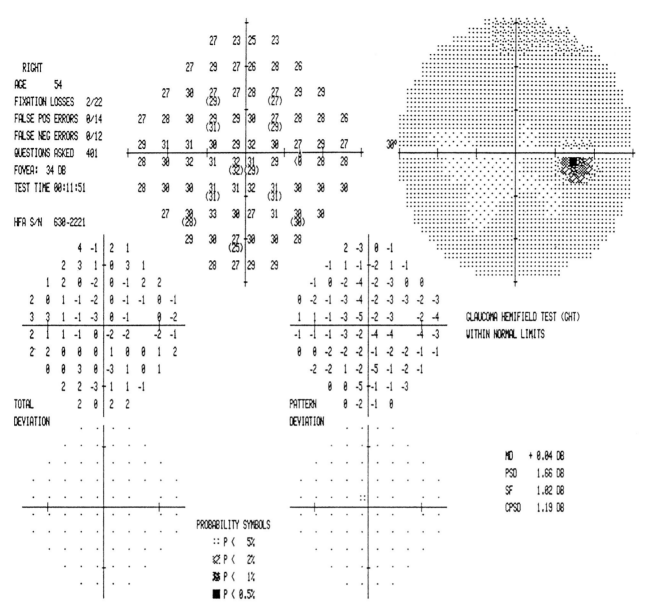

Figure 8.4 The visual field as measured by automated static perimetry. Modern automated static perimeters determine retinal threshold at an array of points and can display the results in a variety of ways. The user determines what points to test and what strategy to use to test them. This figure displays the results of a 30-2 threshold test from the Humphrey Field Analyzer. The test consists of an array of 76 points centered around the fovea with a spacing of six degrees and offset from the axes by three degrees. The numerical grid at the center top represents the retinal threshold expressed in decibels for each test point. Since the decibel scale is a relative scale representing attenuation of the maximum available stimulus intensity, high numbers (above 30 dB, depending upon age) represent good sensitivity (greater attenuation = dimmer stimulus = greater sensitivity). The 'graytone' display on the upper right is a graphical representation of the threshold values, with lighter symbols used for areas of better sensitivity and progressively darker symbols used to represent decreasing sensitivity. The plot on the middle left, labeled 'total deviation', is an array of the differences of the patient's measured threshold values from those exhibited by age-corrected normals, and the lower plot symbolically shows the probability of obtaining the value exhibited by the patient in the reference population. The pattern deviation plot represents a software correction applied to the field for any factors that affect all the points, allowing focal defects to be more readily displayed. A probability plot is displayed for the pattern deviation as well. This figure is an example of a visual field displaying no defects in a patient with mild elevation of intraocular pressure and normal-appearing optic nerves.

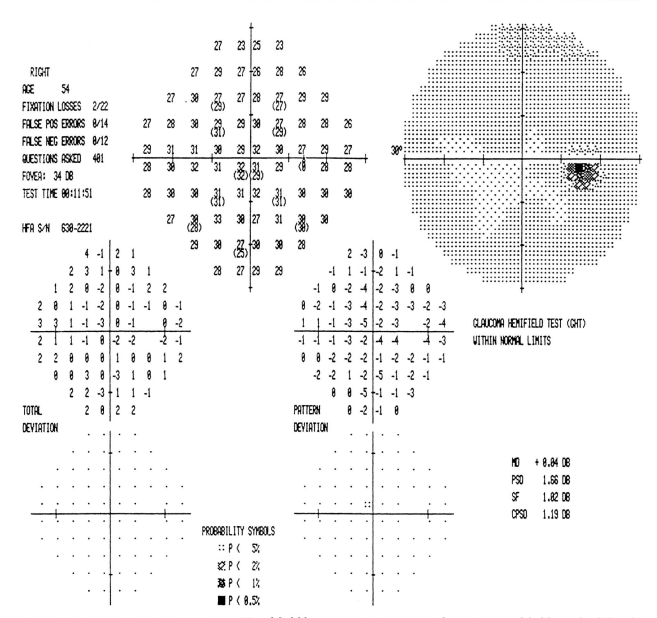

Figure 8.5 Asymmetrical visual field loss. Visual field loss occurs in two ways. The entire visual field may be diffusely affected, causing a loss of sensitivity at all points, manifested as lower threshold values. Many factors acting on the field can produce diffuse loss, including incorrect refraction at the time of the test so that the patient was not properly focused on the bowl, media opacities such as cataract which reduce the amount of light entering the eye, small pupils, inattentiveness and false-negative responses, and diffuse optic nerve damage. This set of visual fields illustrates a difference in mean sensitivity between the two eyes, indicative of asymmetric damage.

The right eye, the same as Figure 8.4, shows no defect and the mean deviation when compared to age-corrected normals is +0.04 dB. The left eye shows no significant focal defect, but a mean deviation of −1.58 dB, indicating a mild overall reduction in sensitivity, not only compared to the reference population but also more importantly when compared to the fellow eye. The intraocular pressures were 16 mmHg in the right eye and 23 mmHg in the left. In addition, there was a mild increase in the cup/disc ratio in the left eye. This mild reduction in sensitivity in the left eye would not usually be considered clinically significant, except when all the data are considered. It is consistent with mild diffuse depression and with early glaucomatous damage and consequently therapy was started in the left eye.

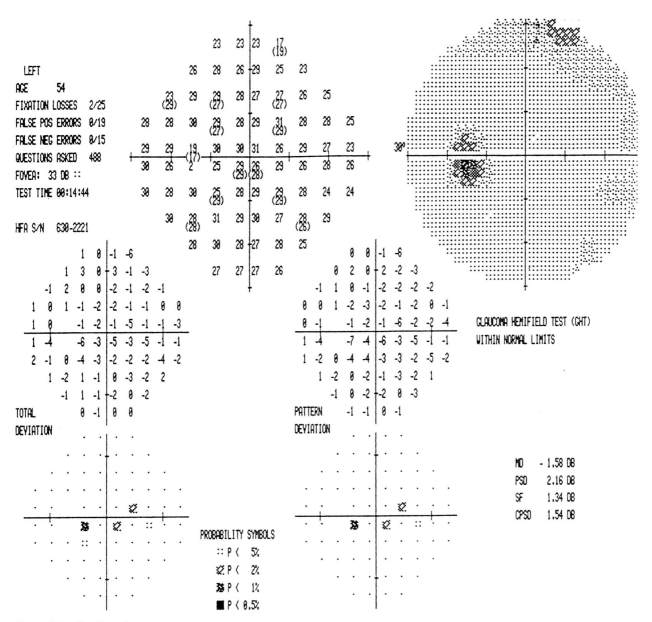

Figure 8.5 *Continued.*

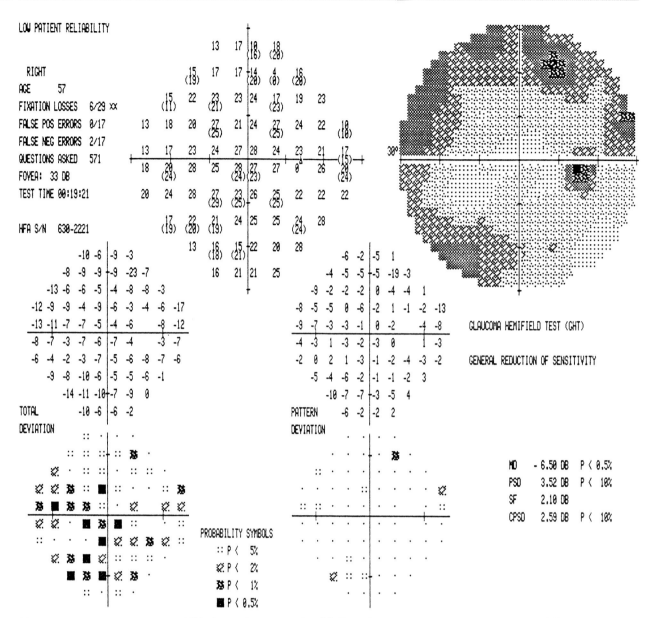

Figure 8.6 Diffuse depression. This is another example of diffuse depression occurring in a patient followed for many years with increased intraocular pressure which had been under treatment. The ocular media are clear, the patient's pupils were dilated for the examination, he was refracted following dilatation to insure the proper distance lens, and the full +3.00 add was used to make sure he was properly focused at the test distance. The mean deviation is −6.50 dB, a value expected to occur in less than 0.5% of the age-corrected normals (i.e. 99.5% of the normals had higher values than this patient), consistent with diffuse optic nerve damage.

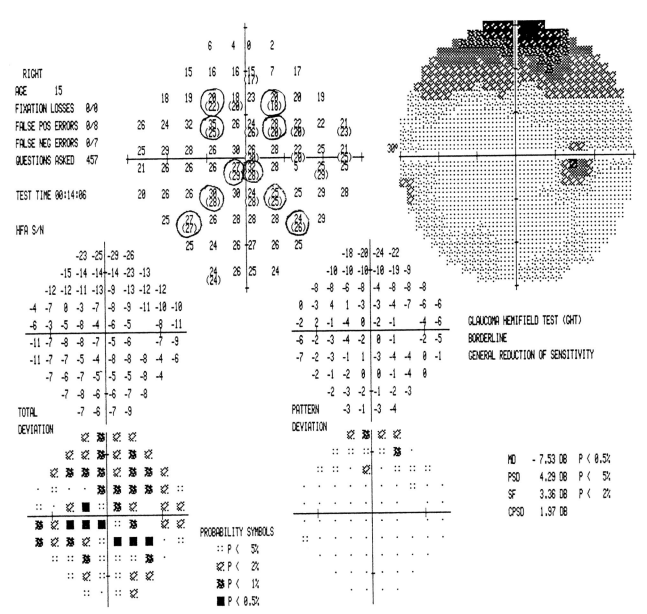

Figure 8.7 Fluctuation. The results of psychophysical tests, such as visual field testing, are subject to a certain degree of variability. Indeed, threshold is defined as that stimulus intensity that has a 50% probability of being seen. This in itself will give rise to varying results as points are retested. Test–retest variability in static perimetry is measurable, has known normal values and has clinical significance. Although an unreliable patient who does not know how to perform the test will show variability in results, unreliability is measured in other ways (e.g. fixation losses, false-positive and false-negative responses), and a large spread in repeat measures in an otherwise reliable field has other significance. It has been shown that, as retinal sensitivity decreases, the variability of threshold in that region increases. It has also been shown that increasing fluctuation may precede the development of a visual field defect, thus giving its measurement particular clinical importance. This figure illustrates ten points (circled) that always have threshold measured twice. The difference of each measurement from the average value is squared, then the squares are summed, averaged across the field and the square root taken. Other factors are applied to account for point location in the field, and the result expressed as the short-term fluctuation value, or 'sf'. This patient has angle-recession glaucoma with intraocular pressure in the low 30s. The field demonstrates diffuse depression, but more importantly an increased sf value of 3.36, expected in less than 2% of the reference population. The high value is derived from two points in the superior arcuate area – one showing measurements of 35 and 25 dB and the other 28 and 20 dB. These large differences in repeat measurements (10 and 8 dB, respectively) point to disturbed portions of the visual field that will most likely go on to develop paracentral and arcuate defects.

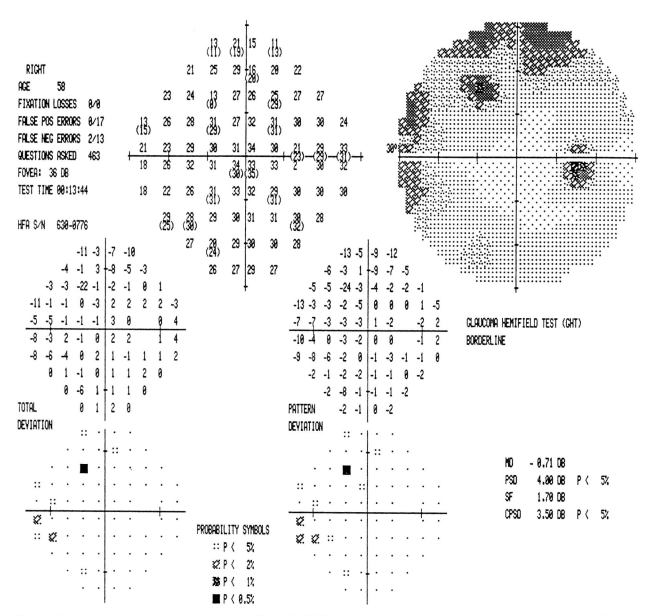

Figure 8.8 Isolated paracentral defects. As indicated in Table 8.2, isolated paracentral defects occur as the initial glaucoma defect in about 40% of patients. This patient shows an isolated defect in the superior paracentral region of 22 dB below normal. Note also the wide fluctuation in repeat measurements of this point (13 dB and then 0 dB). Untreated intraocular pressure was in the upper 20s in this eye.

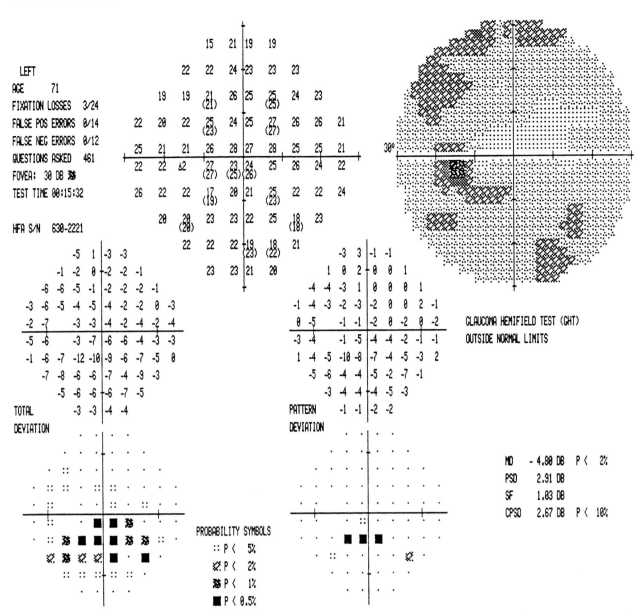

Figure 8.9 Asymmetry across the horizontal meridian. Asymmetry across the horizontal meridian is an important sign of optic nerve disease. The glaucoma hemifield test is a software option as part of the statistical analysis package for the Humphrey Field Analyzer that compares the differences of mirror-image clusters of points on opposite sides of the horizontal from the reference population to determine asymmetry. This is an example of an asymmetric disturbance in the inferior portion of the visual field of a glaucoma patient with an abnormal glaucoma hemifield test. This patient shows an early inferior arcuate enlargement of the blind spot. Note also from the probability map of the pattern deviation that threshold values of 19 dB (or more) occur in the periphery of the superior hemifield in 95% of the age-corrected normals, but a value of 19 dB would be expected in the inferior arcuate area less than 0.5% of the time.

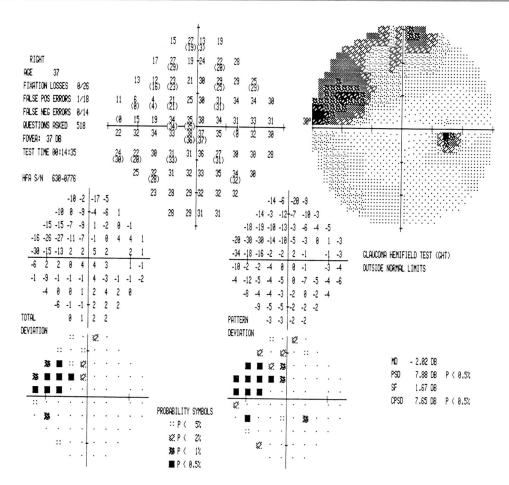

Figure 8.10　Nasal steps.
Nasal steps are very common in glaucoma, representing an asymmetry in threshold across the horizontal midline at the nasal periphery of the measured field. They are the first defects in about half the glaucoma patients. This patient shows a dense superior nasal step.

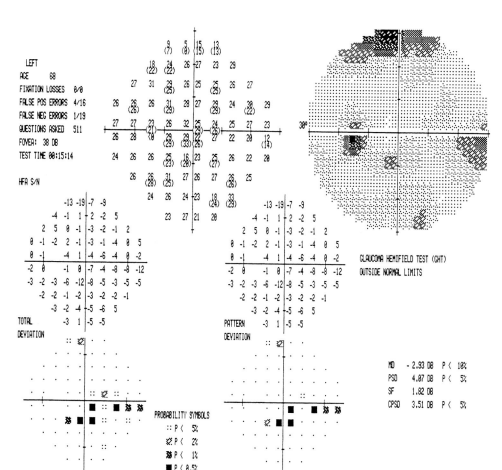

Figure 8.11　Early glaucomatous damage in the inferior hemifield. This is another example of early glaucomatous damage in the inferior hemifield. An inferior nasal step combined with inferior paracentral defects indicates damage to the superior arcuate nerve fibers.

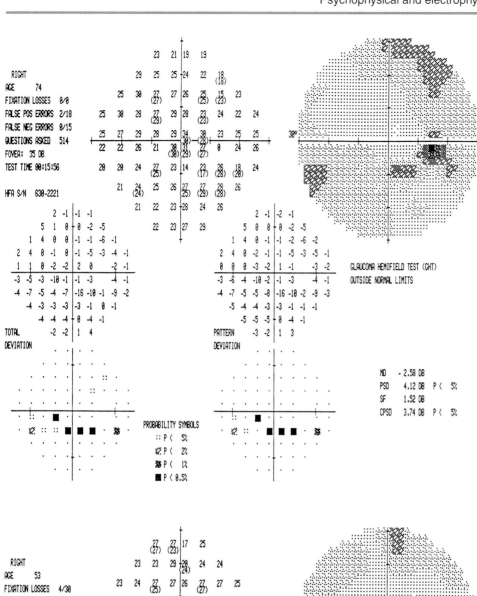

Figure 8.12 An inferior arcuate scotoma. This example of early glaucoma damage shows an inferior arcuate scotoma which does not reach the nasal periphery.

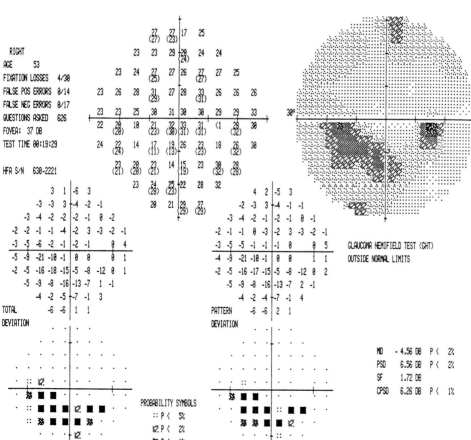

Figure 8.13 A broad inferior arcuate scotoma. This patient has had open-angle glaucoma for many years. He has extensive damage in the fellow eye and has lost fixation. This is an example of a broader inferior arcuate scotoma (compared to Figure 8.12) which connects to the blind spot.

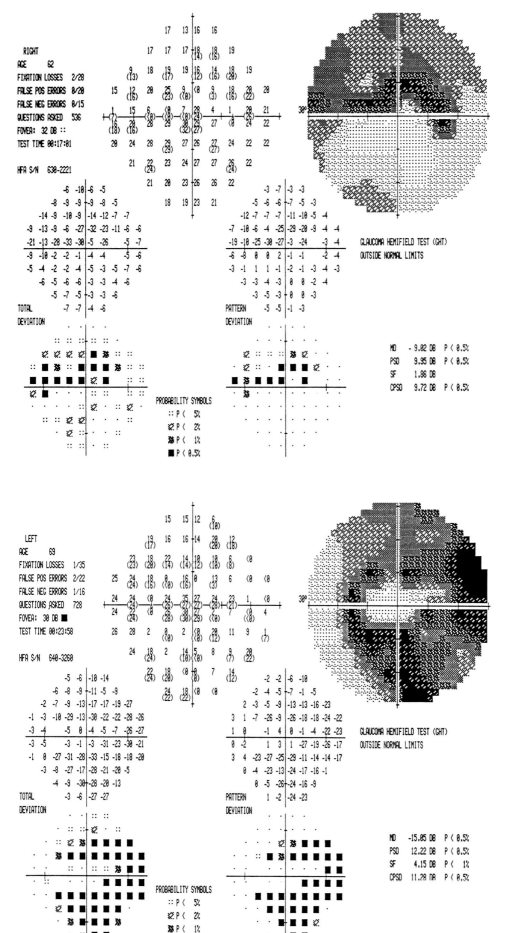

Figure 8.14   A complete loss of a bundle of axons. Extension of the optic cup to the rim of the disc will result in loss of nerve fibers corresponding to that portion of rim. This patient with low-tension glaucoma developed extension of the cup to the inferior pole of the disc and this superior nerve-fiber bundle defect. This represents loss of a complete bundle of axons, is very deep, and breaks through to the nasal periphery. This could possibly represent an ischemic infarction of a portion of the optic nerve.

Figure 8.15   A 'double arcuate' scotoma. This is an example of a 'double arcuate' scotoma, which results from extension of the cup to both poles of the disc. Note that the inferior loss is worse than the superior.

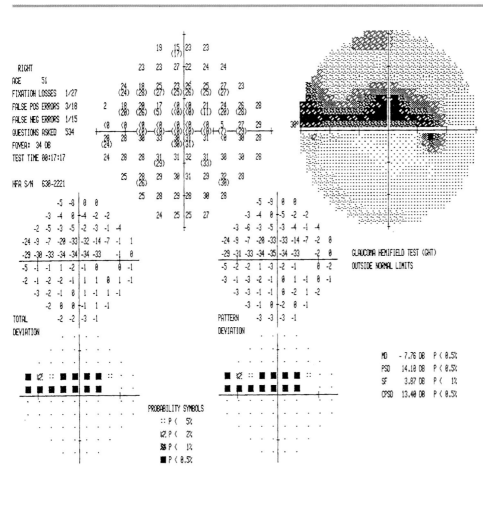

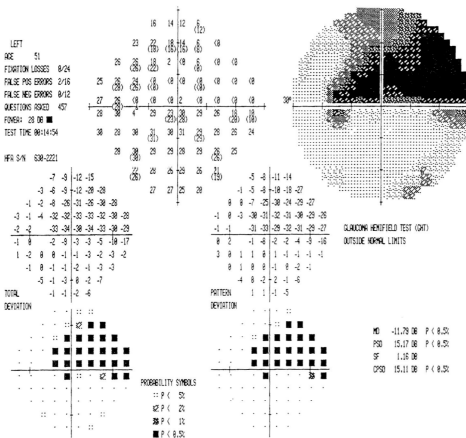

Figure 8.16 Complete nerve-fiber bundle defects. Complete nerve-fiber bundle defects are not common as the initial defects in glaucoma patients. This pair of visual fields from the right and left eyes of this 51-year-old African-American woman were the patient's first visual fields. Initial pressures were in the upper 20s. Note the asymmetry, with the left eye worse than the right.

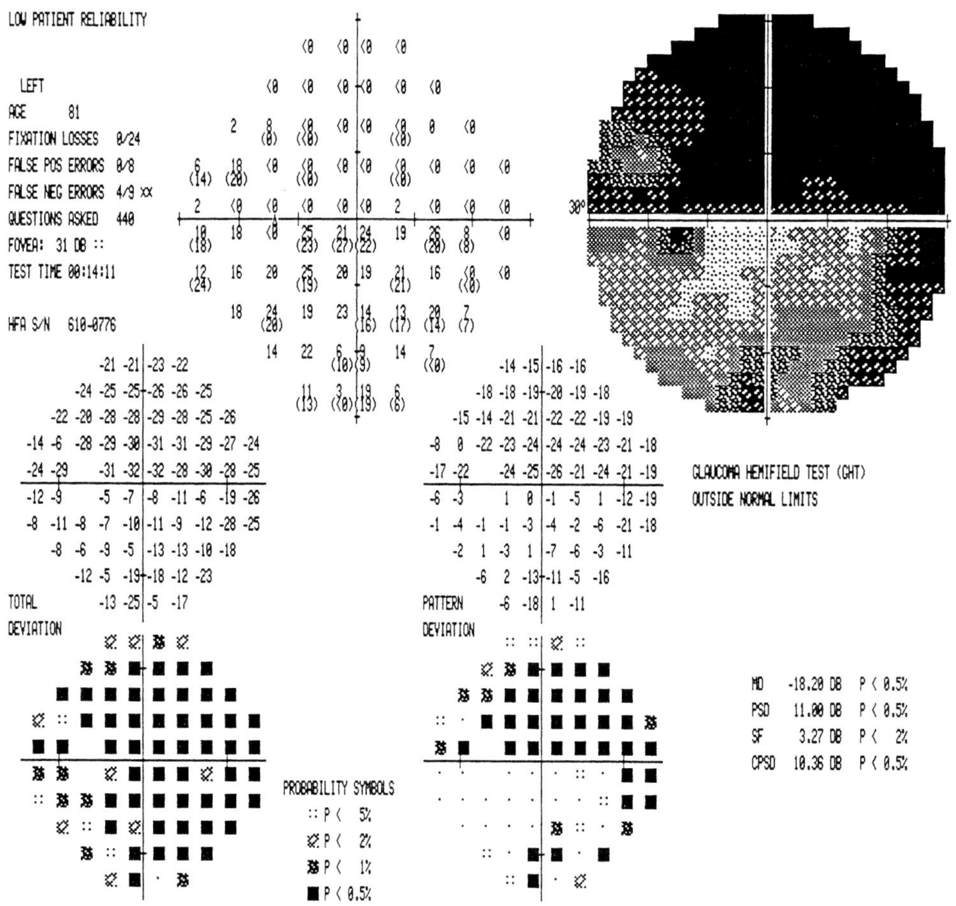

Figure 8.17 Superior altitudinal defect. Complete loss of the inferior pole of the nerve will give rise to a superior altitudinal defect, illustrated here. Although commonly seen following ischemic optic neuropathy, this defect gradually enlarged over time in this patient with low-tension glaucoma (see Figure 8.26).

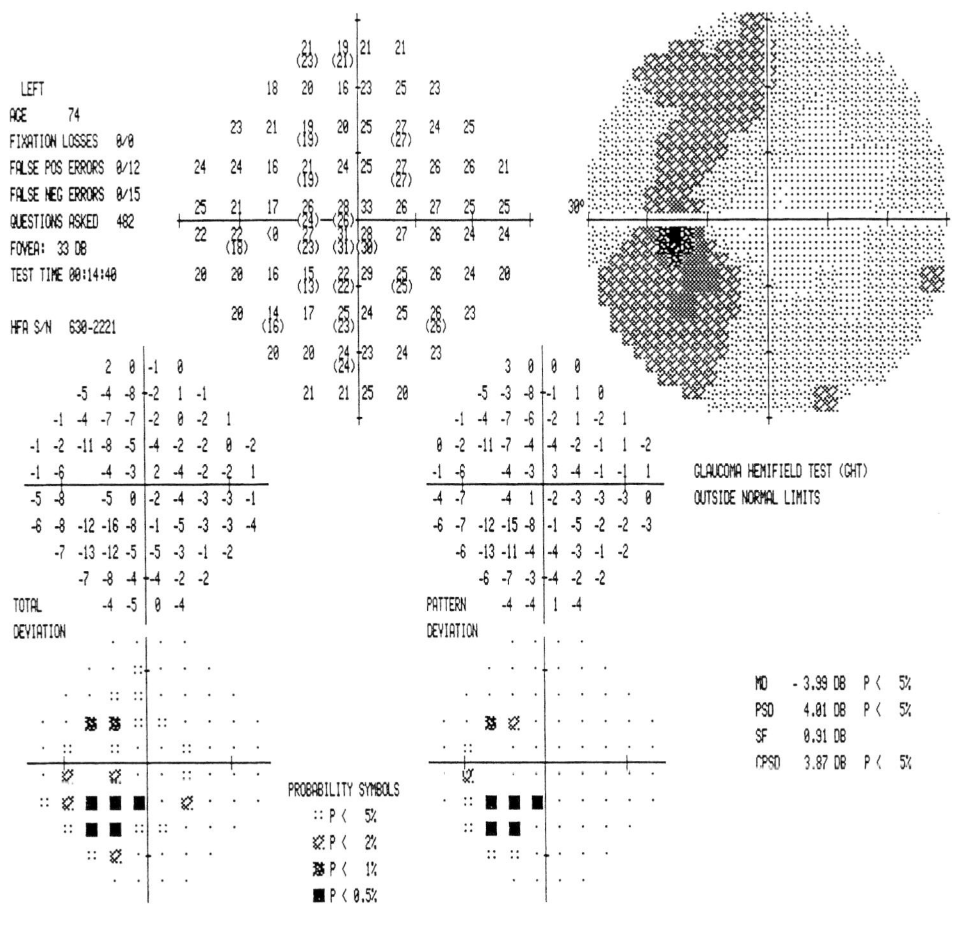

Figure 8.18 Isolated temporal defects. Isolated temporal defects occur about 3% of the time as initial glaucoma defects. This patient shows temporal defects above and below the horizontal midline. Note that the statistical software gives more significance to the inferior disturbances, indicating that some depressions in the superior field of older people is not unusual.

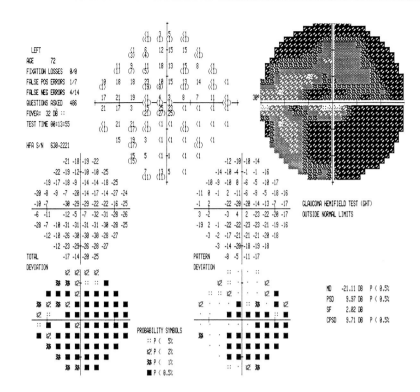

Figure 8.19 Far-advanced glaucomatous optic neuropathy. Progressive loss of nerve fibers results in greater visual field loss, usually affecting the macular fibers and the nasal retina last, leaving central and temporal islands as the end-stage before complete visual loss. This is an example of a patient with far-advanced glaucomatous optic neuropathy, with small islands remaining centrally, temporally and in the superior arcuate area.

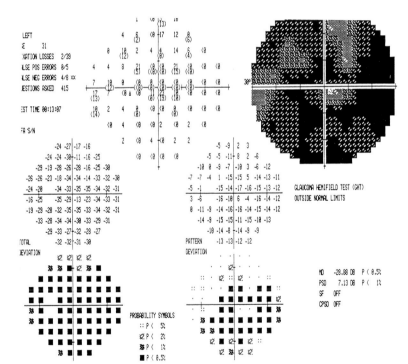

Figure 8.20 High intraocular pressure. Very high intraocular pressure can lead to extensive loss which may become symptomatic. This visual field showing extensive damage was obtained upon initial presentation of a young male with intraocular pressure in the 50s. He noted visual loss and went for an eye examination. His visual acuity was reduced to 20/70. The fellow eye had minimal loss with pressures in the 30s and 20/20 vision. He was found to have abnormal anterior chamber angles, indicating a juvenile-onset type of glaucoma. Following filtering surgery, his visual acuity returned to 20/25 and some of the visual field loss returned.

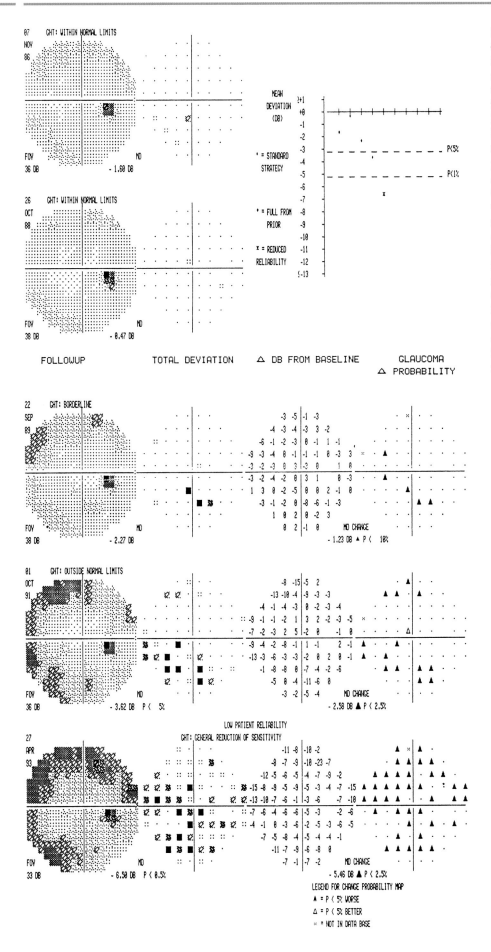

Figure 8.21 The progression of visual field defects. Visual fields may show progression over time in a variety of ways. If initially normal, they may go on to diffuse loss or the development of isolated depressions. This series of fields over a 7-year period was obtained in an African-American man with ocular hypertension which was under treatment. It shows a gradual but steady decrease in retinal sensitivity affecting the field uniformly (the last field is the same as Figure 8.6). A review of optic nerve photographs (particularly comparing the earliest to the latest) shows a concentric enlargement of the cup over time with the neuroretinal rim still intact.

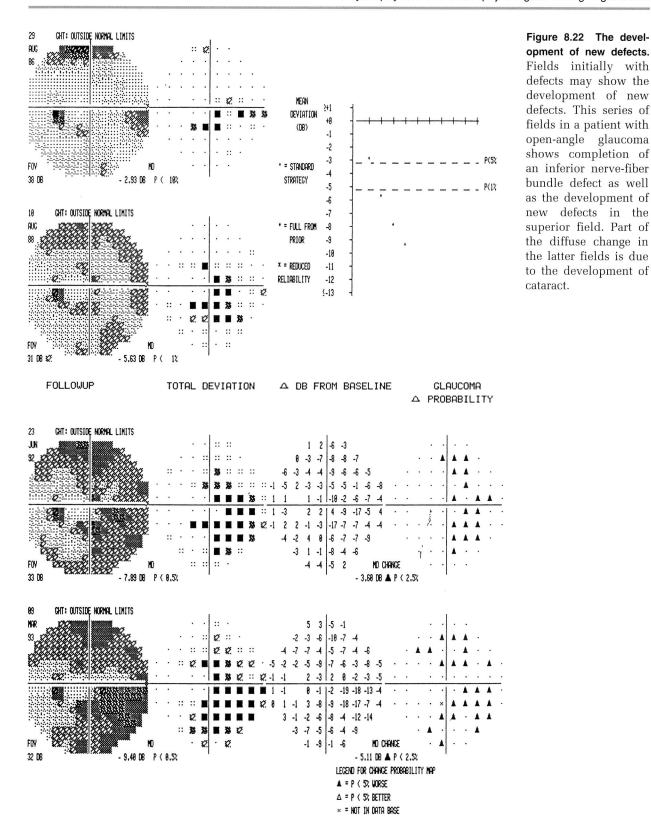

Figure 8.22 The development of new defects. Fields initially with defects may show the development of new defects. This series of fields in a patient with open-angle glaucoma shows completion of an inferior nerve-fiber bundle defect as well as the development of new defects in the superior field. Part of the diffuse change in the latter fields is due to the development of cataract.

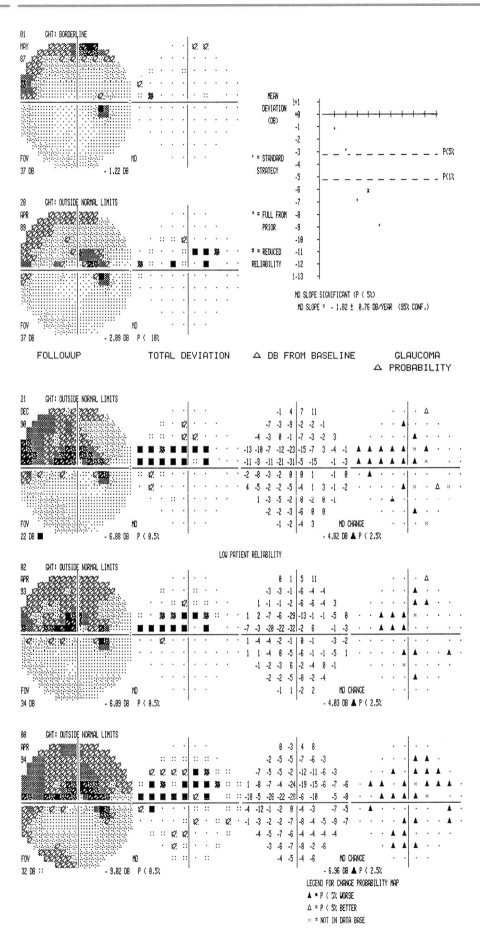

Figure 8.23 Widening and deepening of single nerve-fiber bundle defects. Visual fields may progress by widening and deepening of single nerve-fiber bundle defects. This series of visual fields is from the patient in Figure 8.14. Initially the field was normal and then she developed disturbances in the superior arcuate area. These coalesced and extended over time to involve the entire bundle of axons and a good portion of the superior field.

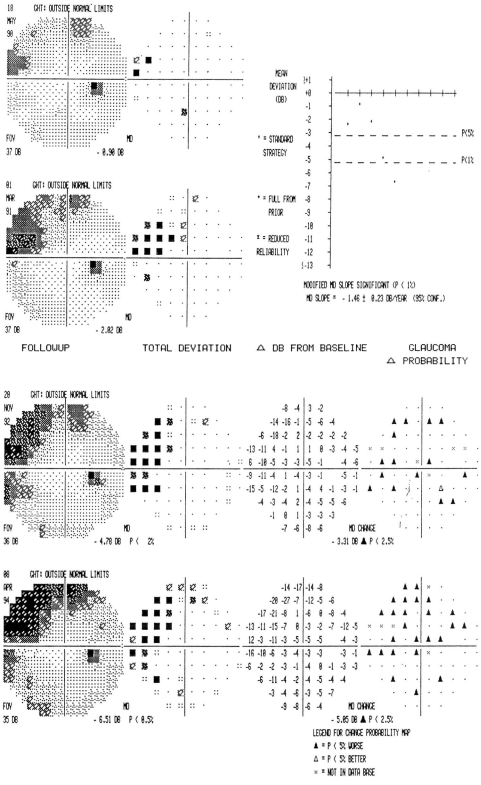

Figure 8.24 Gradual enlargement of the superior nasal step. This series of visual fields was obtained from the fellow eye of the same patient in Figure 8.20. Note the gradual enlargement of the superior nasal step. He has undergone filtering surgery in this eye as well.

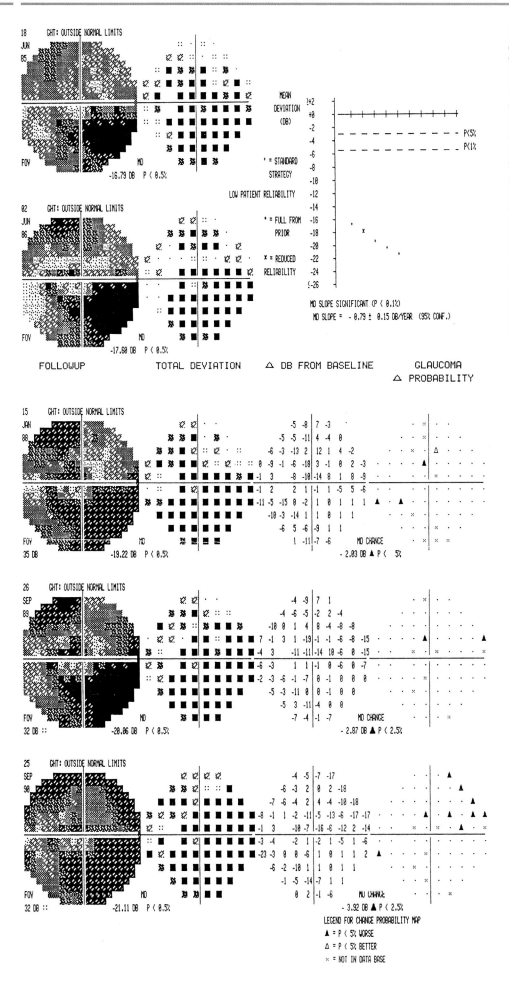

Figure 8.25 A steady decline of 1 dB per year. This is the series of visual fields of the patient in Figure 8.19. Note the extension of the inferior nerve-fiber bundle defect and the development of new defects in the superior hemifield. The statistical software plots the mean deviation over time as a graph on the right side of the top of the printout, and performs statistical tests for significant change over time. This series shows a steady decline of about 1 dB per year, which was highly significant.

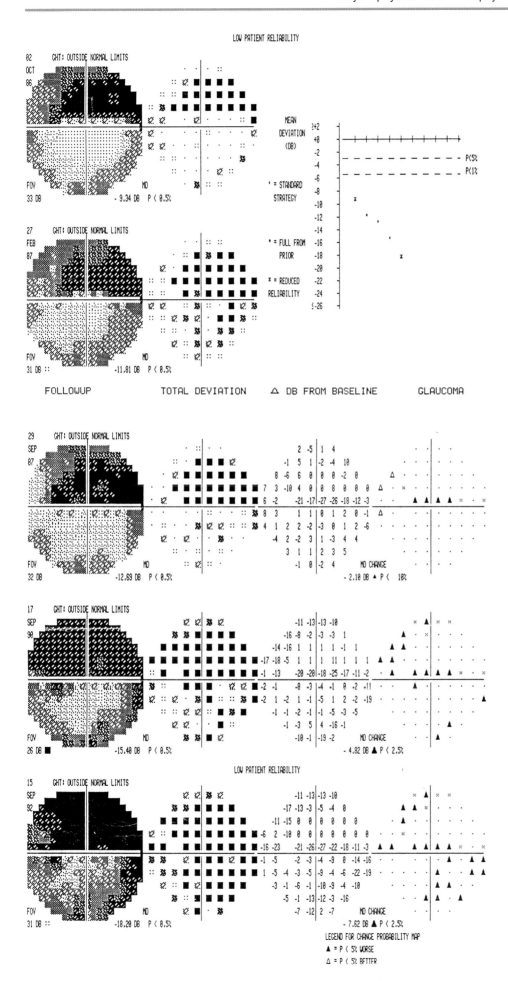

Figure 8.26 Extension of a dense superior nerve-fiber bundle defect. This series illustrates the extension of a dense superior nerve-fiber bundle defect to a complete altitudinal defect over a 6-year period.

Further reading

Anctil JL, Anderson JR. Early foveal involvement and generalized depression of the visual field in glaucoma. Arch Ophthalmol 1980; 102: 363

Atkin A, Bodis-Wollner I, Wolkstein M, et al. Abnormalities of central contrast sensitivity in glaucoma. Am J Ophthalmol 1979; 88: 205–11

Atkin A, Wolkstein M, Bodis-Wollner I, et al. Interocular comparison of contrast sensitivity in glaucoma patients and suspects. Br J Ophthalmol 1980; 64: 858–62

Aulhorn E, Harms H. Early visual field defects in glaucoma. In: Leydhecker W, ed. Glaucoma: Tutzing Symposium 1966. Basel: S Karger, 1967: 151

Austin D. Acquired colour vision defects in patients suffering from chronic simple glaucoma. Trans Ophthalmol Soc UK 1974; 94: 880

Bengtsson BB. A new rapid threshold algorithm for short-wave automated perimetry. Invest Ophthalmol Vis Sci 2003; 44: 1388–94

Breton ME, Wilson TW, Wilson RP, et al. Temporal contrast sensitivity loss in primary open-angle glaucoma and glaucoma suspects. Invest Ophthalmol Vis Sci 1991; 32: 2931–41

Budenz DL, Rhee PP, Feuer WJ, et al. Sensitivity and specificity of the Swedish interactive threshold algorithm for glaucomatous visual field testing. Ophthalmology 2002; 109: 1052–8

Caprioli J. Automated perimetry in glaucoma. Am J Ophthalmol 1991; 112: 235–9

Choplin NT, Edwards RP. Visual Field Testing with the Humphrey Field Analyzer. Thorofare, NJ: SLACK, 1995

Delgado MF, Nguyen NT, Cox TA, et al. Automated perimetry: a report by the American Academy of Ophthalmology. Ophthalmology 2002; 109: 2362–74

Drance SM. The glaucomatous visual field. Br J Ophthalmol 1972; 56: 186

Drance SM, Lakowski R, Schulzer M, Douglas GR. Acquired color vision changes in glaucoma: use of a 100-hue test and Pickford anomaloscope as predictors of glaucomatous field change. Arch Ophthalmol 1981; 99: 829

Feghali JG, Bocquet X, Charlier J, et al. Static flicker perimetry in glaucoma and ocular hypertension. Curr Eye Res 1991; 10: 205–12

Glovinsky Y, Quigley HA, Brum B, et al. A whole-field scotopic retinal sensitivity test for the detection of early glaucoma damage. Arch Ophthalmol 1992; 110: 486–90

Goldberg I, Graham SL, Klistorner AI. Multifocal objective perimetry in the detection of glaucomatous field loss. Am J Ophthal 2002; 133: 29–39

Graham SL, Klistorner AI, Goldberg I. Clinical application of objective perimetry using multifocal visual evoked potentials in glaucoma practice. Arch Ophthalmol 2005; 123: 729–39

Gunduz K, Arden GB, Perry S, et al. Color vision defects in ocular hypertension and glaucoma: quantification with a computer-driven color television system. Arch Ophthalmol 1988; 106: 929–35

Harrington DO. The Bjerrum scotoma. Am J Ophthalmol 1965; 59: 646

Hart WM Jr, Yablonski M, Kass MA, Becker B. Quantitative visual field and optic disc correlates early in glaucoma. Arch Ophthalmol 1978; 96: 2206

Heijl A, Lindgren G, Olsson J. A package for the statistical analysis of visual fields. In: Greve E and Heyl, eds. Seventh International

Visual Field Symposium. Dordrecht: Minitinus Nijoff/Dr W Junk Publishers, 1987: 153–68

Hitchings RA, Spaeth GL. The optic disc in glaucoma. I. Classification. Br J Ophthalmol 1976; 60: 778

Iwata K. Retinal nerve fiber layer, optic cupping, and visual field changes in glaucoma. In: Bellows JG, ed. Glaucoma: Contemporary International Concepts. New York: Masson, 1979: 139

Johnson CA. Recent developments in automated perimetry in glaucoma diagnosis and management. Curr Opin Ophthalmol 2002; 13: 77–84

Johnson CA, Adams AJ, Casson EJ, et al. Blue-on-yellow perimetry can predict the development of glaucomatous visual field loss. Arch Ophthalmol 1993; 111: 645–50

Johnson CA, Adams AJ, Casson EJ, et al. Progression of glaucomatous visual field loss as detected by blue-on-yellow and standard white-on-white perimetry. Arch Ophthalmol 1993; 111: 651–6

Kirsch RE, Anderson DR. Clinical recognition of glaucomatous cupping. Am J Ophthalmol 1973; 75: 442

Maffei L, Fiorentini A. Electroretinographic response to alternating gratings before and after section of the optic nerve. Science 1981; 211: 953

Motolko M, Drance SM, Douglas GR. The early psychophysical disturbances in chronic open-angle glaucoma: a study of visual functions with asymmetric disc cupping. Arch Ophthalmol 1982; 100: 1632

Nadler MP, Miller D, Nadler DJ, eds. Glare and Contrast Sensitivity for Clinicians. New York: Springer-Verlag, 1990

Parisi V, Bucci M. Visual evoked potentials after photostress in patients with primary open-angle glaucoma and ocular hypertension. Invest Ophthalmol Vis Sci 1992; 33: 436–42

Pederson JE, Anderson JR. The mode of progressive disc cupping in ocular hypertension and glaucoma. Arch Ophthalmol 1980; 102: 1689

Phelps CD, Remijan RW, Blondeau P. Acuity perimetry. Doc Ophthalmol Proc Ser 1981; 26: 111

Quigley HA, Addicks EM, Green W. Optic nerve damage in human glaucoma. III. Quantitative correlation of nerve fiber loss and visual field defect in glaucoma, ischemic optic neuropathy, disc edema, and toxic neuropathy. Arch Ophthalmol 1982; 100: 135

Quigley HA, Homan RM, Addicks EM, et al. Morphologic changes in the lamina cribrosa correlated with neural loss in open-angle glaucoma. Am J Ophthalmol 1983; 95: 673

Quigley HA, Sanchez RM, Dunkelberger GR, et al. Chronic glaucoma selectively damages large optic nerve fibers. Invest Ophthalmol Vis Sci 1987; 28: 913–20

Sample PA, Weinreb RM, Boynton RM. Acquired dyschromatopsia in glaucoma. Surv Ophthalmol 1986; 31: 54–64

Sample PA, Ahn DS, Lee PC, et al. High-pass resolution perimetry in eyes with ocular hypertension and primary open-angle glaucoma. Am J Ophthalmol 1992; 113: 309–16

Schmeisser ET, Smith TJ. Flicker visual evoked potential differentiation of glaucoma. Optometry Vis Sci 1992; 69: 458–62

Shih Y, Huang Z, Chang C. Color pattern-reversal evoked potential in eyes with ocular hypertension and primary open-angle glaucoma. Documenta Ophthalmol 1991; 77: 193–200

Stamper RL, Hsu-Winges C, Sopher M. Arden contrast sensitivity testing in glaucoma. Arch Ophthalmol 1982; 100: 947

Trick GL. Retinal potentials in patients with primary open angle glaucoma: physiological evidence for temporal frequency tuning defect. Invest Ophthalmol Vis Sci 1985; 26: 1750

Weinstein GW, Arden GB, Hitchings RA, et al. The pattern electroretinogram (PERG) in ocular hypertension and glaucoma. Arch Ophthalmol 1988; 106: 923–8

9 Primary open-angle glaucoma

Jennifer S Weizer, Paul P Lee

INTRODUCTION

The 2004 revision of the American Academy of Ophthalmology's (AAO) Preferred Practice Pattern (PPP) for primary open-angle glaucoma (POAG) defines the disease as a multifactorial optic neuropathy in which there is a characteristic acquired loss of optic nerve fibers. [It is a] 'chronic, generally bilateral but often asymmetrical disease, which is characterized (in at least one eye) by all of the following: (1) evidence of glaucomatous optic nerve damage from either or both ... the appearance of the disc or retinal nerve fiber layer ... or ... the presence of characteristic abnormalities in the visual field; (2) adult onset; (3) open, normal-appearing anterior chamber angles; and (4) absence of known other (e.g., secondary) causes of open angle glaucoma.' Since practice guidelines (particularly those of the AAO with regards to ophthalmic disease) are likely to carry significant legal weight, if not necessarily scientific heft, due to their reflection of expert opinion consensus, this reflects the current definition of POAG. It is most notable that intraocular pressure is not part of the definition, and that the presence of both optic nerve and visual field abnormalities is not required. Specifically, patients with 'early' glaucoma are, by definition, those without any detectable visual field loss on standardized white-on-white automated static perimetry. The diagnosis of open-angle glaucoma is therefore based on the presence of optic nerve damage, as manifested by either disc or field abnormalities. Importantly, this represents a significant departure from historical associations of glaucoma with intraocular pressure but better reflects the finding that 30–50% of patients with glaucoma in the United States (and higher in Asia) do not have elevated pressures above 21 mmHg.

In addition, this definition incorporates scientific findings that visual field loss generally occurs only after 30–50% of retinal ganglion cells have already been damaged. In the past few years particular attention has been focused on the detection of early glaucomatous damage to prevent field loss. While technological advances in the field of nerve fiber layer imaging are making exciting strides, newer technologies to detect early functional glaucomatous damage are becoming more useful as they become more refined. For example, short-wavelength automated perimetry may detect glaucomatous field damage several years earlier than more commonly used white-on-white automated field testing. Frequency doubling perimetry has been shown to correlate with future standard visual field loss, and is also potentially useful as a glaucoma screening tool.

EPIDEMIOLOGY

Prevalence

Several population-based studies conducted over the past 25 years have illuminated our understanding of the incidence and prevalence of POAG within defined populations in the United States and other countries. However, it is important to interpret these reports in light of the AAO definition of glaucoma. For example, a diagnosis of glaucoma in the Beaver Dam Eye Study required that at least two of three criteria were met: abnormal visual field, optic disc, or intraocular pressure. The impact of such definitions on our understanding of the population prevalence rates of glaucoma can be felt if one re-analyzes the Beaver Dam findings. Adding those cases that had only a visual field abnormality or optic nerve finding (even with the requirement of a history of medical or surgical treatment of glaucoma with either abnormality) would raise the total prevalence of POAG in the study by 31%. Similarly, the Rotterdam Study in the Netherlands defined glaucoma on the basis of a combination of visual field and optic nerve findings or an intraocular pressure greater than 21.

In this study, however, more basic data were not given to allow one to re-analyze the rates. Without additional data, understanding the rates of POAG in this population, given the AAO definition of POAG, becomes problematic. In the Barbados Eye Study of Blacks, definite POAG required the presence of both optic disc and visual field abnormalities. Adding 'suspect OAG' participants defined as those with 'less complete' data (and thus potentially including those with only one of the two criteria or more equivocal findings in both criteria) would increase the rate of POAG in this population by 55%! Indeed, only the Baltimore Eye Survey, in contrast, provides a definition based on either optic nerve head findings or visual field abnormalities, of varying strengths, consistent with the AAO definition. Recent prevalence studies have estimated that 2.22 million Americans have open-angle glaucoma as defined by some abnormality of visual function (generally fields), and that number is expected to reach 3.36 million by the year 2020. However, using the AAO definition of glaucoma, many more Americans could be diagnosed as having glaucoma. Thus, readers and policy-makers should carefully assess how POAG is defined to understand the epidemiological magnitude of this disease.

Risk factors

Nevertheless, across each of these studies, certain general risk factors were evident, regardless of the definition of glaucoma. These risk factors can be thought of in two major categories: risk factors that affect the development of POAG, and risk factors that hasten its progression once the disease has developed. These factors include age, race, and gender of the patient, family history, central corneal thickness, intraocular pressure characteristics, and perhaps myopia and certain systemic medical diseases.

However, there is likely to be overlap between these categories, especially in the case of elevated intraocular pressure, which affects disease incidence as well as progression.

Age, race, and gender

First, the higher the age of the population, the more prevalent open-angle glaucoma was found to be. The relationship between age and prevalence of POAG from the four major prevalence studies mentioned above is summarized in Table 9.1. Second, comparing across the studies, increased skin pigmentation is also associated with a higher prevalence of glaucoma, as shown in Table 9.1. Less well settled is the third issue of gender disparities in prevalence. In the Barbados and Rotterdam studies, men were noted to have a higher prevalence than women, as high as an average of 3.6% across all age groups in the Rotterdam study.

Intraocular pressure

In subsequent analysis of many of these data sets as well as other independent studies, additional risk factors other than age and race (and perhaps gender) were identified. A widely acknowledged risk factor for POAG is the degree of elevation of the intraocular pressure. Work from the Baltimore Eye Survey has shown that, even among normals, the higher the intraocular pressure, the less nerve tissue (as measured by rim area) exists. Certainly, in every population-based study, the higher the intraocular pressure, the greater the rate of POAG.

The fluctuation of intraocular pressure in both the short term (daily) and the long term (over years) has been found to be important in the risk of developing worsening of glaucoma. This is a potentially critical insight, because analysis of the Olmsted County data showed that over 20 years the risk of

Table 9.1 Effect of age on prevalence of POAG			
Study	**Race**	**Age (years)**	**Prevalence rate (%)**
Rotterdam	Not specified	55–59	0.2
		85–89	3.3
Baltimore Eye Survey	White	40–49	0.9
	White	> 80	2.2
	Black	40–49	1.23
	Black	> 80	11.26
Barbados	Black	40–49	1.4
		> 80	23.2
Beaver Dam	White	43–54	0.9
		> 75	4.7

blindness was not related to the intraocular pressure level (although the levels achieved were generally in the high teens). As described in greater detail below, the achieved level of intraocular pressure is an important consideration in the care of patients.

Family history of glaucoma

Another risk factor is the presence of glaucoma in a primary relative of the patient or, sometimes, in any family member; family history has been historically thought to be one of the highest predictors of risk. In an analysis of the Barbados and Baltimore Eye Studies, adjusting age and race for a positive family history revealed a high relative risk, but perhaps less than has traditionally been noted (again, keeping in mind the difference in definitions between the two studies). Table 9.2 summarizes the risk of positive family history on the prevalence of POAG from two major studies.

Central corneal thickness

A new risk factor has been added to the most recent PPP for POAG. Central corneal thickness has been shown in many recent studies, including the Ocular Hypertension Treatment Study, not only to affect the accuracy of intraocular pressure measurements, but also to perhaps act as its own intrinsic risk factor for glaucoma damage. Many studies have shown that central corneal thickness less than 540 μm leads to falsely low intraocular pressure measurements, whereas central corneal thickness greater than 555 μm falsely elevates pressure readings. Ehlers et al. estimated that intraocular pressure is under- or overestimated by approximately 5 mmHg for every 70 μm difference in central corneal thickness from a population mean of 545 μm. Adjusting measured intraocular pressure for central corneal thickness may alter one's management approach for a given POAG patient.

Other risk factors

Other conditions that have been implicated as increasing the risk for the development of POAG require additional analysis. An open mind and future appropriate studies will allow these other factors to be understood as to their relative roles in POAG. Thus, other ocular conditions, such as high myopia, may also carry a higher risk of POAG. The presence of systemic medical conditions such as diabetes and hypothyroidism may be associated with an increased risk for POAG.

Hypertension, which has been thought to be a risk factor for open-angle glaucoma in various studies, has been equally forcefully rejected in other studies. Its likely role may, according to findings from the Barbados study, be best understood by its relationship to perfusion pressure within the eye. Articles have identified that perfusion pressure differentials (i.e. hypotension) is an important risk factor for glaucomatous progression as well as for the presence of glaucoma. The effect of hypertension is thus confounded by the balance between perfusion pressure as reflected in the mean arterial pressure, the end-diastolic pressure, and intraocular pressure, and the effects of medical treatment for hypertension. For example, Hayreh et al. have shown that hypertensive patients on certain forms of anti-hypertensive medications had very low nocturnal arterial pressures, such that they were at greater risk of progression of optic neuropathy presumably due to nocturnal hypoxia or hypoperfusion of the optic nerve. Seen in this light, our understanding of hypertension as a risk factor has grown to allow us to develop a more complex and potentially more accurate understanding of the hemodynamic consequences of hypoperfusion and to expand our larger understanding of the potential mechanisms underlying optic nerve damage. However, as end-organ damage to the vasculature

Table 9.2	Effect of positive family history on prevalence of POAG			
Study	**Adjustments**	**Risk factor**	**Odds ratio**	**95% confidence interval**
Barbados	Age	Men	7.03	4.33–11.41
		Women	3.43	2.23–5.28
Baltimore	Age and race	POAG in parent	1.33	0.68–2.59
		POAG in sibling	2.89*	1.65–5.10
		POAG in child	1.14	0.26–5.03
		POAG in any first-degree relative	1.84*	1.21–2.80

*Statistically significant ($p < 0.05$).

increases with a longer duration of hypertension, one might expect a change in the relationship between perfusion pressure and hypertension due to decreased perfusion.

Other associations have been found not to be present, including alcohol intake, smoking, and possibly migraine headache. Yet, as with hypertension in the past, further study may allow us to better understand the potential contributions of nutrition and environmental conditions to increasing or decreasing the risk of developing POAG. Such interactions are likely to become even more important as we better understand the mechanisms underlying glaucoma in various ocular structures.

PATHOPHYSIOLOGY OF GLAUCOMA

Several mechanisms are likely to underlie the final common pathway of optic nerve dysfunction and ganglion cell death. Indeed, 'open-angle glaucoma' may be more accurately thought of as a syndrome rather than one single disease, with subsets of patients with different mechanisms exerting the primary influence on damage to intraocular structures.

Evidence from the epidemiology of the disease provides key insights for investigation. Possibilities include: (1) direct damage to the optic nerve due to pressure effects on the connective tissue or the nerve fibers; (2) indirect effects of pressure in compromising vascular flow to the optic nerve; (3) susceptibility of the affected cells and connective tissue to damage; (4) direct vascular flow compromise; and (5) interactions between susceptibility, intraocular pressure, perfusion pressure and vascular supply (or on vascular supply itself) as ameliorated by the perfusion pressure relative to the intraocular pressure.

However, these findings may not apply to many or most patients with POAG as defined today. Thus, there is a need for continued investigation and analysis in this area. An interesting implication of this finding is the potential role that it highlights for systemic conditions such as hypothyroidism and diabetes mellitus which have been associated with a greater risk of glaucoma. Decreased cardiac output or reduced arterial pressure may make individuals more susceptible to perfusion-deficit damage, while microvascular damage to capillaries and small blood vessels may act directly to heighten the likelihood of ischemia.

Blood flow and hemodynamics

When additional issues related to vascular perfusion are examined, several other interesting studies add to our understanding. While many of these findings are controversial or have been at odds with other published studies, they offer interesting insights

into potential factors. For example, Schulzer et al. found that they could classify two distinct groups of patients with glaucoma on the basis of hemodynamic and hematological characteristics. One group demonstrated some systemic sensitivity to stimuli causing vasospasm, while another group showed indirect indicators of vascular disease, including abnormal coagulation. Interestingly, the smaller former group (25% of study patients) demonstrated a correlation between peak intraocular pressure and severity of field defect, while the latter (75% of patients) did not. For reasons to be discussed below, peak intraocular pressure may not be the most accurate measure of the effect of intraocular pressure on the eye, yet this study suggests that studies that do not distinguish between these two possible (and perhaps more) subgroups in hemodynamic studies may be 'washing out' a true effect through cross-contamination of study populations. Indeed, an independent study from Japan found that 17–25% of patients with POAG also had a vasospastic response, a rate similar to the Schulzer study. However, even though 12 control patients had a similar 25% rate of vasospastic response, these patients were 4–8 years younger than the POAG subjects.

Other authors have also found deficits in the velocity of blood flow in various elements of the intraocular circulation, including the retinal, central retinal artery, and optic nerve head circulation. In the optic nerve head circulation study, the authors demonstrated increased red blood cell aggregability due to decreased deformability, a finding similar to those of Schulzer et al. in the majority of their patients.

The structural characteristics of the vascular system have also been implicated in the development or worsening of POAG damage. In one review of optic disc photographs of 34 eyes with advanced field loss, the presence of a temporal cilioretinal artery was found to be protective of preserving central field and acuity. In other work, Schwartz postulated that areas of defect in the microcirculation of the disc are associated with both ocular hypertension and POAG and with worsening of POAG status.

A fourth area of analysis has centered on understanding pulsatile ocular blood flow through a variety of means. Since the vast majority of pulsatile flow travels through the choroidal (and thus ophthalmic artery) circulation (from which the optic nerve head circulation derives), measurements of flow are only rough measures of choroidal and ophthalmic artery flow. Nevertheless, while some studies have found deficits in flow in POAG patients as well as differential effects on flow with different therapies, other studies have not found such differences in flow. Yet what is clear across studies is that a wide variation exists among individuals in the ability to autoregulate pulsatile ocular blood flow, especially at night. Decreased blood flow nocturnally or while supine (possibly due to increased intraocular pressure related to increased episcleral venous pressure in this position) may suggest particular susceptibility in certain patients or at certain times.

Finally, recent work has pointed towards retinal vessel diameter as a marker for associated glaucomatous damage. While causation is unclear, other work suggesting that lower end-arteriolar pressure predicts the progression from ocular hypertension to glaucoma, based on the pressure attenuation index.

While partially clarifying the role played by vascular factors in the pathogenesis of glaucomatous optic neuropathy, the above studies have also pointed out its complexity. It is now more apparent that understanding ocular perfusion requires a consideration of not only ocular blood flow parameters and their autoregulation (or lack thereof), but also an appreciation of systemic vascular factors, systemic diseases, and the potential role played by ocular and systemic medications. Vascular factors are only part of the equation in understanding ocular perfusion, however. While such factors may be especially important in the nearly half of patients with glaucoma who will have an intraocular pressure reading in the normal range on any one pressure examination, it is clear that intraocular pressure is also critical, since it generates much of the resistance to flow and perfusion.

Intraocular pressure

Intraocular pressure retains a critical role in the pathogenesis of glaucoma, since it is one part of the equation that determines the relative health of the optic nerve. Traditional work regarding the trabecular meshwork remains critical, since impaired outflow leading to elevated intraocular pressure may result in the optic nerve damage that characterizes glaucoma, either structurally from direct pressure effects or indirectly through compromised perfusion. The mechanisms of decreases in outflow facility underlying the pressure elevation have become better understood over the past few years. Several important avenues of investigation offer the potential for not only a better understanding of trabecular meshwork function (and dysfunction) but also potential new avenues for treatments. First, cytoskeletal changes mediated by key changes in actin and myosin pathways have been shown to be instrumental in altering the ability of trabecular meshwork cells to modulate fluid transport across the meshwork. Tan and others have shown that disruptions of the cytoskeletal structure of interference with the actin–myosin interactions can significantly increase outflow through the trabecular meshwork. Aquaporin mechanisms as well as other intermediate pathways such as rho kinase

(affected by the statin class of drugs) may act through these or related mechanisms to alter fluid transport in those with glaucoma. Second, greater attention has been paid to uveoscleral outflow as a potentially underrecognized pathway of fluid egress from within the eye. If outflow is similar in humans to the 35–50% seen in primate models, then we can anticipate much greater attention in the future to this pathway. Third, the family of matrix metalloproteinases and other factors associated with tissue injury and stress offer important insights into chronic damage mechanisms in the trabecular meshwork (and potentially elsewhere).

The next effect of these mechanisms is that outflow from the eye is impaired, resulting in pressure dysfunction. Evidence is mounting that the most important characteristic of intraocular pressure for the development and progression of glaucoma may not be the peak or average intraocular pressure; rather, it is the variation in intraocular pressure that may be most crucial. For example, David et al. and Asrani et al. found that the diurnal variation in intraocular pressure was higher in ocular hypertensives and those with glaucoma than in normal patients, confirming the findings of a series of studies by Drance, Katavisto, and Kitazawa. Indeed, Oliver et al. found that patients in Olmsted County, MN, who went blind from glaucoma did not differ appreciably from those who maintained vision in terms of their mean intraocular pressure over 20 years.

Studies of progression after intervention also found an important role for the variation of pressure. For example, Elsas et al. found that the variation in intraocular pressure was significantly greater in eyes prior to laser trabeculoplasty than it was after trabeculoplasty, with variation decreasing from 33% of the average intraocular pressure to less than 10%. In another study, Saiz et al. found that those patients who underwent successful trabeculectomy had not only lower peak intraocular pressures but also significantly lower amplitudes of diurnal variation in intraocular pressure than before surgery. The Advanced Glaucoma Intervention Study investigators showed that over the long term patients who consistently had intraocular pressures of 18 or less were far less likely to have visual field progression than those whose pressures fluctuated more widely.

From a biophysical standpoint, it is reasonable that variation in intraocular pressure may be responsible for mechanical effects in the optic nerve head leading to glaucomatous optic atrophy. The human body adapts amazingly well to static pressure loads, but it is the repeated loading and unloading of stress that causes breakdowns in structural properties (as in metal fatigue in airliners subject to repeated takeoffs, landings, and pressurizations). Such variation may be important in leading to repeated episodes of relative ischemia that may over time cause injury to the optic nerve fibers, ultimately resulting in glaucomatous damage. The preferential loss of larger ganglion cells early in glaucoma may reflect the influence of this factor as well as others. Lamina cribrosa pores are larger in the polar regions of the optic nerve head (where the larger axons pass), with thinner septae between these pores than in other areas of the nerve head. The repeated stress of changing intraocular pressure (causing mechanical deformation of the laminar plates) may lead to breakdown of the septae, loss of support for the axons, and axonal damage, as well as causing damaging episodes of relative ischemia. The susceptibility of these large lamina cribrosa pores may thus also help explain why larger diameter optic discs are more prone to glaucomatous damage. Burgoyne and others have developed innovative measures to assess the compliance and resistance of the lamina cribrosa to and fluctuations in intraocular pressure.

Other optic nerve head characteristics

Several risk factors in optic nerve head appearance that make glaucomatous progression more likely have been reported. Not only are large optic discs more likely to develop glaucoma, but those discs with thinner neuroretinal rim areas are more likely to show progression of glaucomatous damage. Also, optic discs with a larger beta zone of peripapillary atrophy (the whitish area located immediately adjacent to the peripapillary scleral ring and characterized by visible underlying choroidal vessels and sclera) are more likely to show visual field progression than discs with a smaller beta zone. This larger beta zone is often associated with optic disc hemorrhage, another sign of glaucomatous progression.

Genetic analyses

Two new areas of research may be of particular promise. First, the pursuit of localizing the gene(s) that are related to POAG proceeds apace. Several genes that affect one's susceptibility to glaucoma have already been identified. Mutations in the TIGR/myocilin gene are present in many cases of juvenile or early-onset POAG. Optineurin gene mutations are present in some families with normal-tension glaucoma. Mutations in another gene, CYP1B1, have been linked to patients with congenital glaucoma, and many more genes possibly affecting glaucoma continue to be studied. With the promise of molecular genetics, a greater grasp of the elements that cause POAG to develop may follow. Second, several investigators are now exploring the concept that apoptotic mechanisms of preprogrammed cell death may underlie a significant proportion of glaucomatous nerve fiber and cell loss. Such cell death may either be triggered by or made more susceptible to certain environmental conditions. Indeed, genetic analysis has begun to identify genotypic susceptibility to glaucomatous cell death as a major factor in the development of POAG. Not everybody with the abnormal gene will necessarily develop glaucoma, but having the gene may put one at higher risk. Understanding the environmental factors around the ganglion cell will be important in better defining how to address factors related to apoptosis.

Other potential factors

Investigators have also sought to explore the link to immune system function and the role of chronic infections as potential additional mechanisms for glaucoma. Intriguing evidence of heightened immune responses and potential autoimmune mechanisms exist for subsets of patients with glaucoma. The role played by infections, as with *Helicobacter pylori* for gastric ulcers, remains to be proven in glaucoma.

MAKING THE DIAGNOSIS OF POAG

As noted in the definition of POAG, four elements are needed to make the diagnosis: (1) the patient must be of adult age (with younger patients being defined as having juvenile-onset glaucoma, though without necessarily any significant differences in treatment philosophy); (2) the anterior chamber angles must be 'open' by gonioscopy (see Chapter 5); (3) there must be no known secondary cause for the glaucoma (see Chapter 10); and (4) there must be optic nerve damage, manifested by either optic disc or nerve fiber layer changes consistent with glaucoma (see Chapter 6) or characteristic visual field abnormalities (see Chapter 8). It is important to note that, of the patients who progressed to glaucoma in the Ocular Hypertension Treatment Study, half of them progressed in terms of disc characteristics alone, while less than 10% were found to progress in terms of visual fields alone. To assist the clinician in determining what changes are 'characteristic of' or 'consistent with' POAG, the AAO provides illustrative examples of each. For visual fields, the definition explicitly encompasses arcuate defects, nasal steps, paracentral scotomata, or generalized depression. For disc or retinal nerve fiber layer appearance, the AAO explicitly includes thinning or notching of the disc rim, progressive change over time, and nerve fiber layer defects. For a full discussion and illustrations of these and other characteristics, please refer to the chapters noted above.

As the sophistication of diagnosing POAG continues to develop, new diagnostic guidelines may be proposed. Even with the PPP guidelines in place, clinician subjectivity and variations in observation remain an issue when diagnosing the presence and severity of POAG. In the future, methods of diagnosis based on objective instrument measurements of intraocular pressure, optic nerve head characteristics, and visual field damage may become more widespread, especially as glaucoma detection instrument technology continues to make further strides. For example, the importance of central corneal thickness measurements has led corneal pachymetry to be added to the PPP in its most recent version for the evaluation of suspected glaucoma.

Patients with POAG typically present either with no symptoms referable to glaucoma or with advanced loss in one or both eyes. In the Olmsted County data from the 1960s to the 1970s, 3% of patients presented with blindness in at least one eye. Furthermore, patients in the United Kingdom with lower socioeconomic status were likely to present with more visual field damage. Because the initial assessment requires that POAG be a diagnosis of exclusion, the history and examination should be carefully oriented towards eliminating other causes of apparent glaucomatous loss. Thus, issues such as use of steroids of any kind, history or signs of trauma or uveitis should be sought.

To assist physicians in using the new definition and meeting the practice guideline requirements, the AAO Preferred Practice Patterns for POAG lists elements of history and examination that should be included in the initial assessment of glaucoma patients. These are summarized in Table 9.3.

Consensus is currently lacking among eye care providers in the classification of open-angle glaucoma.

Also, key steps in providing care for glaucoma patients, such as gonioscopy, optic nerve assessments, and establishment of target pressures, are often not performed regularly in the United States. The AAO Preferred Practice Patterns provide a first step in the process of developing a consensus, which will mature and improve as more evidence-based studies substantiate expert opinions. These standard definitions and disease severity staging systems, along with the development of new technology for better patient care, offer the potential to guide physician behavior and improve treatment and resulting outcomes for POAG patients.

In caring for patients with POAG, careful assessment and documentation of the optic nerve is an essential element of care. The Melbourne group demonstrated that half of those who had glaucoma (97% of whom had visual field loss) but did not know they had glaucoma had been seen in the prior year by an eye care provider. The authors felt that this failure was due to inadequate attention to the optic nerve on examination by providers.

TREATMENT PRINCIPLES

General goals

The traditional goal of glaucoma therapy on the part of eye care providers is to stabilize optic nerve damage and to prevent additional damage. Occasionally, reversal or improvement in optic disc cupping

---

Table 9.3 Recommendations for the initial assessment of a glaucoma patient

Elements of history	Elements of examination
Review ocular, family, and systemic history	Best corrected visual acuity
Review any available old records (visual fields, disc photographs, etc.)	Pupillary examination with attention to afferent pupillary defect
Ocular and systemic medications used	Intraocular pressure measurement prior to gonioscopy and dilation
Previous ocular surgery, if any	
Previous medications used and review of known systemic and local reactions	Complete anterior segment slit lamp examination
Time of last use of glaucoma medications	Gonioscopy
Severity of glaucoma in family members, including history of glaucomatous visual loss	Evaluation of central corneal thickness
	Evaluation of optic disc and nerve fiber layer, with documentation of optic nerve appearance
Assessment of the impact of visual function on activities of daily living	Evaluation of fundus for other abnormalities that might account for any visual field defects
	Visual field examination by automated static threshold technique or by kinetic or static manual technique

following adequate lowering of intraocular pressure has been reported by several authors, particularly in cases of early glaucoma among younger patients. Figure 9.1 demonstrates a case of significant recovery of visual field following aggressive treatment of POAG. These illustrations are the pre- and postoperative fields of a patient with advanced POAG who underwent a successful trephination with postoperative intraocular pressures of between 6 and 8 mmHg. Thus, perhaps our long-term goal of glaucoma treatment for the future should be to improve and restore significant amounts of visual functioning, as measured by a variety of means.

It is vital that treatment be tailored to the needs of the individual patient in partnership with the physician. Issues including compliance with therapy, patient understanding of the disease, cost of treatment, potential side-effects, and impact of therapy on the patient's quality of life should be explicitly incorporated into the patient's care plan. It is not sufficient to limit discussions to intraocular pressure, visual field, and optic nerve status; discussions about the implications of POAG and its care need to be addressed with the patient.

In looking at treatment from a 'patient-centered' perspective, we have significantly more information today on the impact of having glaucoma and glaucoma treatment. First, as shown in the Collaborative Initial Glaucoma Treatment Study (CIGTS), patients report significant amounts of emotional distress upon being informed of their diagnosis, including fears of blindness. Second, from the Early Manifest Glaucoma Trial (EMGT), we know that patient self-reported visual functioning, as measured by the NEI-VFQ questionnaire, has a significant decrease when visual field loss exceeds −4 dB of mean deviation loss or at visual acuities of 20/100. Subsequent to that point, visual functioning declines steadily as visual field worsens, as measured by patient self-report on the NEI-VFQ. Third, an unanswered question is the extent to which issues not measured by the NEI-VFQ or other questionnaires may be present in patients without any visual field loss. Indeed, patient 'side-effects' and 'symptoms' were present at diagnosis with glaucoma in the CIGTS. Such issues are often present and should be assessed at office visits, and such effects were present in those who underwent glaucoma surgery and those using medical therapy in the CIGTS. Fourth, analysis from the Salisbury Eye Evaluation population-based study demonstrates that there is no 'cutoff' or 'inflection point' in the measured ability of patients to perform tasks such as reading, walking through a room, recognizing faces, or other important activities relative to visual acuity, contrast sensitivity, or visual field. Therefore, the choice of a 'disability' level is an arbitrary political decision, not one based on patient ability to function.

Lowering of intraocular pressure

Considering the definition of POAG, our current ability to modulate the course of the disease is still relatively limited. At the present time, the only available treatment for POAG is to reduce the intraocular pressure. Whether this functions to improve perfusion or ocular blood flow or has a direct mechanical benefit on the optic nerve, or both, is not clear. The evidence that lower intraocular pressure is more effective in preventing visual field loss can be indirectly seen in the results of the Moorfields Primary Treatment Trial and the Scottish Glaucoma Trial, in which initial trabeculectomy lowered intraocular pressure more than medicine did, and was also associated with less loss of field on follow-up. Similarly, the lower intraocular pressure obtained with initial laser trabeculoplasty in the Glaucoma Laser Trial was associated with less visual field loss than in the medication-first group.

Several recent clinical trials have directly shown the importance of lowering intraocular pressure, whether accomplished by medicines, laser, or surgery (Table 9.4). The Early Manifest Glaucoma Trial demonstrated that treating early glaucoma patients with medicine and argon laser trabeculoplasty reduced their risk of progression by half compared to observation. The Collaborative Initial Glaucoma Treatment Study reported that both medical and surgical treatments resulted in similar long-term reductions in visual field loss. In the Advanced Glaucoma Intervention Study, patients with average intraocular pressures of less than 14 mmHg had a lower rate of visual field progression than patients with higher pressures. Further, those patients with intraocular pressures consistently under 18 mmHg were highly unlikely to experience progression. Also, a comparison of surgical sequences (performing either argon laser trabeculoplasty or trabeculectomy as the initial surgical procedure) showed that, while intraocular pressure was lowered by either sequence, black patients tended to have better visual function outcomes from argon laser trabeculoplasty first, while white patients tended to have better visual function outcomes from trabeculectomy first. Finally, in the Ocular Hypertension Treatment Study, lowering the intraocular pressure in ocular hypertensive patients halved the risk of progression to POAG. This study also highlighted central corneal thickness as a powerful risk factor for the development of POAG in these patients.

Once a diagnosis of POAG is made, the AAO PPP states that a 'target pressure' should be defined – i.e. the upper limit of what would be considered an 'acceptable' pressure for that particular eye. This target pressure is only an estimate and can be subject to revision based on the patient's clinical course. In selecting the target pressure, it should be at least 20% lower than the baseline intraocular pressure range and should be set lower for those eyes that have

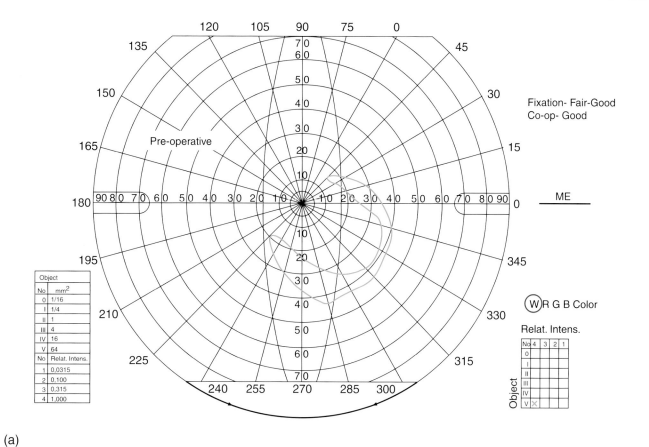

(a)

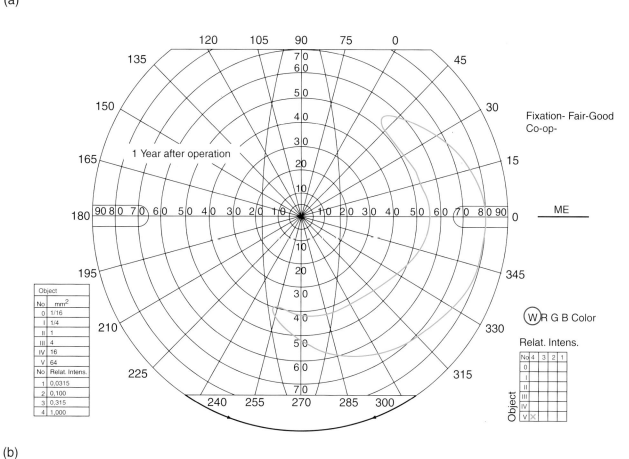

(b)

Figure 9.1 Series of visual fields in a glaucoma patient. The visual field of this patient just prior to filtration surgery is shown in (a). The subsequent fields, (b–e), show considerable improvement attributed to the excellent intraocular pressure control obtained by the surgery. (Courtesy of Pei-Fei Lee, MD.)

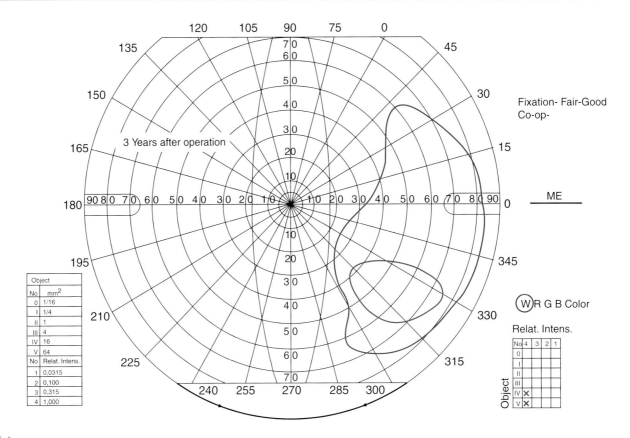

(c)

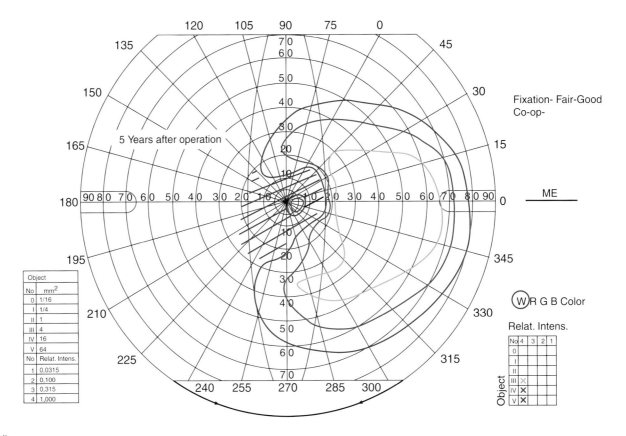

(d)

Figure 9.1   *Continued.*

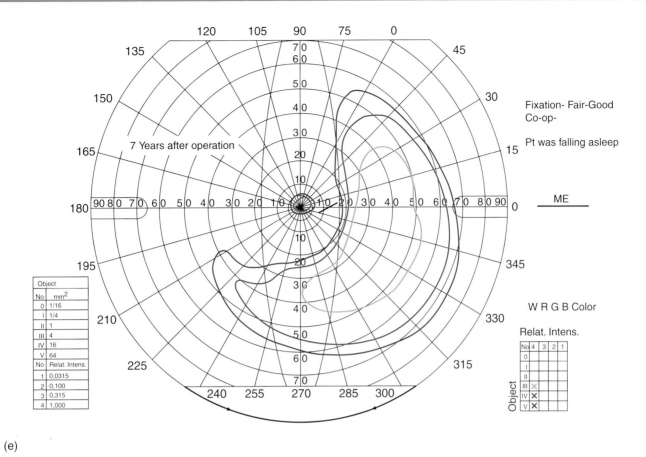

(e)

Figure 9.1 *Continued.*

Table 9.4 Recent clinical trials in glaucoma	
Clinical trial	**Results**
Early Manifest Glaucoma Trial (EMGT)	Treating early glaucoma patients with medicine and argon laser trabeculoplasty reduced risk of progression by half compared to observation
Collaborative Initial Glaucoma Treatment Study (CIGTS)	Both medical and surgical treatments resulted in similar long-term reductions in visual field loss
Advanced Glaucoma Intervention Study (AGIS)	Patients with average intraocular pressure less than 14 had lower rate of visual field progression than patients with higher pressures. Also, Blacks had better visual outcomes from argon laser trabeculoplasty before trabeculectomy, while Whites had better visual outcomes from trabeculectomy before argon laser trabeculoplasty
Ocular Hypertension Treatment Study (OHTS)	Lowering intraocular pressure in ocular hypertensives halved the risk of progression to POAG. Also, central corneal thickness was identified as important risk factor for development of POAG

more pre-existing damage. Additional factors to consider that may argue for an even lower target intraocular pressure are the presence of strong risk factors (see above), the history of loss in the fellow eye at certain intraocular pressure ranges, and the rapidity of damage (if known).

While the PPP takes no position on either the performance of diurnal curves as an aid to understanding progression risk or the likelihood of developing glaucoma or the utility of ocular hemodynamic assessments, these are potentially useful adjuncts to guide therapy.

Follow-up and monitoring

In order to determine whether the target pressure is appropriate, patients need periodic monitoring of their optic nerve status, both directly through evaluation of the disc and nerve fiber layer and indirectly through the performance of periodic visual fields. Detecting optic nerve head appearance change over time is complicated by the need for comparison with remote stereo disc photographs, which may not be available in many instances. A national database of stereo disc photographs of glaucoma patients would perhaps be helpful in giving eye care providers a basis on which to compare present optic disc appearances. If disc damage occurs at or below a target pressure, then the target pressure must be reset, again starting with at least an additional 20% reduction from the current intraocular pressure.

The interval between follow-up visits to the physician is determined by attainment of the target intraocular pressure (or failure to do so) and the presence or absence of disease progression. For example, if the target intraocular pressure has been achieved and no progression is noted, control for longer than 6 months suggests that follow-up every 3–12 months should be sufficient. For more recent control (< 6 months), follow-up in 1–6 months is warranted. However, if the target intraocular pressure needs to be reset because of progression at or below the initial target, follow-up should occur in 1 week to 3 months. For those eyes in which the target has not yet been achieved, follow-up should occur between 1 day and 1 month (for progression) or 3 months (if no progression). These recommendations are summarized in Table 9.5.

During follow-up visits, the history should include interval ocular and systemic medical history, an inquiry into local or systemic problems with medication, verification of the appropriate use of medications, and general assessment of the impact of the condition and treatment on daily living. Each examination should include measurements of visual acuity and intraocular pressure in both eyes, as well as a slit-lamp examination. For periodic optic nerve evaluations, if the target intraocular pressure has been achieved and no progression is noted, control for longer than 6 months suggests that follow-up disc evaluations every 6–18 months should be sufficient. For more recent control (< 6 months), follow-up in 6–12 months is warranted. However, if the target intraocular pressure needs to be reset because of progression at or below the initial target, follow-up disc evaluation should occur in 2–6 months. For those eyes in which the target has not yet been achieved, follow-up should occur between 1 and 6 months (for progression) or 2 to 6 months (if no progression). For interval visual fields, if the target intraocular pressure has been achieved and no progression is noted, control for longer than 6 months suggests that follow-up every 6–24 months should be sufficient. For more recent control (< 6 months), follow-up in 6–24 months is warranted. However, if the target intraocular pressure needs to be reset because of progression at or below the initial target, follow-up fields should occur in 3–12 months. For those eyes in which the target has not yet been achieved, follow-up should occur also between 3 and 12 months.

The AAO makes clear that these are timing ranges that need to be adjusted to fit the needs of each individual patient. Thus, for example, if acceptable compliance is lacking, then physicians need to adjust the treatment regimen to enhance the utility of the therapy for the patient. Similarly, if problems develop with certain medications, switching patients to new medications will necessitate more frequent follow-up visits, just as if a new target pressure was set.

Table 9.5 Recommendations for follow-up visits

Progression of disease	Status	Duration of control	Recommended interval
Progressive optic nerve and/or visual field damage	Not at target pressure	n/a	1 day to 1 month
No progression	Not at target pressure	n/a	1 day to 3 months
Progressive optic nerve and/or visual field damage at initial target pressure; requires resetting target	Requires resetting target	n/a	1 week to 3 months
Progression documented at prior visit	New target recently achieved	Less than 3 months	1 month to 3 months
No progression	At target pressure	Less than 6 months	1 month to 6 months
No progression	At target pressure	More than 6 months	3 months to 12 months

New therapeutic approaches

The current widespread use of newer topical therapeutic agents for POAG (see Chapter 15) continues to aid in the development of more effective therapies for glaucoma. However, therapeutic approaches that directly address the pathophysiological basis of POAG are needed. From recent work on understanding how glaucomatous damage occurs, several intriguing approaches and possibilities exist.

Recent work targeting neuronal damage has shown that glutamate in high levels is toxic to retinal ganglion cells and that glutamate transporter proteins are reduced in animal models of glaucoma. Thus, the possibility now exists of potentially reversing at least some glaucomatous damage through classes of drugs such as glutamate receptor blockers (such as phencyclidine), as well as calcium channel blockers, nitric oxide synthase inhibitors, nerve growth factors, and free-radical scavengers and antioxidants. Statin medication traditionally used to lower cholesterol has recently been demonstrated to be possibly protective against the development of POAG. Renewed interest in the transport capabilities of the endothelial cells of the trabecular meshwork now offers new insights and potentially new classes of drugs for reducing the abnormal outflow resistance that underlies the mechanism for elevated pressure in many patients with POAG. Finally, research on apoptosis and mechanisms of cell death provides hope that 'neuroprotective' drugs will one day be able to prevent the death of retinal ganglion cells initiated by uncontrolled intraocular pressure or other underlying causative agents.

SUMMARY

Our understanding of all forms of glaucoma has grown enormously in the past 25 years. Perhaps nowhere is this more evident than in how we view POAG. Today, POAG is a multifactorial optic neuropathy. It has been said by many authors that POAG is most likely to represent a spectrum of conditions that we currently label with one name. From the work on ocular perfusion and hemodynamics, to intraocular pressure diurnal variation, to gene analysis, to optic nerve head structure, it is the diversity present in the population that often contributes to our still somewhat 'fuzzy' thinking about POAG. From a scientific viewpoint, the future looks enormously promising for new understanding and new treatments.

From a clinical standpoint, care today is much more defined. The American Academy of Ophthalmology's Preferred Practice Pattern lays out specific recommendations to assist physicians in caring for their patients with POAG. Even more importantly, care today reflects modern notions of a physician–patient partnership. No longer are intraocular pressure, visual field, and optic disc status the holy grail of patient relationships. Rather, understanding and addressing the condition of POAG within the context of a patient's life is now the central focus.

Further reading

The Advanced Glaucoma Intervention Study (AGIS): 7. The relationship between control of intraocular pressure and visual field deterioration. The AGIS Investigators. Am J Ophthalmol 2000; 130: 429–40

American Academy of Ophthalmology. Preferred Practice Pattern: Primary Open Angle Glaucoma. San Francisco: AAO, 2003

Asrani S, Zeimer R, Wilensky J, et al. Large diurnal fluctuations in intraocular pressure are an independent risk factor in patients with glaucoma. J Glaucoma 2000; 9: 134–42

Bosem ME, Lusky M, Weinreb RN. Short-term effects of levobunolol on ocular pulsatile flow. Am J Ophthalmol 1992; 114: 280–6

Burgoyne CF, Quigley JA, Thompson HW, et al. Early changes in optic disc compliance and surface position in experimental glaucoma. Ophthalmology 1995; 102: 1800–9

Claridge KG, Smith SE. Diurnal variation in pulsatile ocular blood flow in normal and glaucomatous eyes. Surv Ophthalmol 1994; 38 (Suppl): s198–s205

Cohen SL, Lee PP, Herndon LW, et al. Using the arteriolar pressure attenuation index to predict ocular hypertension progression to open-angle glaucoma. Arch Ophthalmol 2003; 121: 33–8

David R, Zangwill L, Briscoe D, et al. Diurnal intraocular pressure variations: an analysis of 690 diurnal curves. Br J Ophthalmol 1992; 76: 280–3

Dielemans I, Vingerling JR, Wolfs RCW, et al. The prevalence of primary open angle glaucoma in a population-based study in the Netherlands. Ophthalmology 1994; 101: 1851–5

Drance SM. The significance of the diurnal tension variations in normal and glaucomatous eyes. Arch Ophthalmol 1960; 64: 494–501

Ederer F, Gaasterland DA, Dally LG, et al. The Advanced Glaucoma Intervention Study (AGIS): 13. Comparison of treatment outcomes within race: 10-year results. Ophthalmology 2004; 111: 651–64

Ehlers N, Bramsen T, Sperling S. Applanation tonometry and central corneal thickness. Acta Ophthalmol 1975; 53: 34–43

Elsas T, Junk J, Johnsen H. Diurnal intraocular pressure after successful primary laser trabeculoplasty. Am J Ophthalmol 1991; 112: 67–9

Epstein DL. Will there be a remedy to reverse the changes in the trabecular meshwork and the optic nerve? A personal point-of-view on glaucoma therapy. J Glaucoma 1993; 2: 138–40

The Eye Diseases Prevalence Research Group. Prevalence of open angle glaucoma among adults in the United States. Arch Ophthalmol 2004; 122: 532–8

Girkin CA, McGwin G, McNeal SF, et al. Hypothyroidism and the development of open angle glaucoma in a male population. Ophthalmology 2004; 111: 1649–52

Glaucoma Laser Trial Research Group. The Glaucoma Laser Trial (GLT) and Glaucoma Laser Trial Follow-up Study: 7. Results. Am J Ophthalmol 1995; 120: 718–31

Gordon MO, Beiser JA, Brandt JD, et al. The Ocular Hypertension Treatment Study: baseline factors that predict the onset of primary open angle glaucoma. Arch Ophthalmol 2002; 120: 714–20

Gutierrez P, Wilson MR, Johnson CJ, et al. Influence of glaucomatous visual field loss on health-related quality of life. Arch Ophthalmol 1997; 115: 777–84

Hamard P, Jamard J, Dufaux J. Blood flow rate in the microvasculature of the optic nerve head in primary open angle glaucoma. A new approach. Surv Ophthalmol 1994; 38(Suppl): s87–s94

Harris A. Non-invasive assessment of ocular hemodynamics in glaucoma: a review of the literature. Bloomington, IN: Indiana University, 1995

Hattenhauer MG, Johnson DH, Ing HH, et al. Probability of filtration surgery in patients with open-angle glaucoma. Arch Ophthalmol 1999; 117: 1211–15

Hayreh SS, Zimmerman MB, Podhajsky P, Alward WLM. Nocturnal arterial hypotension and its role in optic nerve head and ocular ischemic disorders. Am J Ophthalmol 1994; 117: 603–24

Hyman LG, Komaroff E, Heijl A, et al. Treatment and vision-related quality of life in the early manifest glaucoma trial. Ophthalmology 2005; 112: 1505–13

James CB. Effect of trabeculectomy on pulsatile ocular blood flow. Br J Ophthalmol 1994; 78: 818–22

Janz NK, Wren PA, Lichter PR, et al. Quality of life in newly diagnosed glaucoma patients: The Collaborative Initial Glaucoma Treatment Study. Ophthalmology 2001; 108: 887–97

Janz NK, Wren PA, Lichter PR, et al. The Collaborative Initial Glaucoma Treatment Study: interim quality of life findings after initial medical or surgical treatment of glaucoma. Ophthalmology 2001; 108: 1954–65

Jay JL, Allan D. The benefit of early trabeculectomy versus conventional management in primary open angle glaucoma relative to severity of disease. Eye 1989; 3: 528–35

Jonas JB, Martus P, Horn FK, et al. Predictive factors of the optic nerve head for development or progression of glaucomatous visual field loss. Invest Ophthalmol Vis Sci 2004; 45: 2613–18

Kass MA, Heuer DK, Higginbotham EJ, et al. The Ocular Hypertension Treatment Study: a randomized trial determines that topical ocular hypotensive medication delays or prevents the onset of primary open angle glaucoma. Arch Ophthalmol 2002; 120: 701–13

Katavisto M. The diurnal variations of ocular tension in glaucoma. Acta Ophthalmol 1964; 78: 1–30

Kitazawa Y, Horie T. Diurnal variation in intra-ocular pressure in primary open angle glaucoma. Am J Ophthalmol 1975; 79: 557–66

Klein BE, Klein R, Sponsel WE, et al. Prevalence of glaucoma: the Beaver Dam Eye Study. Ophthalmology 1992; 99: 1499–504

Klein BE, Klein R, Meuer SM, Goetz LA. Migraine headache and its association with open angle glaucoma: the Beaver Dam Eye Study. Invest Ophthalmol Vis Sci 1993; 34: 3024–7

Klein BE, Klein R, Ritter LL. Relationship of drinking alcohol and smoking to prevalence of open angle glaucoma. Ophthalmology 1993; 100: 1609–13

Klein BE, Klein R, Jensen SC. Open angle glaucoma and older-onset diabetes. Ophthalmology 1994; 101: 1173–7

Kountouras J, Zavos C, Chatzopoulos D. Induction of apoptosis as a proposed pathophysiological link between glaucoma and *Helicobacter pylori* infection. Med Hypotheses 2004; 62: 378–81

Lee PP. The effect of Preferred Practice Patterns on malpractice actions. J Glaucoma 1992; 1: 286–9

Lee SS, Schwartz B. Role of the temporal cilioretinal artery in retaining central visual field in open angle glaucoma. Ophthalmology 1992; 99: 696–9

Leske MC, Connell AMS, Schachat AP, Hyman L, the Barbados Eye Study Group. The Barbados Eye Study: prevalence of open angle glaucoma. Arch Ophthalmol 1994; 112: 821–9

Leske MC, Connell AMS, Wu S-Y, et al. The Barbados Eye Study Group. Arch Ophthalmol 1995; 113: 918–24

Leske MC, Heijl A, Hussein M, et al. Factors for glaucoma progression and the effect of treatment: the early manifest glaucoma trial. Arch Ophthalmol 2003; 121: 48–56

Lichter PR, Musch DC, Gillespie BW, et al. Interim clinical outcomes in the Collaborative Initial Glaucoma Treatment Study comparing initial treatment randomized to medications or surgery. Ophthalmology 2001; 108: 1943–53

Lutjen-Drecoll E, Gabelt BT, Tian B, Kaufman PL. Outflow of aqueous humor. J Glaucoma 2001; 10(5 Suppl 1): S42–4

Martin KR, Levkovitch-Verbin H, Valenta D, et al. Retinal glutamate transporter changes in experimental glaucoma and after optic nerve transaction in the rat. Invest Ophthalmol Vis Sci 2002; 43: 2236–43

Mastropasqua L, Lobefalo L, Mancini A, et al. Prevalence of myopia in open angle glaucoma. Eur J Ophthalmol 1992; 2: 33–5

McGwin G, McNeal S, Owsley C, et al. Statins and other cholesterol-lowering medications and the presence of glaucoma. Arch Ophthalmol 2004; 122: 822–6

Medeiros FA, Sample PA, Weinreb RN. Frequency doubling technology perimetry abnormalities as predictors of glaucomatous visual field loss. Am J Ophthalmol 2004; 137: 863–71

Migdal C, Gregory W, Hitchings R. Long-term functional outcome after early surgery compared with laser and medicine in open angle glaucoma. Ophthalmology 1994; 101: 1651–7

Mitchell P, Leung H, Wang JJ, et al. Retinal vessel diameter and open-angle glaucoma: the Blue Mountains Eye Study. Ophthalmology 2005; 112: 245–50

Oliver JE, Hattenhauer M, Herman D, et al. Blindness and glaucoma: a comparison of patients progressing to blindness from glaucoma with patients maintaining vision. Am J Ophthalmol 2002; 133: 764–72

Polo V, Larrosa JM, Pinilla I, et al. Predictive value of short-wavelength automated perimatry: a 3-year follow-up study. Ophthalmology 2002; 109: 761–5

Quigley HA. Open angle glaucoma. N Engl J Med 1993; 328: 1097–106

Rankin SJA, Walman BE, Buckley AR, Drance SM. Color doppler imaging and spectral analysis of the optic nerve vasculature in glaucoma. Am J Ophthalmol 1995; 119: 685–93

Rezaie T, Child A, Hitchings R, et al. Adult-onset primary open angle glaucoma caused by mutation in Optineurin. Science 2002; 295: 1077–9

Saiz A, Alcuaz A, Maquet JA, de la Fuente F. Pressure-curve variations after trabeculectomy for chronic primary open angle glaucoma. Ophthalmic Surg 1990; 21: 799–801

Schoff EO, Hattenhauer MG, Ing HH, et al. Estimated incidence of open angle glaucoma in Olmsted County, Minnesota. Ophthalmology 2001; 108: 882–6

Schultz JS. Initial treatment of glaucoma: surgery or medications: III. Chop or drop? Surv Ophthalmology 1993; 37: 293–305

Schulzer M, Drance SM, Carter CJ, et al. Biostatistical evidence of two distinct chronic open angle glaucoma populations. Br J Ophthalmol 1990; 74: 196–200

Schumer RA, Podos SM. The nerve of glaucoma. Arch Ophthalmol 1994; 112: 37–44

Schwartz B. Circulatory defects of the optic disk and retina in ocular hypertension and high pressure open angle glaucoma. Surv Ophthalmol 1994; 38 (Suppl): s23–s34

Sharir M, Zimmerman TJ. Initial treatment of glaucoma: surgery or medications: II. Medical therapy. Surv Ophthalmol 1993; 37: 293–305

Sheffield VC, Stone EM, Alward WLM, et al. Genetic linkage of familial open angle glaucoma to chromosome 1q21-q31. Nat Genet 1993; 4: 47–50

Sherwood MB, Migdal CS, Hitchings RA. Initial treatment of glaucoma: surgery or medications: I. Filtration surgery. Surv Ophthalmol 1993; 37: 293–305

Smith KD, Tevaarwerk GJM, Allen LH. Case reports: reversal of poorly controlled glaucoma on diagnosis and treatment of hypothyroidism. Can J Ophthalmol 1992; 27: 345–7

Smith KD, Arthurs BP, Saheb J. An association between hypothyroidism and primary open angle glaucoma. Ophthalmology 1993; 100: 1580–4

Sommer A, Tielsch JM, Katz J, et al. Relationship between intraocular pressure and primary open angle glaucoma among white and black Americans. Arch Ophthalmol 1991; 109: 1090–5

Susanna R, Sheu W. Comparison of latanoprost with fixed-combination dorzolamide and timolol in adult patients with elevated intraocular pressure: an eight-week, randomized, open-label, parallel-group, multicenter study in Latin America. Clin Ther 2004; 26: 755–68

Tan JC, Peters DM, Caufman PL. Recent developments in undestanding the pathophysiology of elevated intraocular pressure. Curr Opin Ophthalmol 2006; 17: 168–74

Tezel G, Wax MB. The immune system and glaucoma. Curr Opin Ophthalmol 2004; 15: 80–4

Tezel G, Yang J, Wax MB. Heat shock proteins, immunity and glaucoma. Brain Res Bull 2004; 62: 473–80

Tian B, Geiger B, Epstein DL, Kaufman PL. Cytoskeletal involvement in the regulation of aqueous humor outflow. Invest Ophthalmol Vis Sci 2000; 41: 619–23

Tielsch JM, Sommer A, Katz J, et al. Racial variations in the prevalence of primary open angle glaucoma: the Baltimore Eye Survey. J Am Med Assoc 1991; 266: 369–74

Tielsch JM, Katz J, Sommer A, et al. Family history and risk of primary open angle glaucoma. Arch Ophthalmol 1994; 112: 69–73

Tielsch JM, Katz J, Sommer A, et al. Hypertension, perfusion pressure, and primary open angle glaucoma. Arch Ophthalmol 1995; 113: 216–21

Trew DR, Smith SE. Postural studies in pulsatile ocular blood flow: II. Chronic open angle glaucoma. Br J Ophthalmol 1991; 75: 71–5

Usuai T, Iwata K. Finger blood flow in patients with low tension glaucoma and primary open angle glaucoma. Br J Ophthalmol 1992; 76: 2–4

West SK, Rubin GS, Broman AT, et al. How does visual impairment affect performance on tasks of everyday life? The SEE Project. Salisbury Eye Evaluation. Arch Ophthalmol 2002; 120: 774–80

Wiggs JL, Haines JL, Pagliniauan C, et al. Genetic linkage of autosomal dominant juvenile glaucoma to 1q21-q31 in three affected pedigrees. Genomics 1994; 21: 299–303

Wiggs JL, Auguste J, Allingham RR, et al. Lack of mutations in Optineurin with disease in patients with adult-onset primary open angle glaucoma. Arch Ophthalmol 2003; 121: 1181–3

Wolf S, Arend O, Sponsel WE, et al. Retinal hemodynamics using scanning laser ophthalmoscopy and hemorheology in chronic open angle glaucoma. Ophthalmology 1993; 100: 1561–6

Wong EY, Keeffe JE, Rait JL, et al. Detection of undiagnosed glaucoma by eye health professionals. Ophthalmology 2004; 111: 1508–14

10 Secondary open-angle glaucomas

Jonathan Myers, L Jay Katz

INTRODUCTION

The secondary open-angle glaucomas comprise a number of conditions in which intraocular pressure (IOP) becomes elevated through a variety of mechanisms other than primary dysfunction of the trabecular meshwork. Often the term 'glaucoma' is applied even in the absence of optic nerve damage. The glaucoma is often characterized by the addition of the descriptive term referring to the condition responsible for the elevated IOP. Primary open-angle glaucoma is discussed in Chapter 9, and the angle-closure glaucomas are discussed in Chapter 11.

PIGMENTARY GLAUCOMA

Pigmentary glaucoma is a secondary open-angle glaucoma in which released iris pigment interferes with trabecular meshwork function, leading to elevated intraocular pressure. A flaccid peripheral iris, bowing posteriorly, is believed to rub against the zonular fibers, damaging the iris pigment epithelium. Radial, slit-like iris transillumination defects are typical (Figure 10.1). Risk factors for development of pigmentary dispersion syndrome include myopia, male sex, white race and young age. Blacks and Asians rarely develop pigmentary dispersion; this may be due to their thicker, less flaccid irides. With increasing age, increasing relative pupillary block may play a protective role as aqueous in the posterior chamber accumulates and keeps the peripheral iris away from the zonular fibers.

Released pigment is carried by aqueous flow into the anterior chamber. Pigment may be phagocytozed by corneal endothelial cells, creating a Krukenberg spindle (Figure 10.2). Pigment may also be deposited in circumferential iris furrows and on the posterior lens surface (Figure 10.3).

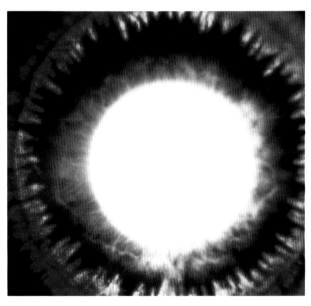

Figure 10.1 Transillumination defects seen using the red reflex. Characteristically in the peripheral half of the iris, they correspond to the location and orientation of the zonular fibers. Mild cases may have very few transillumination defects; these may increase or decrease with time.

Aqueous flow carries the pigment to the trabecular meshwork which is typically heavily pigmented for 360° (Figures 10.4 and 10.5). Pigment deposition anterior to Schwalbe's line is seen in the inferior 180° (Figure 10.6).

Approximately one-third of patients with pigment dispersion syndrome will go on, over 15 years, to develop pigmentary glaucoma. Treatment of pigmentary glaucoma includes the full spectrum of pharmacological, laser and surgical modalities. Miotics work well to lower pressures both by opening the trabecular meshwork and by pulling the iris away from zonular fibers, reducing pigment release. However, many of these young patients are intolerant of miosis-induced headaches

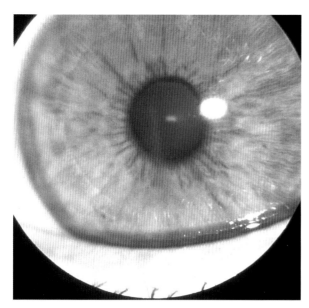

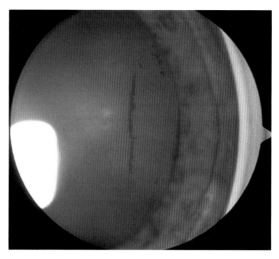

Figure 10.3 Pigment deposition. Pigment deposition on the posterior surface of the lens is highly suggestive of pigment dispersion syndrome and pigmentary glaucoma.

Figure 10.2 The Krukenberg spindle. The Krukenberg spindle, a vertical deposition of pigment in the lower central cornea, is apparently shaped by convection currents in the anterior chamber.

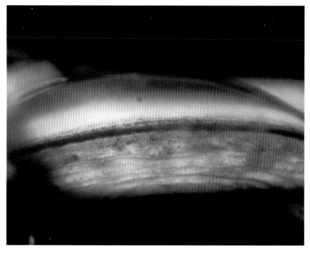

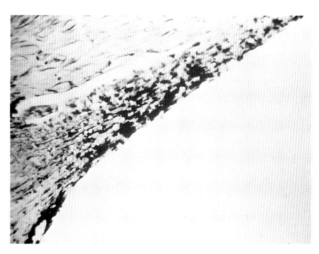

Figure 10.5 Histopathologic section showing trabecular meshwork laden with pigment. Endothelial cells coating the trabecular beams in the meshwork phagocytoze the pigment. Experiments have shown that, when enough pigment is released, overloaded endothelial cells move off the beams and disintegrate. Trabecular collapse with loss of filtering intratrabecular spaces follows, leading to decreased facility of outflow and increased intraocular pressure.

Figure 10.4 Heavy pigmentation. Heavy pigmentation of the trabecular meshwork and other angle structures is seen circumferentially. Typical posterior bowing of the peripheral iris on gonioscopy is seen here.

and blurred vision. Longer-release preparations, such as pilogel and ocuserts, reduce these symptoms adequately for some patients. These patients are also at increased risk for retinal detachment with miotics. For these reasons many clinicians start with aqueous suppressants such as beta blockers, and more recently apraclonidine and dorzolamide. Adrenergic agents and prostaglandin analogs are also effective.

Laser peripheral iridotomy has been advanced as a prophylactic therapy, although no studies have yet demonstrated its efficacy. This procedure relieves reverse pupillary block and may reduce iris chafe and pigment release (Figure 10.7).

Laser trabeculoplasty has been shown to be very effective. Lower laser powers are sufficient as the trabecular meshwork pigment absorbs the energy well. However, long-term results show more than half of patients losing treatment effect within 5 years. Conventional filtering surgery yields good results in pigmentary glaucoma. Results are similar to those obtained in patients

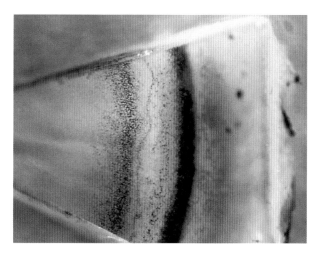

Figure 10.6 Pigment deposition on angle structures. Specimen showing pigment deposition on angle structures, including those anterior to Schwalbe's line.

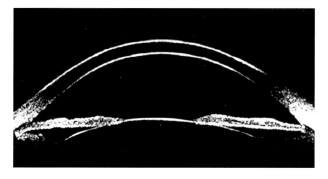

(a)

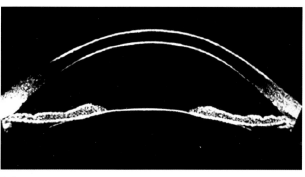

(b)

Figure 10.7 Ultrasound biomicroscopic images. Reverse pupillary block occurs when a blink forces a small amount of aqueous into the anterior chamber, past a floppy iris laying against the lens. This slight increase in anterior chamber volume and pressure bows the iris back against the lens and zonular fibers, increasing the block and increasing the contact which leads to pigment release. The iridotomy relieves this block, allowing the iris to come forward from the lens (b). This may prevent further pigment release and the development of glaucoma if done early in the disease process.

with primary open-angle glaucoma. Antimetabolites should be used cautiously, as these young, myopic patients are more prone to hypotensive maculopathy.

EXFOLIATION SYNDROME

Exfoliation syndrome is a common cause of secondary open-angle glaucoma in many populations. Signs of exfoliation syndrome may be seen in over 20% of patients in Iceland and Finland, accounting for as much as half of the glaucomatous population. In the USA, the incidence is much lower but patients with exfoliation syndrome still make up about 10% of those with glaucoma, perhaps even more of the ocular hypertensives. With age, the incidence of exfoliation syndrome increases, and this may contribute to its association with female gender. Findings are more often unilateral in American studies, but bilaterality increases with longer follow-up.

The classic finding in exfoliation syndrome is the grayish-white flaky material on the anterior lens capsule (Figures 10.8 and 10.9). This material may also be seen at the pupil margin, corneal endothelium, trabecular meshwork, zonular fibers and ciliary body; after cataract extraction it appears on the posterior capsule, intraocular lens and vitreous face as well. This same material has been found in the conjunctiva, orbital blood vessels, skin, myocardium, lung, liver, gallbladder, kidney and cerebral meninges, usually localized to connective tissue.

Abrasive exfoliation material on the anterior lens capsule leads to the release of pigment from the posterior surface of the iris. Peripupillary transillumination defects and loss of the pigmented ruff may be evident (Figures 10.10 and 10.11). Pigment deposition is seen throughout the anterior chamber and angle (Figure 10.12). Pigment and exfoliation material within the trabecular meshwork are thought to lead to the increased IOP associated with exfoliation syndrome.

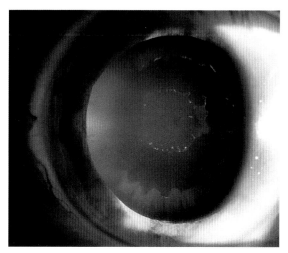

Figure 10.8 Exfoliation material on the anterior lens capsule. Deposition of exfoliative material is often in a bull's-eye configuration consisting of a central disc, mid-peripheral clearing and a more irregular peripheral ring of deposits.

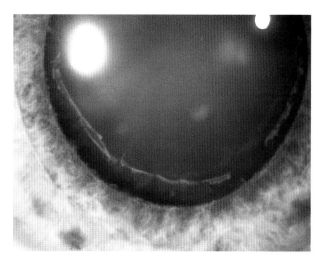

Figure 10.9   Exfoliation material.   Seen on dilatation only; central disc deposition absent.

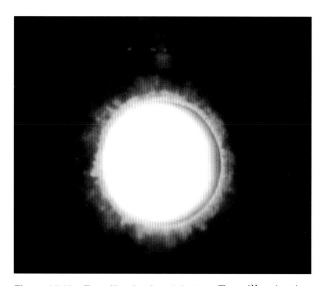

Figure 10.10   Transillumination defects.   Transillumination defects in exfoliation syndrome are typically near the pupil margin.

Affected eyes show poor dilatation with mydriatics for a number of reasons. Iris ischemia leads to neovascularization and posterior synechiae. Chronic miotic therapy reduces mydriasis and allows the lens iris diaphragm to move forward, contributing to the formation of synechiae. Narrow angles are common and secondary angle closure may result. Exfoliation material deposition in the iris stroma may increase rigidity. Intraocular pressure spikes secondary to pigment dispersion are common with dilatation. Zonular fibers in affected eyes are weakened; lens dislocation may occur with minimal surgical manipulation, or spontaneously (Figure 10.13). These factors make cataract extraction more difficult, increasing the likelihood of vitreous loss.

Glaucoma in exfoliation syndrome is associated with higher IOPs and increased treatment failures when compared to primary open-angle glaucoma.

Miotic therapy increases trabecular meshwork outflow and may reduce pigment release, but also contributes to posterior synechiae and reduced dilatation. Laser trabeculoplasty is effective, but transient IOP spikes following treatment may be more common and more severe compared to primary open-angle glaucoma. Some patients show reduced IOPs following lens extraction; this is thought to be secondary to reduced pigment release since the exfoliation material is still produced. The success with trabeculectomy is similar to that seen in primary open-angle glaucoma.

APHAKIC AND PSEUDOPHAKIC GLAUCOMAS

Increased IOP is a well-known complication of cataract extraction. Reported incidences vary depending on sample size and technique; increased IOPs may be less common with extracapsular cataract extraction and phacoemulsification than with intracapsular approaches. Many etiologies lead to postoperative pressure elevations and are best considered by time of onset.

Within the first week, many of the materials dispersed during surgery can lead to elevated pressures. Alpha-chymotrypsin frequently results in reduced facility of outflow in the first 2 days following intracapsular cataract extraction. Retained viscoelastic material is a source of trabecular obstruction manifesting in the first postoperative day. Increased IOPs are seen with all current viscoelastics; no definitive difference in incidence has been shown among them. The viscoelastic Orcolon was withdrawn from the market because of pressure spikes. Meticulous removal at the time of surgery may reduce the frequency of this complication. Hyphema following surgery also blocks outflow and can lead to elevated IOP. Debris, inflammation and trabecular edema may also play roles in acutely elevated pressures postoperatively. Pre-existing glaucoma increases the frequency and severity of acute postoperative pressure elevations. These complications are best treated medically with aqueous suppressants and topical steroids. Fibrin clots may be treated with intracameral injection of tissue plasminogen activator (Figure 10.14). Surgical evacuation of viscoelastic or blood is reserved for pressures which do not respond to medical therapy and threaten the optic nerve.

After the first week, other factors may lead to glaucoma. Vitreous in the anterior chamber may reduce aqueous outflow. Hyphema, related to wound construction or intraocular lens position, may occur. Ghost-cell glaucoma results from long-standing hyphema or vitreous hemorrhage leading to degenerated erythrocytes, which are less flexible and block trabecular channels. Retained lens particles become hydrated and more prominent, blocking

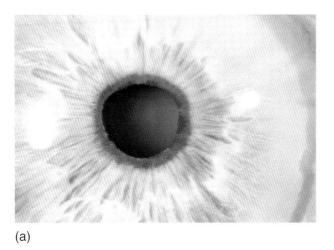
(a)

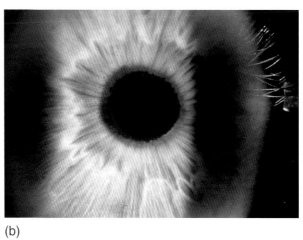
(b)

Figure 10.11   Clinically unilateral exfoliation syndrome and glaucoma.   This patient with clinically unilateral exfoliation syndrome and glaucoma shows absence of the pigmented ruff at the pupil margin in the affected eye (a) and a normal ruff in the unaffected eye (b).

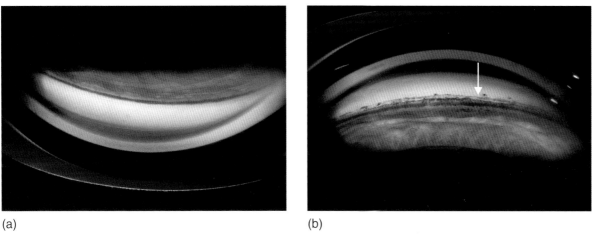
(a)   (b)

Figure 10.12   Anterior chamber angle with pigment deposition in exfoliation syndrome.   Pigment is unevenly deposited over angle structures (a) in the superior angle. Sampaolesi's line, a wavy line of pigment anterior to Schwalbe's line, is present inferiorly (b). This pattern of pigmentation differs from that seen in pigmentary glaucoma which is typically more homogeneous and often limited to the trabecular meshwork.

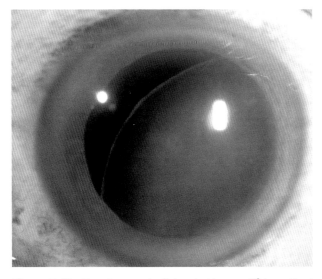

Figure 10.13   Spontaneously dislocated lens.   This patient with exfoliation syndrome has a spontaneously dislocated lens in the absence of trauma.

the trabecular meshwork. Postoperative inflammation related to retained lens particles, intraocular lens position, vitreous traction and surgical trauma may become more manifest. Corticosteroid-induced glaucoma must be considered as a common source of increased IOP in postoperative patients on topical steroids. Discontinuation of steroids or a therapeutic challenge of the fellow eye with topical steroids will often aid in the diagnosis.

Late pressure elevations, occurring months to years following surgery, may also be secondary to inflammation and hemorrhage. *Propionibacterium acnes* endophthalmitis may lead to chronic inflammation with increased pressures. Intraocular lenses may be a source of inflammation and hyphema in the UGH (Uveitis, Glaucoma, Hyphema) syndrome (Figures 10.15 and 10.16). Anterior chamber lenses may directly damage the trabecular meshwork. Vitreous in the anterior chamber may still block outflow. Following YAG laser capsulotomy,

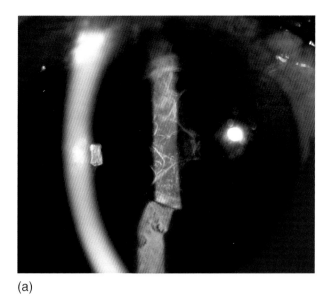
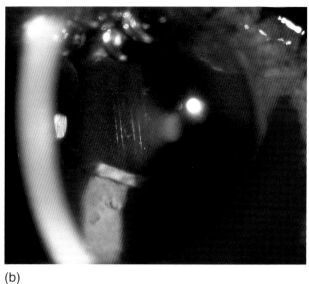

(a)   (b)

Figure 10.14   Fibrin clots.   Fibrin clot over posterior chamber intraocular lens with elevated intraocular pressure following combined guarded filtration procedure and cataract extraction (a). Same eye (b) following intracameral injection of tissue plasminogen activator. Visual acuity improved dramatically; intraocular pressure dropped from 38 to 10, and remained well controlled.

inflammation may lead to quite significant pressure elevations, whose frequency is greatly reduced by pretreatment with a topical α_2 agonist, such as apraclonidine.

Angle-closure glaucoma related to intraocular lenses is discussed in Chapter 11.

CORTICOSTEROID-INDUCED GLAUCOMA

The use of corticosteroids in any form may lead to the development of a secondary open-angle glaucoma. Increased IOP has been demonstrated with topical, periocular, inhalational and systemic steroids as well as with increased endogenous steroids in adrenal hyperplasia and Cushing's syndrome (Figure 10.17). Past steroid use and glaucoma may simulate the presentation of normal-tension glaucoma, as the optic nerve damage and visual field loss may have occurred when the IOP was elevated when the steroids were being used, and returned to normal levels once steroid use terminated. Topical steroids are more likely to elevate IOP than systemic steroids. IOPs rise more frequently and more severely with the more potent steroids and with greater dosing. Pressure elevation typically manifests 2–6 weeks after the initiation of steroids. Patients with primary open-angle glaucoma respond much more frequently and severely to steroids with elevated IOP. Depending on steroid dose, duration and diagnostic criteria, over 90% of patients with primary open-angle glaucoma may have pressure elevations with steroids compared to 5–10% of normals. Other risk factors for steroid responsiveness include ocular hypertension, angle-

recession glaucoma (in either eye), primary relative of patient with primary open-angle glaucoma, pigmentary glaucoma, myopia, diabetes and history of connective tissue disease, but not exfoliative glaucoma.

Corticosteroids result in the accumulation of glycosaminoglycans in the trabecular meshwork, reducing outflow facility. Theories for the mechanism of this accumulation of glycosaminoglycans include increased production as well as reduced clearance, mediated either by nuclear steroid receptors or by membrane stabilization.

The diagnosis may be made either by withdrawing steroid therapy and observing reduced pressures or by challenging the fellow eye in topical steroid cases. IOPs usually return to baseline within 1–2 months, but may remain high in patients who have been on steroids for long periods of time. Elevated pressures following periocular injection of steroids may require the excision of depot steroids. Aqueous suppressants and miotics can be effective in treating the elevated pressure. Argon laser trabeculoplasty may be useful, although less effective than in primary open-angle glaucoma, pigmentary glaucoma and exfoliative glaucoma.

POST-TRAUMATIC GLAUCOMAS

Ocular trauma remains a common cause for emergency room visits and hospital admissions, being most frequent among young males. Causes vary with age: play-related accidents in young children, sports and assaults in young adults, and work and domestic accidents or abuse in older adults.

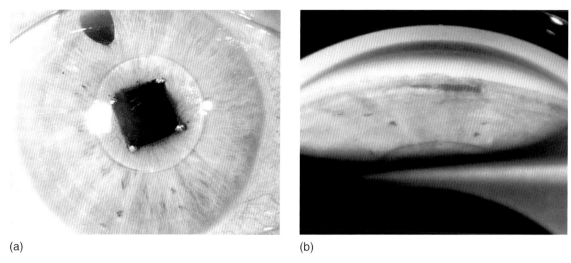

(a)   (b)

Figrue 10.15

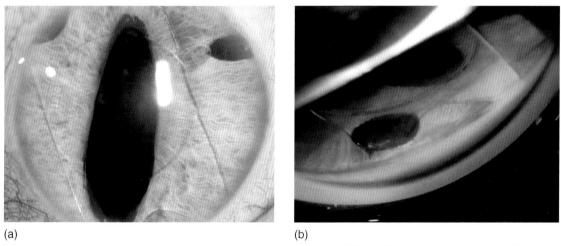

(a)   (b)

Figures 10.15 and 10.16   UGH syndromes.   Right (Figure 10.15(a) and (b)) and left (Figure 10.16(a) and (b)) eyes of a patient with intraocular lenses and the UGH syndrome in both eyes. This patient had multiple hyphemas over a period of years. In some instances the inflammation was readily apparent but the hyphema was only appreciated on gonioscopy. (a) shows the clinical appearance, while (b) is the goniophotograph.

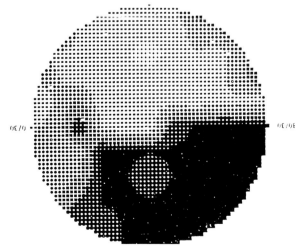

Figure 10.17   Advanced visual field loss.   This is the visual field of a doctor who self-prescribed topical steroids for vernal conjunctivitis for many years without eye examinations developed steroid glaucoma with advanced visual field loss.

The mechanism of trauma often dictates the specific injuries to the eye, almost all may lead to glaucoma. Non-penetrating injuries of the eye secondary to blunt trauma are usually related to the anterior to posterior compression of the eye with secondary equatorial stretching. This stretching may result in pupil sphincter tears, iridodialysis, angle recession, cyclodialysis, trabecular dialysis, disruption of the zonules and retinal dialysis or detachment. Tears in the face of the ciliary body, usually between the circular and longitudinal muscles, may disrupt the major arterial circle of the iris and the arterial and venous connections of the ciliary body resulting in hyphema. Severity may range from a microhyphema, in which the slit-lamp microscope is necessary to appreciate the presence of blood in the anterior chamber, to total hyphema, in which the anterior and posterior chambers are entirely filled with blood (Figures 10.18 and 10.19). Following injury, IOP may be elevated or reduced, depending on the balance of several factors. Aqueous secretion may be acutely reduced; uveoscleral outflow may be increased by an accompanying cyclodialysis; blood may obstruct an injured and inflamed trabecular meshwork. Although red blood cells normally pass through the pores in the meshwork, acute inflammation and swelling of the meshwork combined with excessive amounts of red blood cells and debris may overwhelm the meshwork's capacity. Aqueous suppressants are effective in many cases. Steroids help to reduce inflammation. Miotics are generally avoided as they may predispose to posterior synechiae, further compromise the blood–aqueous barrier and reduce uveoscleral outflow.

Patients with hyphema are generally kept at bedrest and treated with mydriatics and topical steroids. Aminocaproic acid, an antifibrinolytic agent, is also used in some centers to reduce the incidence of rebleeds, which may be severe. Prolonged elevation of IOP may require surgical evacuation of the blood. Timing is dependent on the ability of the nerve to withstand elevated pressures; otherwise healthy nerves may tolerate pressures of up to 50 mmHg for several days. Evacuation may also be necessary because of the development of blood staining of the cornea, especially in those at risk for amblyopia (Figure 10.20). Surgical evacuation is ideally performed near the fourth day post-trauma. This is past the peak incidence of rebleed and allows time for the anterior-chamber blood to clot and retract somewhat from ocular structures, facilitating removal.

Patients with sickle-cell disease are at greater risk for complications from hyphemas. Significant intraocular pressure elevations may occur with even small hyphemas. Sickling has been demonstrated in the anterior chamber blood; this may reduce clearance and increase intraocular pressure. Central retinal arterial obstruction may occur at lower pressures following hyphemas in these patients. Carbonic anhydrase inhibitors are avoided in sickle-cell disease as they may worsen sickling and reduce clearance of blood by increasing aqueous ascorbic acid and by promoting systemic acidosis. African-American patients with hyphemas should be screened for sickle-cell hemoglobin, and positive patients should undergo hemoglobin electrophoresis. All available therapies should be used to keep intraocular pressures below 25 mmHg.

As also discussed elsewhere (see Chapter 11), trauma may also lead to angle-closure glaucoma through a variety of mechanisms. Clots may cover the pupil leading to pupillary block and angle closure.

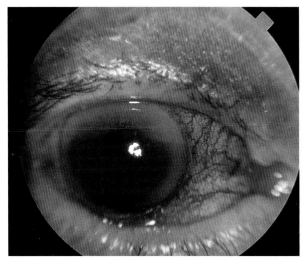

Figure 10.18 Traumatic hyphema. Two fluid levels exist as the red blood cells settle and clot.

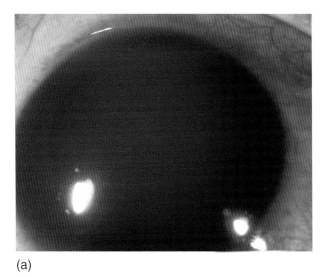

(a)

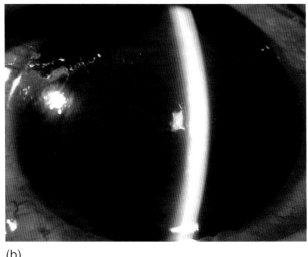

(b)

Figure 10.19 Total hyphema. (a) The incidence of elevated intraocular pressure increases with the amount of blood in the anterior chamber. More than half of those with total hyphemas have significant pressure elevations. (b) With 'blackball' or 'eight-ball' hyphemas, this approaches 100%. Patients with sickle-cell disease may suffer severe pressure elevations with relatively minor hyphemas.

Dislocated lenses may cause pupillary block. Post-traumatic inflammation may lead to extensive peripheral anterior and posterior synechiae. Shallow anterior chambers with penetrating trauma also may create extensive anterior synechiae. Rarely, photoreceptors from a retinal detachment will cause a secondary open-angle glaucoma (Schwartz's syndrome).

Angle-recession glaucoma is an important late complication of ocular trauma. IOPs may remain normal for years to decades and then become severely elevated. Patients must be strongly advised of the need for lifelong, regular follow-up.

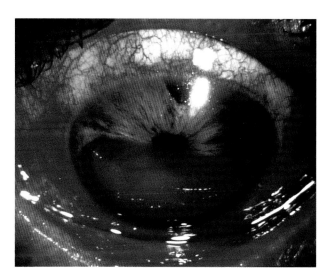

Figure 10.20 Corneal blood staining following a traumatic hyphema. These generally clear over weeks to months, starting at the periphery, following hyphema resolution. In patients in the age group capable of developing ambylophia, incipient blood staining may require surgical evacuation of the blood.

Angle-recession glaucoma is more common in eyes with 180° or more of angle recession, occurring in 6–20% over a 10-year period (Figure 10.21). Angle recession must be considered in unilateral glaucomas. Patients often do not recall the long-past trauma. With time, angle recession also tends to scar, becoming less evident by gonioscopy in apparent severity and extent or even forming peripheral anterior synechiae. The affected areas, although reapproximated, still have non-functioning meshwork, secondary to scarring or their closure by a Descemet's-like membrane. Fellow eyes are at increased risk of developing open-angle glaucoma; 25% were affected in one study.

Angle-recession glaucoma may respond to aqueous suppressants. Miotics and argon laser trabeculoplasty are rarely effective. Long-term success rates for trabeculectomy are worse than in primary open-angle glaucoma; some surgeons use antimetabolites on primary procedures for this reason.

GHOST-CELL GLAUCOMA

Ghost cells are degenerated red blood cells whose leaky membranes have allowed much of the cell's hemoglobin to escape. Residual, degenerated hemoglobin precipitates on the inner cell walls in the form of Heinz bodies. These spherical cells are much less pliable than red blood cells and cannot pass through the intertrabecular spaces. Ghost cells in the anterior chamber result in elevated IOP much more readily than red blood cells. The formation of ghost cells requires the sequestration of red blood cells in the vitreous for several weeks. The source of vitreous hemorrhage does not matter: a bleed from

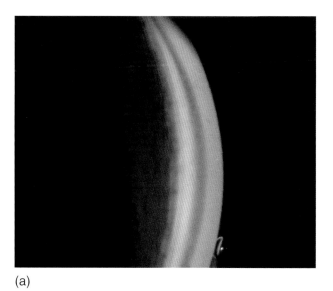

(a)

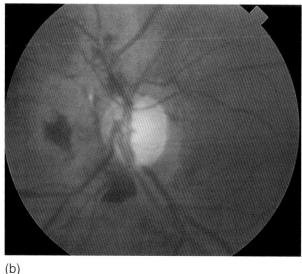

(b)

Figure 10.21 Angle recession. (a) An abnormally wide ciliary body band is seen, as well as bare sclera posteriorly. Fundoscopic examination (b) revealed a glaucomatous optic nerve with markedly increased cupping compared to the fellow eye. Traumatic scars of the retinal pigment epithelium are also seen.

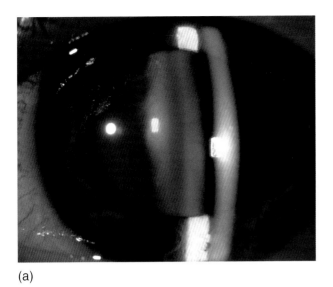

(a)

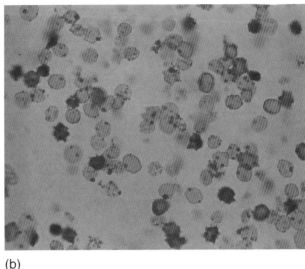

(b)

Figure 10.22   Ghost-cell glaucoma.   This patient with ghost-cell glaucoma had 2+ anterior chamber khaki-colored cells and marked khaki-colored cells in the anterior vitreous (a). Vitrectomy specimen showed ghost cells (b).

diabetic neovascularization of the retina, hemorrhage secondary to trauma or a postsurgical hyphema with spill-over into the vitreous through a compromised vitreous face may evolve into a secondary glaucoma. After several weeks, the degenerated cells migrate into the anterior chamber through a defect in the vitreous face (surgical or traumatic) and obstruct the trabecular meshwork. Tan or khaki-colored cells are seen in the anterior chamber, anterior vitreous, on the trabecular meshwork, and may also form a pseudohypopyon. If the vitreous face is intact, the ghost cells do not reach the anterior chamber and glaucoma does not develop.

Several other blood-related elevations of IOP may be differentiated from ghost-cell glaucoma. Hyphemas may result in acutely elevated pressure, especially in patients with sickle-cell disease. This is secondary to obstruction of the meshwork by red blood cells in the first days following the hyphema. Rarely, an eight-ball, total hyphema may persist long enough to contain ghost cells which add to the trabecular obstruction. Hemolytic glaucoma occurs when the contents of ruptured red blood cells are ingested by macrophages which then obstruct the meshwork. Hemolytic glaucoma is also typically seen in the first days to weeks following the initial hemorrhage. Hemosiderotic glaucoma, in which iron-containing blood breakdown products stain and poison the cells of the trabecular meshwork, occurs much later, often years after the hemorrhage.

Aqueous suppressants often control the intraocular pressure. Miotics are rarely helpful as the meshwork is obstructed; similarly, argon laser trabeculoplasty is not indicated. Anterior chamber lavage with balanced salt solution may resolve the glaucoma. If unsuccessful, or too great a reservoir of ghost cells remains in the vitreous, total vitrectomy,

removing as much hemorrhagic material as possible, is usually effective in resolving the glaucoma.

INFLAMMATORY GLAUCOMAS

Inflammation within the eye alters aqueous humor dynamics and can lead to increased IOP. Acute inflammation may reduce aqueous secretion and increase uveoscleral outflow, reducing IOP. However, inflammatory material, consisting of white blood cells, macrophages, and proteins, may obstruct the trabecular meshwork. Chemical mediators of inflammation may further compromise trabecular function as may trabeculitis (inflammation of the trabecular meshwork itself). Trabecular dysfunction may be transient, clearing with resolution of the inflammation, or may persist with permanent structural changes reducing trabecular outflow facility. Additionally, inflammatory scarring may lead to peripheral anterior synechiae and posterior synechiae resulting in angle-closure glaucoma (see Chapter 11). Chronic uveitis may lead to neovascularization and neovascular glaucoma. Patients may manifest some or all of these findings, the balance dictating the nature of the glaucoma. For example, a patient may present acutely during a uveitic episode with uveitic hypotony, progress to a secondary open-angle glaucoma as white blood cells block the meshwork, develop an angle-closure component as synechiae form, and then be left with a chronic mixed-mechanism secondary glaucoma with residual synechiae and scarring of the meshwork.

Virtually all sources of ocular inflammation can lead to glaucoma. Idiopathic uveitis (Figure 10.23), glaucomatocyclitic crisis (Figure 10.24), Fuch's heterochromic cyclitis (Figure 10.25), lens-related uveitis (Figure 10.26), herpes (Figure 10.27) and

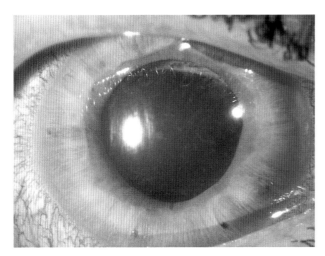

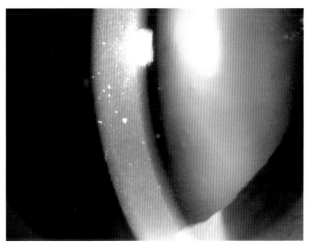

Figure 10.23   Idiopathic uveitis resulting in secondary glaucoma with closed and open-angle components. Note the multiple peripheral iridectomies for previous acute iris bombé. Following resolution of acute attacks the patient had persistent elevation of intraocular pressure in spite of large areas of open anterior chamber angle on gonioscopy.

Figure 10.24   Glaucomatocyclitic crisis (Posner–Schlossman syndrome). Unilateral involvement consisting of fine keratic precipitates in a patient with minimal anterior chamber reaction and markedly elevated intraocular pressure. Following multiple similar attacks, the patient developed chronically elevated intraocular pressure and optic nerve damage requiring trabeculectomy.

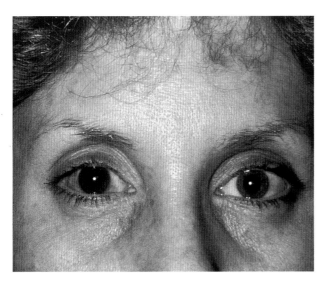

Figure 10.25   Fuch's heterochromic cyclitis Note the much lighter iris color in the involved eye. The triad of heterochromia, uveitis and cataract typically appears in the third to fourth decade. The uveitis is asymptomatic. Open-angle glaucoma is common, increasing with duration of the disease. Friable angle vessels may bleed easily with surgery; however, frank neovascularization of the iris and neovascular glaucoma are uncommon.

sarcoidosis (Figure 10.28) may all result in increased IOP. Other uveitic glaucomas include HLA-B27-related uveitides, pars planitis, sarcoidosis, juvenile rheumatoid arthritis, Behçet's disease, Crohn's disease, syphilis, toxoplasmosis, coccidiomycosis, mumps, rubella, leprosy, sympathetic ophthalmia, Vogt–Koyanagi–Harada syndrome and other less common entities.

Treatment strategies are similar for these entities. Resolution of inflammation is the first goal,

which may require topical or systemic steroids, antibiotics for infectious diseases and lens extraction in lens-related conditions. Increased intraocular pressure secondary to steroid therapy or to increased aqueous production with resolving inflammation may confuse the clinical picture. Cycloplegics are effective through many mechanisms. Dilatation prevents the formation of a small secluded pupil and relieves the discomfort of ciliary spasm. Cycloplegics also improve uveoscleral outflow and stabilize the blood–aqueous barrier. Topical and systemic aqueous suppressants are effective. Miotics should be avoided as these agents cause increased breakdown of the blood–aqueous barrier, making the inflammation worse, and also reduce uveoscleral outflow. Laser trabeculoplasty is generally ineffective and increases inflammation. Filtering surgery is less successful in these patients, especially during acute attacks. Adjunctive use of antimetabolites such as 5-fluorouracil and mitomycin-C may improve results. Drainage tube implants may also be effective. Cyclodestructive procedures can be used in refractory cases, but add to intraocular inflammation and pose significant risks to vision.

GLAUCOMA ASSOCIATED WITH OCULAR TUMORS

Benign and malignant intraocular tumors may cause glaucoma by a variety of mechanisms. Direct infiltration of the trabecular meshwork by the tumor can block aqueous outflow. Free-floating tumor cells may obstruct the meshwork. Hemorrhage may produce a secondary open-angle glaucoma.

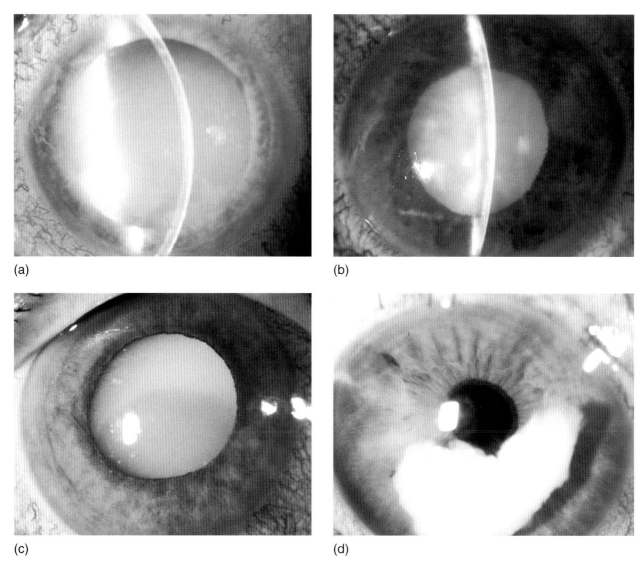

(a)

(b)

(c)

(d)

Figure 10.26 Lens-related glaucoma.   In phacolytic glaucoma, a hypermature lens leaks proteins into the anterior chamber through a grossly intact capsule (a); these proteins and ingesting macrophages block the trabecular meshwork. A swollen, mature cataract may also lead to pupillary block in phacomorphic glaucoma; (b) note the narrow angle present in a patient with phacomorphic glaucoma. A hypermature cataract with liquefied cortex and dense nucleus may also lead to phacolytic glaucoma (c). Retained lens cortex (d) following cataract extraction may increase in size with hydration and lead to glaucoma through trabecular obstruction by lens material. Phacoanaphylaxis exists when lens material is present outside the capsule following surgery or trauma and leads to granulomatous inflammation. A previous history of trauma to the lens or cataract surgery in the fellow eye is typical. Phacoanaphylaxis often leads to significant pressure elevation.

Tumor-related neovascularization of the iris and angle produces glaucoma in some cases. Large posterior masses sometimes press the iris and lens anteriorly, resulting in angle closure (Chapter 11). Tumor-related glaucomas are typically unilateral. Treatment of the glaucoma without diagnosis of the tumor may have serious consequences for the patient. A thorough examination will reveal most intraocular malignancies, especially for clinicians alert to such tip-offs as a sentinel vessel (Figure 10.29).

Uveal melanoma is the most common intraocular malignancy in adults, and is the most common cause of tumor-related glaucoma. Iris melanomas may obstruct the trabecular meshwork by direct invasion or by hemorrhage (Figure 10.30). Ciliary body melanomas may be more difficult to detect, remaining hidden until relatively large. Glaucoma most often results from the tumor pushing the iris anteriorly to close the anterior chamber angle. Glaucoma may also result because of direct extension of the tumor into the trabecular meshwork, iris neovascularization, hyphema or tumor necrosis, causing obstruction of the meshwork by cells and debris. Choroidal melanoma less commonly causes glaucoma. Mechanisms of glaucoma in choroidal melanomas include iris and angle neovascularization most commonly, as well as angle closure, hemorrhage and necrosis.

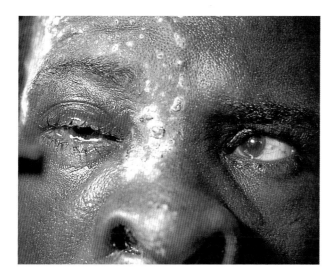

Figure 10.27 Herpes zoster ophthalmicus. Herpes zoster ophthalmicus with characteristic skin lesions affecting the dermatome of the first branch of the facial nerve. The tip of the nose is involved, a harbinger of ocular involvement (Hutchinson's sign). Marked conjunctival injection and a granulomatous uveitis are present. Glaucoma is a frequent complication in herpes zoster and herpes simplex uveitis.

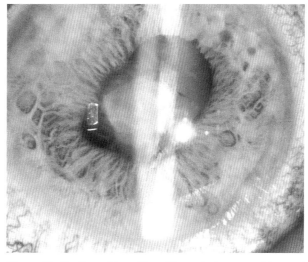

Figure 10.28 Sarcoid uveitis with posterior synechiae and cataract. Up to one-half of patients with sarcoid suffer from uveitis at some point during the disease process. Granulomatous anterior uveitis is a common manifestation, frequently becoming bilateral, recurrent and chronic. Sarcoid nodules on the iris (Busacca's in the crypts, Koeppe's at the pupillary margin) may be seen. Secondary open and closed-angle glaucoma is common. As the disease is more common in Blacks, clinicians must be wary of steroid-induced glaucoma as a complication of treatment.

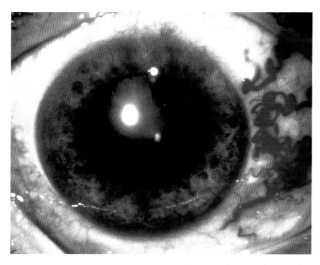

Figure 10.29 Uveal melanoma. Sentinel vessel overlying the sclera in a patient with uveal melanoma.

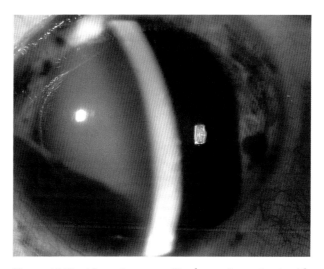

Figure 10.30 Iris melanoma. Hyphema in patient with iris melanoma producing a secondary open-angle glaucoma.

Histologically benign tumors of the iris may also cause glaucoma. Diffuse uveal melanomas may block the meshwork with melanoma cells or pigment. Melanocytomas, most commonly found on the optic disc but also seen in the iris or ciliary body, can produce glaucoma. These tumors have a propensity to undergo necrosis and fragmentation, blocking the trabecular meshwork with debris, producing the so-called melanomalytic glaucoma. Differentiation of these tumors from their malignant counterparts is a crucial step in treatment, often requiring histopathologic study. Intraocular metastases are typically to the uveal tissues. Glaucoma is found more frequently in metastases to the iris and ciliary body (64% and 67%, respectively) than in metastases to the choroid (2%). Common primary tumors include those of the breast and lung, as well as tumors of the gastrointestinal tract, kidney, thyroid and skin. Efforts to identify the primary neoplasm are not always successful. Friable metastases often seed the anterior chamber angle, obstructing the trabecular meshwork (Figures 10.31 and 10.32).

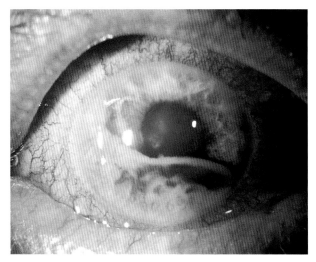

Figure 10.31 **Metastatic tumor.** Metastatic tumor to iris from lung.

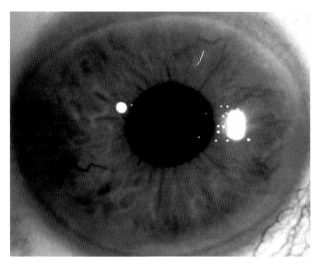

Figure 10.32 **Multiple myeloma.** Multiple myeloma of iris.

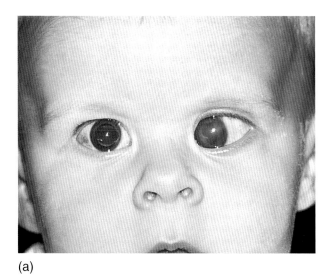

(a)

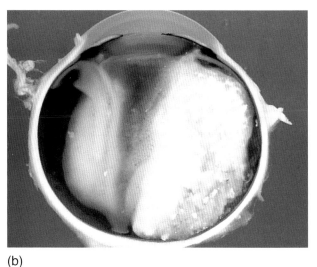

(b)

Figure 10.33 **Retinoblastoma.** Retinoblastoma causing glaucoma (a) (external photo) and (b) gross pathology.

Pseudohypopyons and ring infiltrates are sometimes seen.

Benign reactive lymphoid hyperplasia can directly invade the trabecular meshwork. Large cell lymphoma (reticulum cell sarcoma, histiocytic lymphoma) and leukemia may also infiltrate the meshwork and lead to glaucoma.

Retinoblastoma is the most common intraocular malignancy of childhood. Glaucoma is not uncommon, occurring in 17% of cases in one study (Shields *et al.*). In that study of 303 eyes, the glaucoma was thought to be secondary to iris neovascularization with or without hemorrhage in 72%, angle closure in 26%, and tumor seeding in 2% (Figure 10.33). The less common but benign medulloepithelioma may also cause glaucoma secondary to iris neovascularization, as well as direct invasion of angle structures or obstruction of the meshwork by hyphema and tumor-related debris.

Various ocular tumors are manifested by the phakomatoses. Unilateral glaucoma, congenital or later onset, may be seen in neurofibromatosis of both types (Figure 10.34). Half of all eyes with plexiform neuromas of the upper lid develop glaucoma. The glaucoma associated with encephalotrigeminal angiomatosis (Sturge–Weber syndrome) is discussed below, along with other causes of increased episcleral venous pressure. Congenital glaucoma may also be seen. Oculodermal melanocytosis (nevus of Ota) has been reported to have an incidence of glaucoma of 10%, including angle-closure, open-angle and congenital varieties.

INCREASED EPISCLERAL VENOUS PRESSURE

The Goldmann equation, $Po = F/C + Pev$ (where Po is intraocular pressure, F is aqueous production, C outflow facility and Pev episcleral venous pressure), describes a direct relation of IOP to episcleral venous pressure. Normal episcleral venous pressure is between 9 and 10 mmHg. Increases in episcleral venous pressure lead to increases in

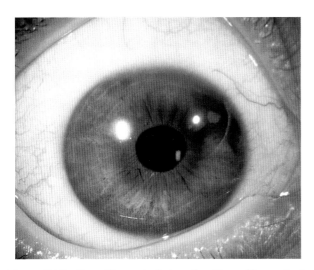

Figure 10.34 Neurofibromatosis type 1. Neurofibromatosis type 1 with Lisch nodules, most prominently superonasal. Lisch nodules, variably pigmented collections of melanocytic spindle cells, are seen bilaterally in all patients over age 16 with neurofibromatosis type 1. Nodules are rare and unilateral in neurofibromatosis type 2.

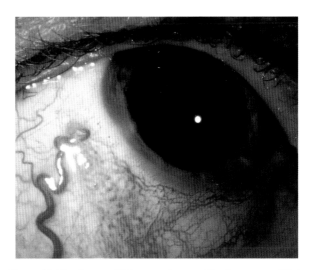

Figure 10.35 Sturge–Weber syndrome with glaucoma. Note dilated conjunctival vessel and episcleral hemangioma.

intraocular pressure. Experimentally, this relationship is slightly less than 1 : 1, possibly due to decreased aqueous inflow or increased uveoscleral outflow with increased IOP. However, any cause of increased episcleral venous pressure may increase IOP. Obstruction of venous drainage along any part of the outflow pathway may lead to increased episcleral venous pressure and increased IOP. Dilated vessels are seen beneath the conjunctiva that do not blanch with epinephrine. Blood may be seen in Schlemm's canal on gonioscopy. Orbital congestion in thyroid ophthalmopathy may increase episcleral and intraocular pressures; this may be responsive to steroids, radiation and decompression. Thrombosis of an orbital vein or the cavernous sinus can produce similar findings. Retrobulbar tumors, jugular vein obstruction and superior vena cava syndrome also lead to increased episcleral pressure.

Arteriovenous anomalies, by exposing the venous system to the greater pressures of the arterial system, result in increased episcleral venous pressure. Sturge–Weber syndrome (Figures 10.35–10.37), carotid cavernous fistulas (Figure 10.38) and orbital varices can in this manner produce glaucoma. Idiopathic cases of increased episcleral venous pressure exist as well (Figure 10.39).

Treatment of the underlying cause of increased venous pressure is ideal but not always possible or worthwhile. Embolization of carotid-cavernous fistulas carries significant risk of central nervous system vascular accident; many close spontaneously. Aqueous suppressants often are helpful. Miotics and laser trabeculoplasty are not often useful, given the typically normal facility of outflow. Trabeculectomy is effective as it bypasses the elevated episcleral venous pressure, but has a higher incidence in these patients of serous and

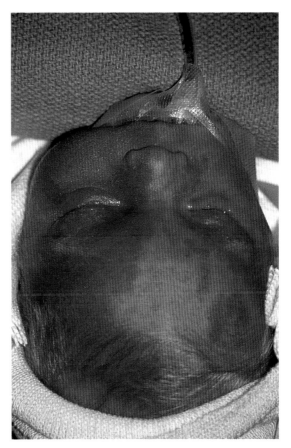

Figure 10.36 Sturge–Weber syndrome in an infant. Infant with Sturge–Weber syndrome undergoing examination under anesthesia. Intraocular pressure was normal. Glaucoma is more common with upper lid involvement by the hemangioma.

hemorrhagic choroidal detachments. Prophylactic partial-thickness scleral flaps with full-thickness sclerostomies have been advocated.

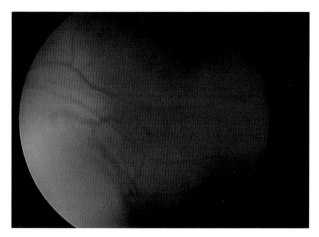

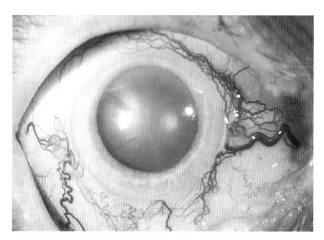

Figure 10.37 Resolving suprachoroidal hemorrhage following trabeculectomy in patient with Sturge–Weber syndrome Although prophylactic partial-thickness scleral windows with full-thickness sclerostomies were performed, a large hemorrhage still occurred.

Figure 10.38 Dilated and tortuous episcleral vessels. A patient with carotid-cavernous fistula and increased intraocular pressure. These patients are also at risk for ocular ischemia leading to neovascular glaucoma, uveal effusions with angle closure, and central retinal arterial and venous obstruction.

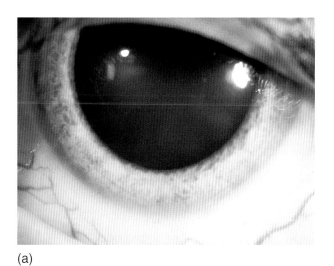

(a)

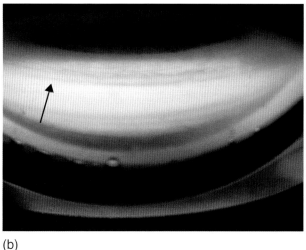

(b)

Figure 10.39 Sporadic, idiopathic elevated episcleral venous pressure. Patient with sporadic, idiopathic elevated episcleral venous pressure shows mildly dilated episcleral vessels (a) and blood in Schlemm's canal on gonioscopy (b). Familial forms of idiopathic elevated episcleral venous pressure exist as well.

Further reading

Campbell DG, Schertzer RM. Pigmentary glaucoma. In: Ritch R, Shields MB, Krupin T, eds. The Glaucomas, 2nd edn. St Louis, MO: Mosby, 1996: 975–92

Campbell DG, Schertzer RM. Ghost cell glaucoma. In: Ritch R, Shields MB, Krupin T, eds. The Glaucomas, 2nd edn. St Louis, MO: Mosby, 1996: 1277–88

Epstein DL. Chandler and Grant's Glaucoma, 3rd edn. Philadelphia, PA: Lea & Febiger, 1986: 332–51; 391–5; 403–7

Farrar SM, Shields MB. Current concepts in pigmentary glaucoma. Surv Ophthalmol 1993; 37: 233–52

Folberg R, Parrish RK II. Glaucoma following trauma. In: Tasman W, Jaeger EA, eds. Duane's Clinical Ophthalmology, revised edn. Philadelphia, PA: Lippincott, 1994: 54C: 1–7

Krupin T, Feitl ME, Karalekas D. Glaucoma associated with uveitis. In: Ritch R, Shields MB, Krupin T, eds. The Glaucomas, 2nd edn. St Louis, MO: Mosby, 1996: 1225–58

Lampink A. Management of the aphakic and pseudophakic patient with glaucoma. In: Higginbotham EJ, Lee DA, eds. Management of Difficult Glaucoma. Boston, MA: Blackwell Scientific, 1994: 144–54

Mermoud A, Heuer DK. Glaucoma associated with trauma. In: Ritch R, Shields MB, Krupin T, eds. The Glaucomas, 2nd edn. St Louis, MO: Mosby, 1996: 1259–76

Ritch R. Exfoliation syndrome. In: Ritch R, Shields MB, Krupin T, eds. The Glaucomas, 2nd edn. St Louis, MO: Mosby, 1996: 993–1022

Shields JA, Shields CL, Shields MB. Glaucoma associated with intraocular tumors. In: Ritch R, Shields MB, Krupin T, eds. The Glaucomas, 2nd edn. St Louis, MO: Mosby, 1996: 1131–42

Tomey KF, Traverso CE. Glaucoma associated with aphakia and pseudophakia. In: Ritch R, Shields MB, Krupin T, eds. The Glaucomas, 2nd edn. St Louis, MO: Mosby, 1996: 1289–324

11 The angle-closure glaucomas

Celso Tello, Jeffrey M Liebmann, Robert Ritch, David S Greenfield

INTRODUCTION

The angle-closure glaucomas are a diverse group of disorders characterized by apposition of the iris to the trabecular meshwork. This results in mechanical blockage of aqueous outflow, progressive trabecular dysfunction, synechial closure and elevated intraocular pressure (IOP) that leads to optic nerve damage and loss of visual function.

Angle closure can be caused by one or a combination of the following: (1) abnormalities in the *relative* sizes or positions of anterior segment structures; (2) abnormalities in the *absolute* sizes or positions of anterior segment structures; and (3) abnormal forces in the posterior segment which alter the anatomy of the anterior segment. Classification of angle closure by the anatomic level of the cause of the block, defined by the structure producing the 'forces' leading to the block, facilitates understanding of the various mechanisms, and appropriate treatment in any particular case becomes an exercise in deductive logic. We have defined four levels of block, from anterior to posterior. Each level of block may have a component of each of the levels preceding it. The appropriate treatment becomes more complex for each level of block, as each level may also require the treatments for lower levels of block.

With high-frequency, high-resolution, anterior segment ultrasound biomicroscopy (UBM), we can image the structures surrounding the posterior chamber, examination of which has been previously limited to histopathological examination. UBM is ideally suited to the study of the angle-closure glaucomas because of its ability to simultaneously image the ciliary body, posterior chamber, iris–lens relationship and angle structures. The currently available commercial unit operates at 50 MHz and provides lateral and axial resolution of approximately 50 μm

and 25 μm, respectively. Tissue penetration is approximately 4–5 mm. The scanner produces a 5 × 5-mm field with 256 vertical image lines (or A-scans) at a scan rate of 8 frames per second. The images shown in this chapter were obtained with the standard 50-MHz transducer.

In this chapter, we evaluate the angle-closure glaucomas with an emphasis on their anatomic basis.

BLOCK ORIGINATING AT THE LEVEL OF THE IRIS

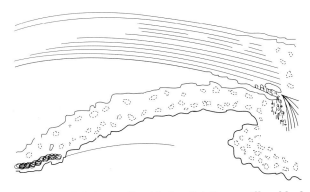

Figure 11.1 Relative pupillary block. Relative pupillary block is the underlying mechanism in approximately 90% of patients with angle closure. Relative pupillary block typically occurs in hyperopic eyes, which have a shorter than average axial length, a more shallow anterior chamber, a thicker lens, a more anterior lens position, and a smaller radius of corneal curvature. In pupillary block, flow of aqueous from the posterior to the anterior chamber is impeded between the anterior surface of the lens and the posterior surface of the iris. Aqueous pressure in the posterior chamber becomes higher than that in the anterior chamber, causing anterior iris bowing, narrowing of the angle, and acute or chronic angle-closure glaucoma.

Supported in part by the New York Glaucoma Research Institute, New York, NY.
The authors do not have a financial interest in any technique or device described in this manuscript.

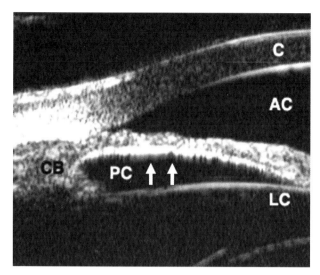

Figure 11.2   Relative pupillary block and angle closure (pupillary block–angle closure), UBM.   In phakic pupillary block–angle closure, the iris has a convex configuration (white arrows) because of the relative pressure differential between the posterior chamber (PC) (the site of aqueous production) and the anterior chamber (AC). The cornea (C), anterior lens capsule (LC), and ciliary body (CB) are visible.

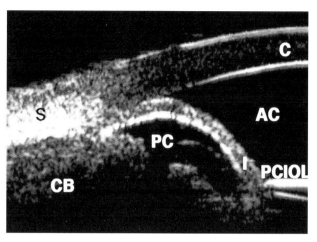

Figure 11.3 Pseudophakic pupillary block, UBM. In pseudophakic pupillary block, resistance to aqueous flow occurs because of posterior synechiae between the iris (I) and posterior chamber intraocular lens (PCIOL) which limit aqueous flow into the anterior chamber causing the iris in this patient to assume a bombé configuration. The angle is closed.

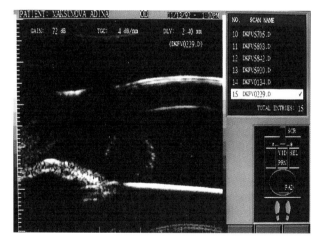

Figure 11.4   Iridovitreal block, UBM.   Occasionally, aqueous access to the anterior chamber can be impeded by vitreous in the posterior or anterior chambers. In this illustration, the round bulge of vitreous prolapse into the anterior chamber is visible and the iris is convex. A posterior chamber intraocular lens is present.

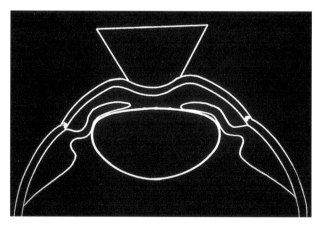

Figure 11.5   Indentation gonioscopy.   Indentation gonioscopy is critical to accurate diagnosis of the angle-closure glaucomas. During indentation, the central corneal curvature is altered, forcing aqueous posteriorly. The iris is pushed against the lens, creating a flap valve effect, which prevents aqueous from moving through the pupil into the posterior chamber. Aqueous is then forced into the angle recess, which opens an appositionally closed angle.

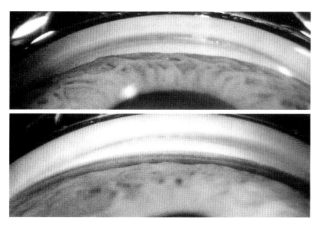

Figure 11.6 Indentation gonioscopy in relative pupillary block. In pupillary block, the peripheral iris is held in its anterior position because of the force of the aqueous behind it (top) (see also Figure 11.1). During indentation, the peripheral iris can move posteriorly because of the minimal resistance of the aqueous behind the iris plane to the force of indentation (bottom). This is very different from other forms of angle closure, such as plateau iris syndrome. (Reprinted from Ritch R, Liebmann JM. Argon laser peripheral iridoplasty. Ophth Surg Lasers 1996; 27: 289–300 (Figure 2).)

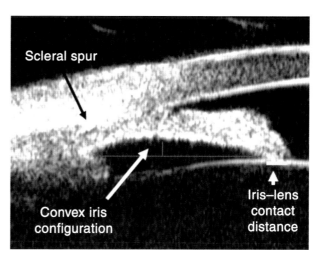

Figure 11.7 Iris–lens contact in pupillary block, UBM. The anatomy of relative pupillary block in a phakic, unoperated patient is illustrated in this ultrasound biomicrograph. Scleral spur is clearly visible, and the trabecular meshwork just anterior to it is in contact with the iris. Note the relatively short region of iris–lens contact. Although there is resistance to flow through the pupillary space, the increased pressure within the posterior chamber compared to the anterior chamber has lifted the remaining iris off the lens surface.

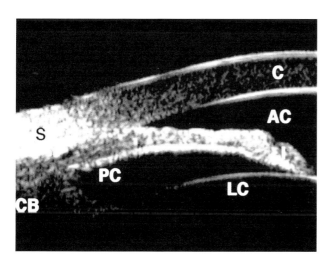

Figure 11.8 Synechiae formation, UBM. Iris apposition to the trabecular meshwork is an indication for laser iridotomy. In this patient, the iris is in contact with the trabecular meshwork. A small, clear, fluid-filled space is present immediately posterior to the region of iridotrabecular contact, indicating that the first location for appositional closure in this eye was in the mid- or upper trabecular meshwork.

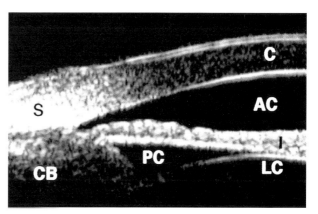

Figure 11.9 Laser iridotomy, UBM. Laser iridotomy is the definitive treatment for pupillary block, and allows aqueous pressures in the anterior and posterior chambers to equalize and the iris to assume a planar configuration. Following laser iridotomy in the patient shown in Figure 11.8, the iris has flattened and the angle has opened. There are no peripheral anterior synechiae present.

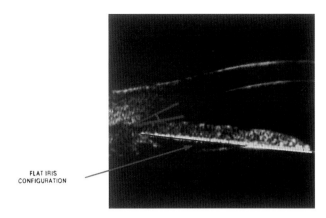

Figure 11.10   Anatomy following laser iridotomy, UBM.   Following iridotomy, the angle in the patient shown in Figure 11.7 has opened. Note the increase in iris–lens contact, as aqueous now bypasses the pupillary space and flows through the iridotomy.

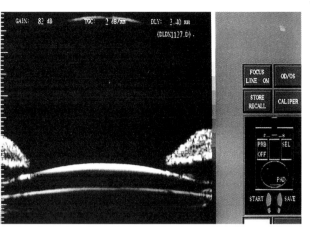

Figure 11.11   Pseudophakic pupillary block, UBM.   An alteration in the relationship between the anterior surface of the posterior chamber intraocular lens and iris occurs following laser iridotomy for pseudophakic pupillary block. In pseudophakic pupillary block, aqueous flows between the posterior chamber intraocular lens and the iris into the anterior chamber and may lift the iris off the surface of the lens.

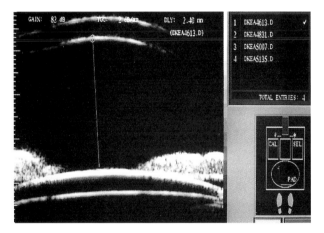

Figure 11.12   Laser iridotomy for pseudophakic pupillary block, UBM.   Following laser iridotomy in the eyes shown in Figure 11.11, the iris moves posteriorly against the intraocular lens as aqueous bypasses the pupil, flows through the iridotomy, and allows the iris to flatten.

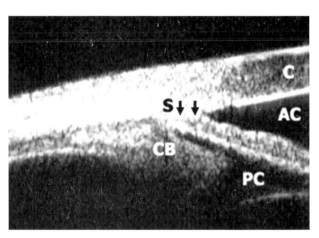

Figure 11.13   Chronic angle closure with synechiae, UBM. Following laser iridotomy for pupillary block–angle-closure glaucoma in this patient, the iris has assumed a flat configuration, consistent with relief of pupillary block, but iridotrabecular apposition persists (arrows), indicating the presence of synechial closure.

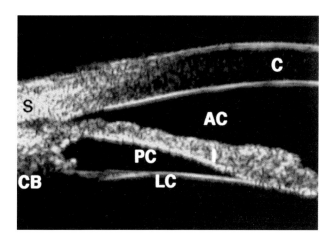

Figure 11.14 Dark-room provocation, UBM. When assessing a patient with a narrow angle for occludability, it is important to perform gonioscopy in a completely darkened room, using the smallest square of light for a slit beam, so as to avoid stimulating the pupillary light reflex. This eye is being scanned under normal room illumination. The angle is open.

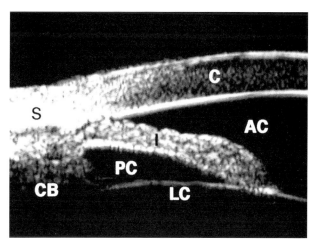

Figure 11.15 Dark-room provocation, UBM. Under dim illumination, the pupil dilates and the peripheral iris moves into the angle causing appositional angle closure. At least two minutes in total darkness should be allowed for the angle to close before assuming that it is not spontaneously occludable. If the angle closes under these conditions, opening the door of the examination room, turning on the light, or increasing the size of the slit beam will allow the pupil to constrict once again, so that the angle configuration in any quadrant can be compared in a light–dark–light situation.

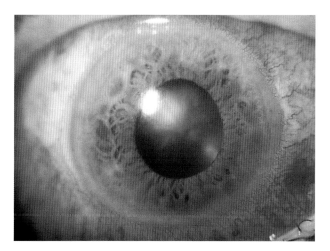

Figure 11.16 Acute angle-closure glaucoma. Acute angle-closure glaucoma is often characterized by ocular injection, blurred vision, and pain. The pupil is often fixed in a mid-dilated position.

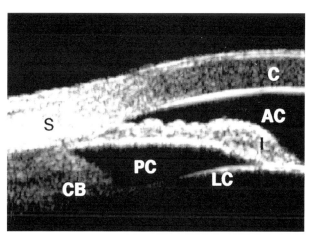

Figure 11.17 Acute angle-closure glaucoma, UBM. During an attack of acute angle closure, the length of iridolenticular contact is typically small, although the resistance to aqueous flow through the pupil is maximal.

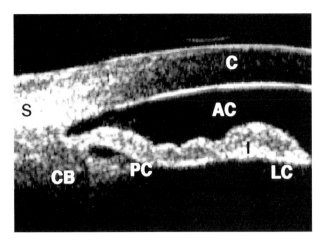

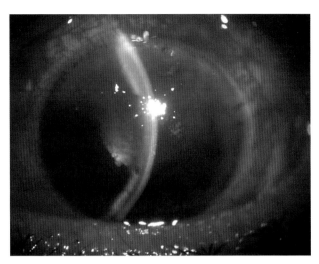

Figure 11.18 Anterior chamber angle configuration after laser iridotomy, UBM. Following laser iridotomy, the angle opens if peripheral anterior synechiae are not present. Following laser iridotomy in the patient described in Figure 11.17, the iris remains in contact with the lens surface and assumes its curvilinear contour. The peripheral iris has flattened following the iridotomy.

Figure 11.19 Acute pseudophakic pupillary block. Prior to treatment in this patient with acute pseudophakic pupillary block, the anterior chamber is shallow and the cornea is edematous. The intraocular pressure is 65 mmHg.

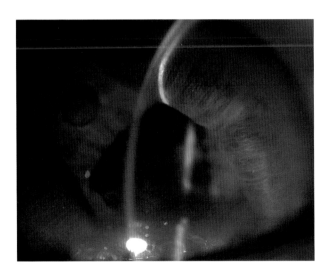

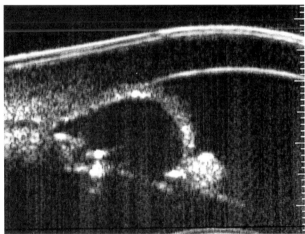

Figure 11.20 Acute pseudophakic pupillary block. In this patient with an anterior chamber intraocular lens and pupillary block, the iris surrounding the intraocular lens has assumed a bombé configuration, while the portion of iris immediately posterior to the intraocular lens remains held in its flat position by the implant itself.

Figure 11.21 Pupillary block with posterior chamber intraocular lens, UBM. In this patient with acute pseudophakic pupillary block angle-closure glaucoma, iris bombé is present and the optic is in relatively normal position. The end of the haptic is visible. (Reprinted from Tello C, Chi T, Shepps G, Liebmann J, Ritch R. Ultrasound biomicroscopy in pseudophakic malignant glaucoma. Ophthalmology 1993; 100: 1330–4 (Figure 4a).)

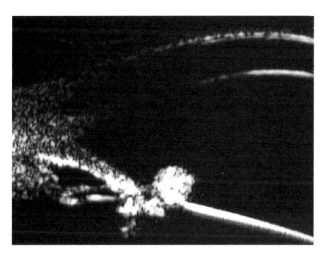

Figure 11.22 Acute pseudophakic pupillary block angle closure, UBM. Following laser iridotomy, the iris configuration has returned to normal, opening the angle in the patient shown in Figure 11.21. (Reprinted from Tello C, Chi T, Shepps G, Liebmann J, Ritch R. Ultrasound biomicroscopy in pseudophakic malignant glaucoma. Ophthalmology 1993; 100: 1330–4 (Figure 4b).)

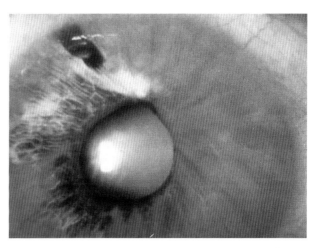

Figure 11.23 Sectoral iris atrophy. Following resolution of an attack of acute angle-closure glaucoma, sectoral iris atrophy may occur from pressure-induced iris ischemia.

BLOCK ORIGINATING AT THE LEVEL OF THE CILIARY BODY

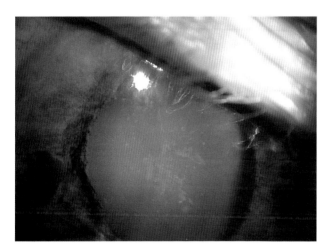

Figure 11.24 Glaukomflecken. Subepithelial lens opacification may occur following acute angle-closure glaucoma and is termed glaukomflecken.

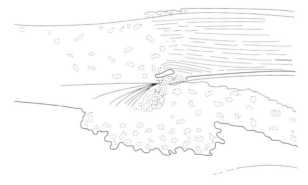

Figure 11.25 Plateau iris syndrome. A large or anteriorly positioned ciliary body can maintain the iris root in proximity to the trabecular meshwork, creating a configuration known as plateau iris.

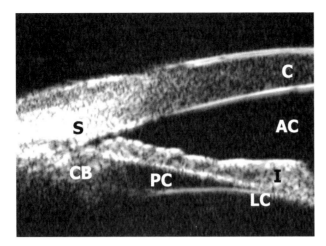

Figure 11.26 Plateau iris syndrome, UBM. In plateau iris syndrome, the physical presence of an anteriorly placed ciliary body (CB) forces the peripheral iris (I) into the angle. In this patient, iridotomy has relieved the contribution of pupillary block to the angle narrowing (the iris contour is planar in this patient), but not the closure related to the abnormal ciliary body position. The angle in this patient is barely open.

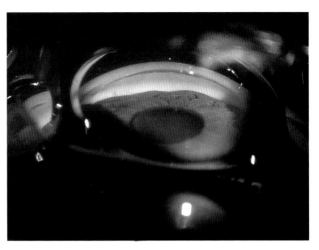

Figure 11.27 Gonioscopy in plateau iris. Gonioscopic appearance of the angle in plateau iris syndrome prior to indentation. (Reprinted from Ritch R, Liebmann JM. Argon laser peripheral iridoplasty. Ophthalmic Surg 1996; 27: 289–300 (Figure 4a).)

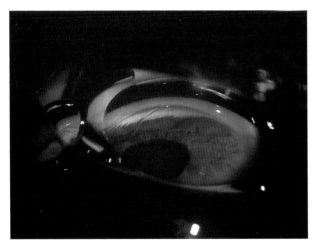

Figure 11.28 Indentation gonioscopy in plateau iris. The physical presence of the lens behind the iris plane holds the iris in position and tries to prevent posterior movement of the central iris. As a result, a sinuous configuration results (sigma sign), in which the iris follows the curvature of the lens, reaches its deepest point at the lens equator, then rises again over the ciliary processes before dropping peripherally. Much more force is needed during gonioscopy to open the angle than in pupillary block, because the ciliary processes must be displaced, and the angle does not open as widely. (Reprinted from Ritch R, Liebmann JM. Argon laser peripheral iridoplasty. Ophthalmic Surg 1996; 27: 289–300 (Figure 4b).)

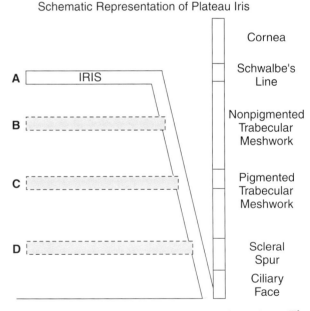

Figure 11.29 Degrees of plateau iris configuration. The extent, or the 'height' to which the plateau rises, determines whether or not the angle will close completely or only partially. In the complete plateau iris syndrome, the angle closes to the upper meshwork or Schwalbe's line, blocking aqueous outflow and leading to a rise in IOP. This situation is far less common than the incomplete syndrome, in which the angle closes only partially, leaving the upper portion of the filtering meshwork open, so that the IOP will not rise. (Reprinted from Lowe RF, Ritch R. Angle-closure glaucoma. Clinical types. In: Ritch R, Shields MB, Krupin T, eds. The Glaucomas, 2nd edn. St Louis: CV Mosby, 1996: 827 (Figure 38-6).)

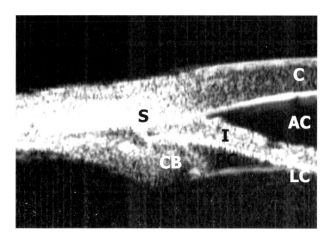

Figure 11.30   Angle closure in plateau iris, UBM. The angle is closed in this patient with plateau iris syndrome. The iris configuration is planar.

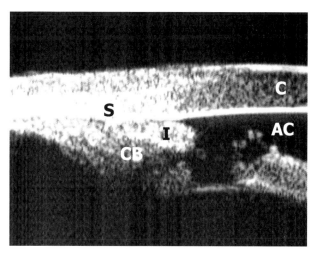

Figure 11.31   Laser iridotomy in plateau iris, UBM. A patent laser iridotomy in the eye shown in Figure 11.30 with plateau iris syndrome and persistent appositional angle closure.

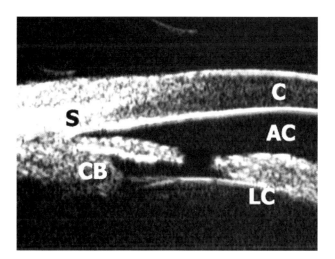

Figure 11.32   Dark-room provocation in plateau iris, UBM. Provocative testing in eyes with plateau iris configuration should be performed following laser iridotomy. Under normal room illumination, the angle in this patient with plateau configuration is narrow, but open.

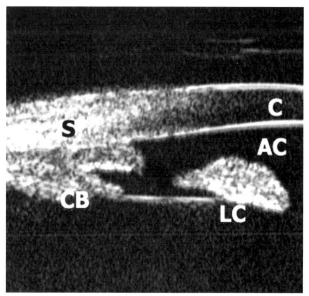

Figure 11.33   Dark-room provocation in plateau iris, UBM. During dark-room provocation and ultrasound scanning, the peripheral iris dilates and appositional angle closure develops.

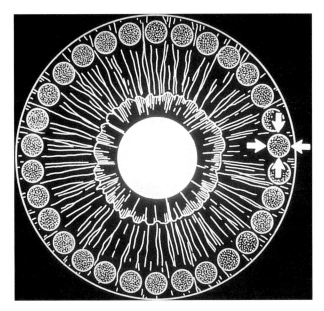

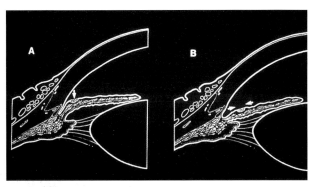

Figure 11.35 Effects of peripheral iridoplasty on the iris. Iridoplasty compacts the iris stroma and pulls it toward the site of the laser application. When the iris which is opposed to the meshwork (A) moves toward the burn, the angle opens (B).

Figure 11.34 Location of laser iridoplasty. The treatment of angle-closure secondary to plateau iris syndrome requires argon laser peripheral iridoplasty. Laser energy (long duration, low power, large spot size) is applied to the extreme iris periphery.

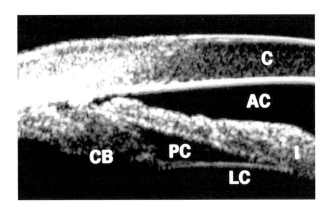

Figure 11.36 Peripheral iridoplasty (pre-treatment), UBM. Angle closure caused by plateau iris syndrome prior to laser iridoplasty.

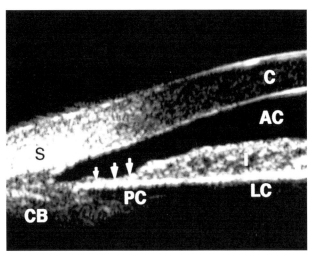

Figure 11.37 Laser iridoplasty (post-treatment), UBM. Following argon laser peripheral iridoplasty, the site of the burn is visible (arrows). The iris stoma has been compacted and the angle is open.

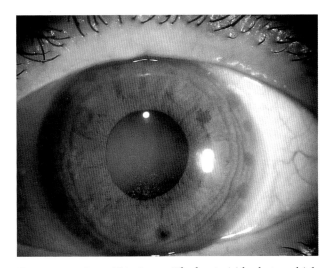

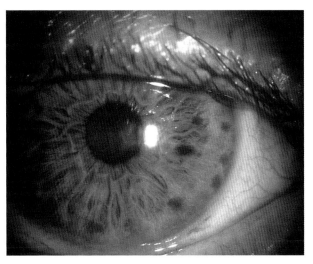

Figure 11.38   Laser iridoplasty. The key to iridoplasty, which can also be used during an acute attack of angle-closure glaucoma unresponsive to medical therapy, or when iridotomy cannot be safely performed because of hazy media, is correct placement of the laser applications, which, in this patient, has produced a ring of hyperpigmented spots corresponding to the treatment sites. This patient has an inferiorly placed laser iridotomy.

Figure 11.39   Laser iridoplasty. Iridoplasty in this patient was performed incorrectly, and laser application sites are visible in the mid-peripheral iris.

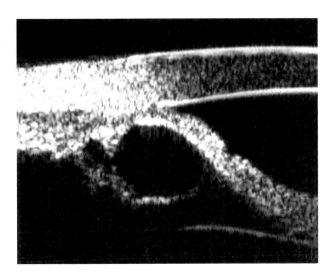

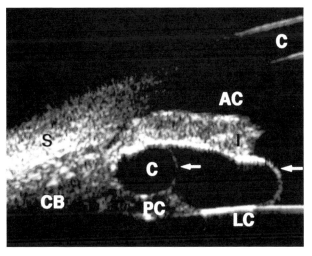

Figure 11.40   Pseudoplateau iris configuration, UBM. Other abnormalities of ciliary body architecture may result in a condition termed pseudoplateau iris. This general term is non-specific and does not differentiate between distinct entities as cyst, tumor, or inflammation. These conditions are usually easily diagnosed, as the angle is closed either in one quadrant or, if cysts are multiple, intermittently. Focal forms of angle closure may be induced by cystic or solid masses involving the iris or the ciliary body. Iridociliary cysts are characterized by an echolucent interior. For example, a pigment epithelial cyst in this patient has caused focal narrowing of the anterior chamber angle in the region of the cyst.

Figure 11.41   Loculated iridociliary cysts, UBM. Pigment epithelial cysts can arise from the pigment epithelium of the iris, the ciliary body, or the junction between them. Iridociliary cysts are the most common form, and some have multiple loculations. The walls of these cysts are indicated (arrows).

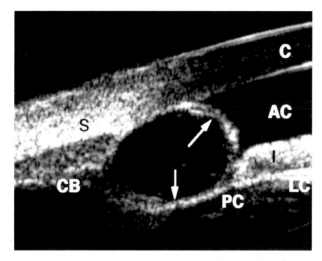

Figure 11.42 Ciliary body cyst, UBM. Abnormal embryogenesis can lead to focal angle closure by true cysts of the ciliary body stroma, as is present in this patient. The pigment epithelium is normal and the ciliary body architecture is distorted.

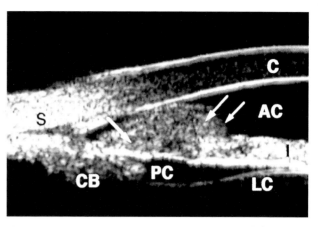

Figure 11.43 Anterior segment tumors, UBM. Primary or metastatic tumors of the iris and/or ciliary body can cause angle closure. This iris tumor is causing mechanical obstruction of the meshwork.

BLOCK AT THE LEVEL OF THE LENS

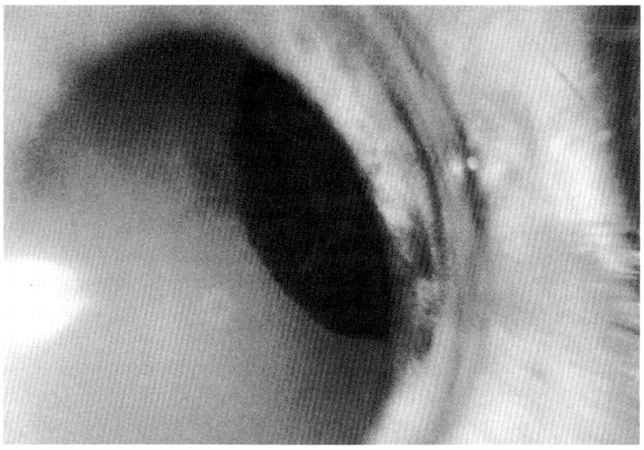

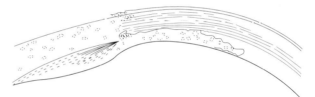

Figure 11.45 Lens-induced angle-closure. Angle-closure glaucoma may be caused by an anteriorly subluxed, dislocated, intumescent lens. In this schematic, the physical presence of an anteriorly positioned, enlarged lens is causing shallowing of the anterior chamber and angle closure.

Figure 11.44 Ciliary body tumor. Ciliary body tumor enlargement can occur, owing to anterior segment inflammation, as shown here.

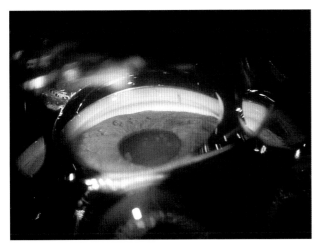

Figure 11.46 Gonioscopy in lens-induced angle closure. Prior to indentation in a patient with lens-induced angle closure, the angle is closed.

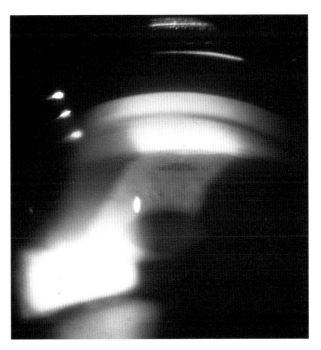

Figure 11.47 Indentation gonioscopy. Because of the enlarged lens, indentation permits only slight opening of the angle.

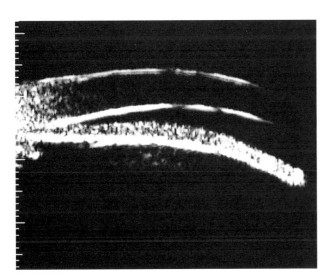

Figure 11.48 Laser iridotomy in lens-induced angle closure, UBM. Ultrasound biomicroscopy following laser iridotomy shows the iris to be in contact with the anterior lens surface, mechanically obstructing the angle.

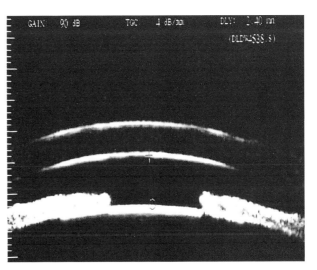

Figure 11.49 Central anterior chamber depth in lens-induced angle closure, UBM. The central anterior chamber is considerably shallower in eyes with lens-induced angle closure than in eyes with angle closure caused by pupillary block or plateau iris syndrome.

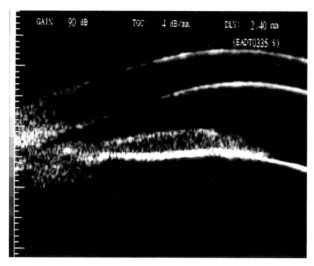

Figure 11.50 Peripheral iridoplasty in lens-induced angle closure, UBM. Following peripheral iridoplasty in the patient shown in Figure 11.48, the angle widened.

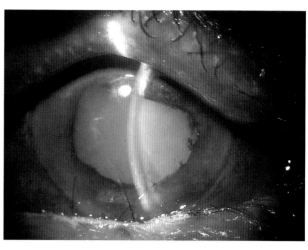

Figure 11.51 Lens intumescence. Occasionally, the lens may become intumescent and cause crowding of the anterior segment.

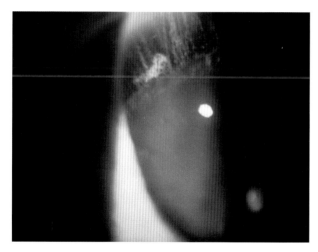

Figure 11.52 Lens subluxation. Alterations in lens position can result in angle-closure glaucoma in a number of ways. Perhaps the most common and underdiagnosed cause of lens subluxation is exfoliation syndrome. In this disorder, zonular laxity permits the lens to move slightly anteriorly, increasing relative pupillary block and leading to angle closure. Eventually zonular dehiscence from the ciliary body may occur, and lead to lens dislocation. In this figure, dehisced zonules can be seen resting on the equatorial lens capsule.

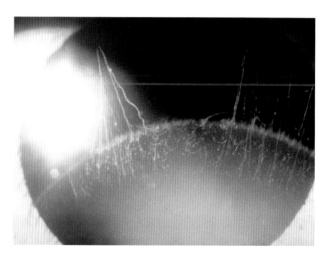

Figure 11.53 Lens dislocation in exfoliation syndrome. In this patient, nearly complete superior zonular dehiscence has allowed the lens to move inferiorly.

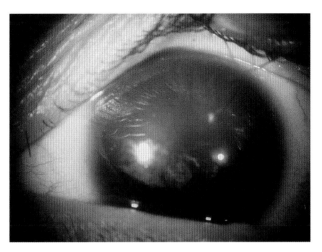

Figure 11.54 Marfan's syndrome. Lens subluxation and dislocation are a common feature of Marfan's syndrome. The most common direction for lens movement is superotemporal. In homocystinuria, the subluxed lens tends to move inferonasally.

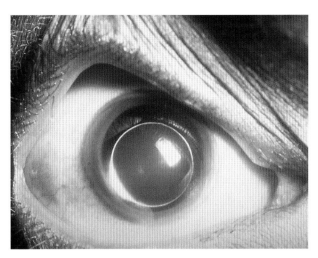

Figure 11.55 Microspherophakia. In microspherophakia, the smaller lens can dislocate into the anterior chamber, where it can become trapped.

BLOCK RELATED TO PRESSURE POSTERIOR TO THE LENS

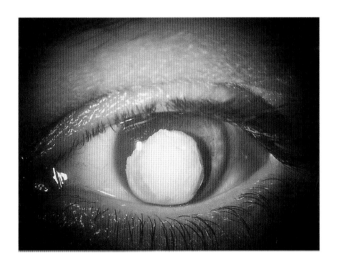

Figure 11.56 Traumatic lens dislocation. Long-standing anterior dislocation can lead to progressive cataract formation.

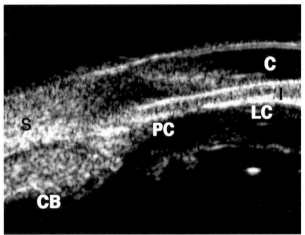

Figure 11.57 Malignant glaucoma, UBM. Malignant glaucoma (ciliary block glaucoma; aqueous misdirection) is a poorly understood clinical entity characterized by angle closure, normal posterior segment anatomy, and patent iridotomy. Most, but not all, cases occur postoperatively. In malignant glaucoma, the lens and iris are forced anteriorly by posterior pressure. In this eye, the anterior lens capsule (LC) is nearly against the corneal endothelium (C).

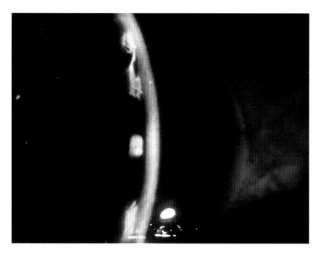

Figure 11.58 Pseudophakic malignant glaucoma. Following uneventful cataract surgery in this patient with undiagnosed angle-closure glaucoma, the anterior chamber shallowed and the pressure rose. Multiple iridotomies failed to restore normal anatomic relationships. (Reprinted from Tello C, Chi T, Shepps G, Liebmann J, Ritch R. Ultrasound biomicroscopy in pseudophakic malignant glaucoma. Ophthalmology 1993; 100: 1330–4 (Figure 1b).)

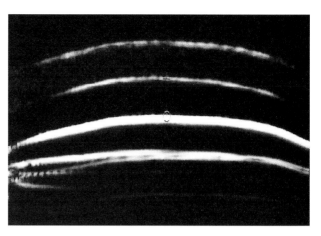

Figure 11.59 Pseudophakic malignant glaucoma, UBM. Ultrasound biomicroscopy prior to treatment. The central anterior chamber is shallow. (Reprinted from Tello C, Chi T, Shepps G, Liebmann J, Ritch R. Ultrasound biomicroscopy in pseudophakic malignant glaucoma. Ophthalmology 1993; 100: 1330–4 (Figure 2d).)

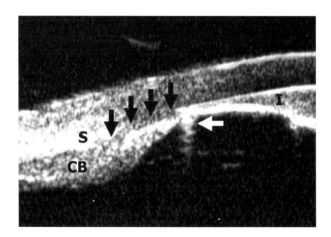

Figure 11.60 Pseudophakic malignant glaucoma, UBM. In the temporal angle, peripheral iridocorneal apposition is present (black arrows). The haptic is visible beneath the iris (white arrow).

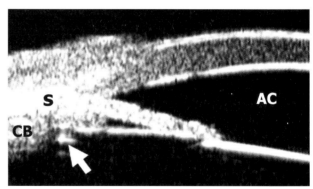

Figure 11.61 Pseudophakic malignant glaucoma, UBM. Immediately following Nd:YAG laser capsulotomy/anterior hyaloidectomy, the anterior chamber is deeper and the haptic has moved posteriorly (arrow).

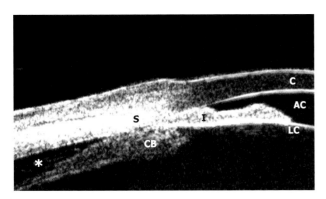

Figure 11.62 Phakic malignant glaucoma, UBM. In this phakic patient with a clinical diagnosis of a malignant glaucoma the angle has closed because of anterior rotation at the ciliary body due to annular ciliary body detachment (asterisk), rather than aqueous misdirection. This distinction is clinically important in as much as the treatment involves vigorous topical and occasional systemic steroids, intensive cycloplegia and possible drainage of the supraciliary fluid. It does not typically respond to Nd:YAG laser surgery. Rarely, suprachoroidal effusion may be caused by topiramate.

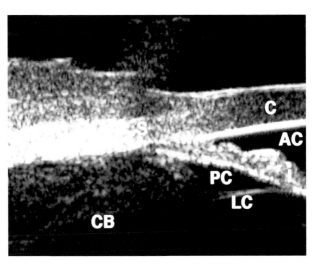

Figure 11.63 Scleritis and angle closure, UBM. In a similar fashion, anterior rotation of the ciliary body may occur following pan retinal photocoagulation, scleral buckling procedures, central retinal vein occlusion, contraction of retrolental tissue, such as in retinopathy of prematurity, or inflammation of adjoining tissues, such as this patient with anterior scleritis with secondary ciliary body edema. Note the overlying thickened conjunctiva.

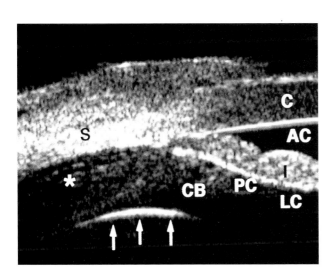

Figure 11.64 Intravitreal gas and angle closure, UBM. Intravitreal expansile gas (arrows) may cause progressive angle closure following vitreoretinal surgery. In this particular case, the ciliary body, iris, and lens have been forced anteriorly, closing the angle.

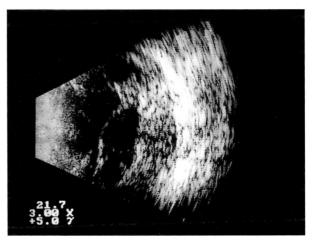

Figure 11.65 Choroidal hemorrhage. Choroidal hemorrhage can result in forward movement of the lens–iris diaphragm and elevated intraocular pressure. Although intraoperative choroidal hemorrhage is relatively rare during glaucoma surgery, delayed choroidal hemorrhage in hypotonus eyes is not. The typical presenting complaint is the abrupt onset of pain, often associated with the Valsalva maneuver, in an eye with known hypotony and choroidal effusion.

ANGLE-CLOSURE GLAUCOMA ASSOCIATED WITH OTHER OCULAR DISORDERS

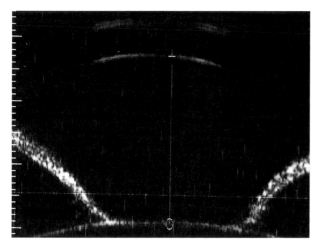

Figure 11.66 Uveitis and glaucoma. Intraocular inflammation can cause angle closure by a variety of mechanisms. In this patient acute angle closure has developed because of a pupil secluded by posterior synechiae. The iris is adherent at the pupillary border, and has assumed a bombé configuration elsewhere.

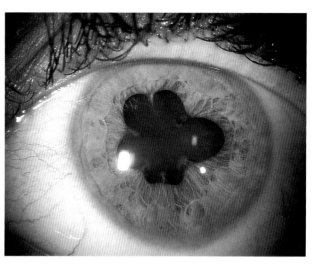

Figure 11.67 Posterior synechiae due to uveitis. Early posterior synechia formation often presages the development of increased pupillary block. Frequent dilatation may prevent complete pupillary block.

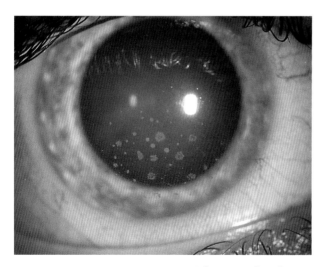

Figure 11.68 Keratic precipitates. When peripheral anterior synechiae are present without pupillary block, other evidence of prior intraocular inflammation should be sought. In this patient with multiple synechiae but an otherwise wide-open angle, old keratic precipitates provide evidence of prior anterior uveitis.

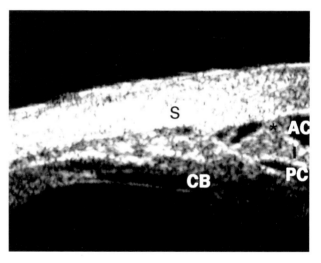

Figure 11.69 Uveitis-related anterior synechiae, UBM. In this patient with sarcoid uveitis, peripheral anterior synechiae have formed in the angle.

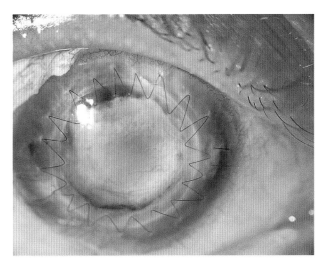

Figure 11.70 Anterior chamber fibrin. Severe inflammatory reactions, such as this fibrin mass on the anterior surface of a recently implanted intraocular lens, may result in pupillary block.

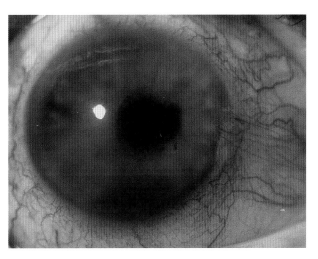

Figure 11.71 Neovascular glaucoma. Neovascularization of the anterior segment causes glaucoma by direct obstruction of the trabecular meshwork by the proliferating neovascular membrane. Neovascular glaucoma, which may be recalcitrant to therapy, is often associated with high intraocular pressures and spontaneous hyphema.

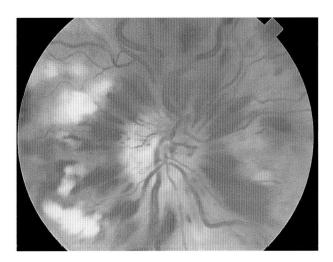

Figure 11.72 Central retinal vein occlusion. The most common cause of iris neovascularization is retinal ischemia. Ischemic central retinal vein occlusion (shown here) and proliferative diabetic retinopathy are the two most common offending disorders.

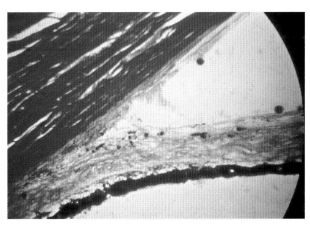

Figure 11.73 Angle neovascularization. As the neovascular membrane proliferates, it slowly covers the angle structures.

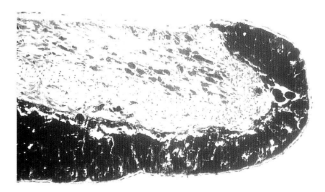

Figure 11.74   Ectropion uveae. Contraction of the membrane pulls the iris into the angle, and may cause ectropion uveae, as shown here.

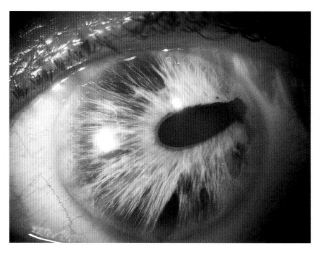

Figure 11.75   Iridocorneal endothelial syndrome. Iridocorneal endothelial syndrome is also associated with a proliferating anterior segment membrane. In this disorder, migration of corneal endothelial and associated basement membrane causes obstruction of the trabecular meshwork and iris abnormalities. Essential iris atrophy, shown here, is characterized by corectopia, melting holes, and stretching holes caused by membrane contraction.

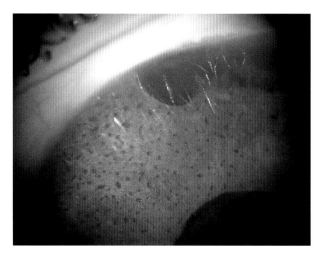

Figure 11.76   Iris–nevus syndrome. Another variant of iridocorneal endothelial syndrome, the iris–nevus syndrome.

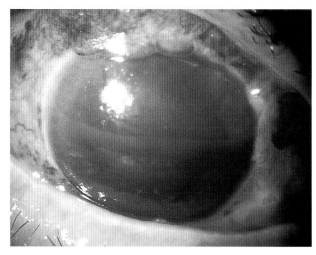

Figure 11.77   Hyphema. Anterior segment trauma can cause angle closure because of uveitis or lens subluxation. In this patient with hyphema, pupillary block caused by the obstruction to aqueous flow by the anterior segment clotted blood is part of the differential diagnosis of the elevated intraocular pressure.

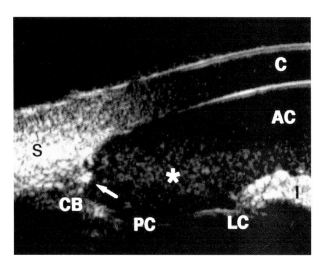

Figure 11.78   Iridodialysis and angle recession, UBM. Blood within the anterior chamber (asterisk) may mask other forms of angle injury, such as iridodialysis and angle recession.

12 Normal-tension glaucoma

Darrell WuDunn, Louis B Cantor

Von Graefe first described the condition we now recognize as normal- or low-tension glaucoma in the 1850s[1-3]. Glaucoma as a disease entity associated with elevated intraocular pressure had been recognized for only approximately 50 years. The notion of glaucoma without elevated intraocular pressure was not well received[4] and still remains an enigma to this day[5]. With the development of tonometry in the early 1900s and more widespread use of ophthalmoscopy to examine the optic disc, normal-tension glaucoma became a more widely recognized and accepted entity. Many names were applied to this condition including pseudoglaucoma, amaurosis with excavation, cavernous optic atrophy, paraglaucoma, arteriosclerotic optic atrophy, low-tension glaucoma, and others. The variety of terms applied to this condition underscores our lack of understanding of the pathophysiology of this disease entity or group of entities, which we have come to call normal-tension glaucoma.

DEFINITION

Since little is known of the etiology and pathophysiology of primary open-angle glaucoma, not to mention normal-tension glaucoma, our ability to define this condition or group of conditions has been unsatisfactory. According to the most recent (2003) American Academy of Ophthalmology Preferred Practice Pattern[6], primary open-angle glaucoma is defined as 'a multifactorial optic neuropathy in which there is a characteristic acquired loss of retinal ganglion cells and atrophy of the optic nerve'. Without mention of intraocular pressure, this definition also includes normal-tension glaucoma. We therefore may define normal-tension glaucoma as an optic neuropathy that has certain characteristics that are within the spectrum of disease we recognize as glaucoma. The hallmark of glaucomatous nerve damage is 'cupping' (Figure 12.1), though

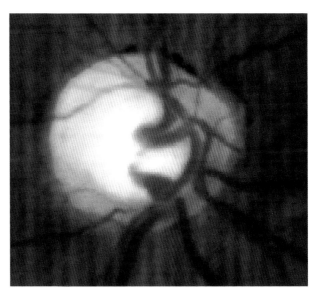

Figure 12.1 Concentric thinning of the neuroretinal rim. Optic disc cupping with concentric thinning of the neuroretinal rim in primary open-angle glaucoma. (Note: A striped pattern is projected on the fundus in this image to enhance topographic analysis.)

even this characteristic is highly variable and may take many forms. The level of intraocular pressure may be considered just one of the possible risk factors for this disease process similar to our thinking for primary open-angle glaucoma. As shall be discussed, however, the optic disc and visual field changes in normal-tension glaucoma may contrast with those in primary open-angle glaucoma, though there is conflicting evidence in this regard which is at least in part due to our inability to define appropriate study populations and therefore to accurately discriminate between the various glaucomas. It may also be the case that we are merely describing a disease process with a broad spectrum that would defy discrimination. Historically, different authors have used different benchmarks for the intraocular pressure in defining their study populations, none of which has proved to be satisfactory. This has gradually led to a change in terminology from low-tension glaucoma to normal-tension glaucoma, implying less emphasis on intraocular pressure while still attempting to describe the clinical features of a type of glaucoma where the level of intraocular pressure is not statistically elevated, based on population norms, though the pressure may still play a role. Despite all of these limitations in our ability to accurately define normal-tension glaucoma, it is still a worthwhile exercise to review the clinical and epidemiological findings which have been described in normal-tension glaucoma compared to primary open-angle glaucoma.

EPIDEMIOLOGY

'Hardness of the eyeball' had been attributed to glaucoma for over a century. Leydhecker et al., in 1958[7], in their landmark study described the intraocular pressure in the general population. Utilizing Schiotz tonometry in 20 000 individuals they observed that the mean pressure in their population was 15.5 mmHg (standard deviation ± 2.57). At that time anyone with an intraocular pressure more than two standard deviations above the mean (20.5 mmHg) was considered suspect for glaucoma, and an intraocular pressure above three standard deviations (24 mmHg) was felt to be diagnostic for glaucoma. Armaly[8], Bankes[9], Linner[10], Perkins[11], Schappert-Kimmijser[12], and others have provided us with ample evidence that elevated intraocular pressure and glaucoma are not synonymous. Continuing epidemiological studies have provided additional evidence to this day. Intraocular pressure is known to be distributed in a non-Gaussian fashion and to be skewed toward higher pressures. Clinical evidence indicates that there are many exceptions to the commonly held notions linking intraocular pressure and glaucoma, both in eyes with high pressure that do not have glaucoma damage and in eyes with low or normal pressures that do have glaucomatous optic nerve atrophy or visual field loss. Recent population-based prevalence studies suggest that perhaps 40–60% of individuals with either optic disc changes consistent with glaucoma, characteristic visual function loss, or both have intraocular pressures within two standard deviations of the population mean[13,14]. Therefore, the entity we call normal-tension glaucoma appears to have at least an equal if not greater prevalence than primary open-angle glaucoma.

Epidemiologic evidence of other risk factors for normal-tension glaucoma compared to primary open-angle glaucoma is incomplete. Age, race, and family history are known risk factors for primary open-angle glaucoma. Age is thought to be a factor in some cases of normal-tension glaucoma.

Senile sclerotic glaucoma, described by Greve and others, occurs mostly in older individuals and is characterized by relatively low intraocular pressures, peripapillary atrophy, and choroidal sclerosis. However, the entity of focal glaucoma based on focal notching of the disc described by Spaeth[15] is characteristically seen in younger individuals than has been described for primary open-angle glaucoma. The role of race remains undefined in normal-tension glaucoma. A positive family history may be noted for normal-tension glaucoma and primary open-angle glaucoma, although it is not clear whether the risk is similar between the different entities.

Evidence is accumulating that thin central corneal thickness may be an important risk factor for normal-tension glaucoma. Several studies have shown that persons with normal-tension glaucoma tend to have thinner central corneas than normals or persons with high-tension glaucoma or ocular hypertension[16–18]. Whether this relates to underestimating true intraocular pressure or to an increased susceptibility of eyes with thinner cornea and sclera remains unresolved. Traditional Goldmann applanation tonometry underestimates intraocular pressure in eyes with thin corneas. This influences not only our risk assessment but also our ability to classify persons with normal-tension glaucoma.

OPTIC DISC FINDINGS

A wide variety of optic disc changes may occur in normal-tension glaucoma. Controversy exists as to whether these changes differ from those seen in primary open-angle glaucoma. Lewis et al.[19] could not distinguish normal-tension glaucoma from primary open-angle glaucoma by disc appearance when attempting to predict visual field loss. Miller and Miller[20] also could not distinguish between the two glaucoma entities in a retrospective review of disc photographs, but they did comment that the connective tissue bundles within the lamina cribrosa were less apparent in normal-tension glaucoma. Levene[21], in his landmark review of low-tension glaucoma, felt that there were similar disc changes in normal-tension glaucoma and primary open-angle glaucoma, although there may be a disproportionate degree of cupping relative to the extent of the visual field loss in eyes with lower pressures and glaucoma. Tuulonen and Airaksinen[22] concluded from their study that eyes with normal-tension glaucoma had larger discs than in primary open-angle glaucoma, where large and small discs were approximately equal. Jonas et al.[23], however, concluded that glaucomatous optic neuropathy was not related to disc size.

The call for a new classification system for glaucoma based on the appearance of the optic disc by Spaeth and others includes descriptions of clinical entities for which a low intraocular pressure may be characteristic. Nicolela and Drance[24] have also presented their impressions that certain disc appearances may be characteristics of specific glaucoma entities, some of which are characterized by low intraocular pressure (Figure 12.2).

The amount of cupping and the topography of the disc rim have been evaluated in normal-tension glaucoma. Caprioli and Spaeth[25] concluded that the disc rim in normal-tension glaucoma eyes is thinner than in eyes with primary open-angle glaucoma, especially along the inferior and temporal margins (Figure 12.3), when compared to primary open-angle glaucoma eyes which were matched for visual field loss. This was consistent with the suggestion by Levene[14] that there was disproportionate cupping

relative to the extent of visual field loss in normal-tension glaucoma. Fazio et al.[26], utilizing computerized disc analysis, concluded that the cupping in normal-tension glaucoma is more broadly sloping with less disc volume alteration than in primary open-angle glaucoma.

A common finding in normal-tension glaucoma is focal notching or acquired pits in the neuroretinal rim. Javitt et al.[27] found a higher prevalence of acquired pits in normal-tension glaucoma compared to primary open-angle glaucoma eyes with similar degrees of visual field loss. Spaeth[15] has referred to this type of disc change as perhaps one of the characteristic types of glaucomatous optic atrophy and suggested that this type of finding be used to develop new ways of classifying glaucoma. Individuals with this pattern of disc change tend to

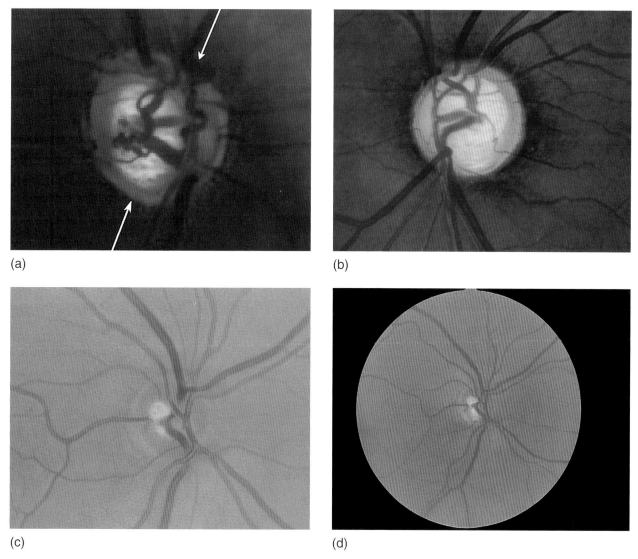

(a) (b) (c) (d)

Figure 12.2 Notching of the rim. (a) 'Focal glaucoma' with typical notching of the neuroretinal rim often found in younger individuals with normal-tension glaucoma. Also note development of collateral shunt vessels. (b) Another example of a large focal notch in the neuroretinal rim, giving a typical 'keyhole' cup. (c) and (d) Development of a focal notch in a normal-tension glaucoma patient over a 15-year period. Note in (c) the vertical extension of the cup towards the 5:30 position. (d) 15 years later, the cup has extended to the disc margin, obliterating the rim, and the patient has developed a corresponding superior arcuate scotoma (e). ((b–e) countesy of Neil T Choplin, MD.)

Continued

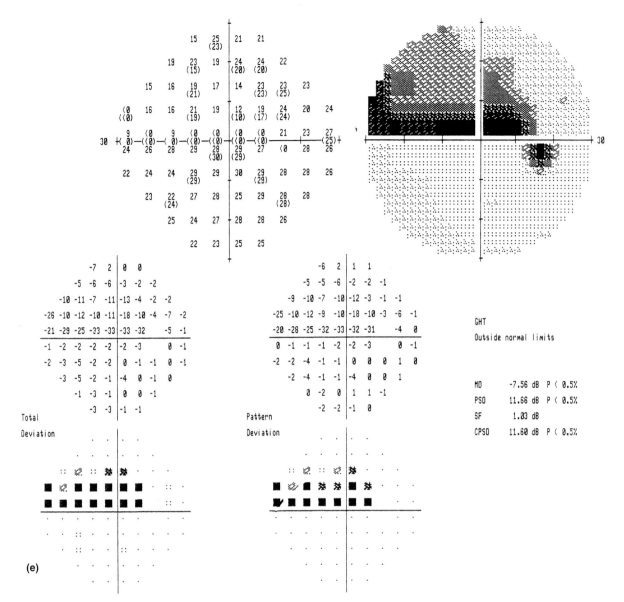

Figure 12.2 *Continued.*

have lower intraocular pressures and tend to be younger and are more often female (Figure 12.4).

Disc hemorrhages (Figure 12.5) have been frequently described as occurring more frequently in normal-tension glaucoma. Kitazawa et al.[28] noted a prevalence of disc hemorrhage of 20.5% in individuals with normal-tension glaucoma. Recurrent disc hemorrhage occurred in 64% of these eyes, which was much higher than in the other groups they studied. Drance[29], in his extensive review article, noted that disc hemorrhages were not rare events. The closer one follows the disc and records the disc appearance, the more hemorrhages will be noted. He estimated the prevalence to be about 20% in normal-tension glaucoma. In addition, he felt that there were possibly two groups of patients: those who hemorrhage and those who do not. Disc hemorrhages were also felt to precede retinal nerve fiber layer loss, topographic changes of the optic disc, and visual field loss. Hendrickx et al.[30],

however, felt that the cumulative incidence of disc hemorrhages were similar in ocular hypertension, primary open-angle glaucoma, and normal-tension glaucoma. With treatment, however, they noted that the incidence of disc hemorrhages decreased in ocular hypertension and primary open-angle glaucoma, but not in normal-tension glaucoma. In addition, recurrent disc hemorrhages tended to be scattered all over the disc in normal-tension glaucoma, but tended to occur at the same site in primary open-angle glaucoma and ocular hypertension, perhaps implying a different etiology for the disc hemorrhage in the different conditions.

Peripapillary atrophy (Figures 12.5 and 12.6) also has been reported to occur more frequently in normal-tension glaucoma than in primary open-angle glaucoma. Buus and Anderson[31] concluded that peripapillary crescents correlated with disc damage and were therefore more common in normal-tension glaucoma than in ocular hypertension.

Peripapillary atrophy

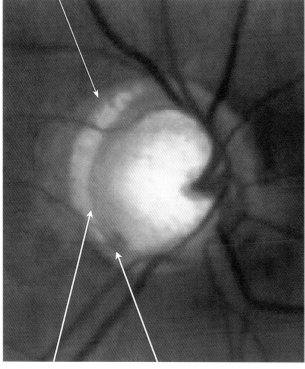

Loss of rim   Resolving disc hemorrhage

Figure 12.3 Loss of inferotemporal rim. Low-tension glaucoma with greatest loss of temporal and inferior rim. Also note peripapillary atrophy.

Loss of temporal rim

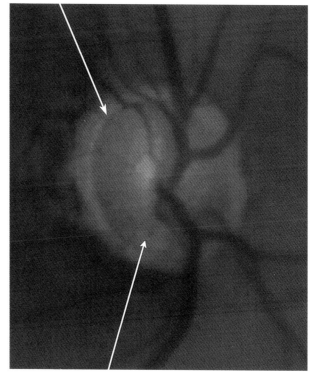

Deep cupping

Figure 12.4 Loss of inferotemporal rim. Loss of temporal and inferior rim with especially deep inferior cupping of the optic disc in normal-tension glaucoma.

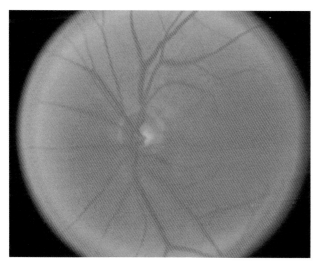

Figure 12.5 Disc hemorrhage. Low-tension glaucoma with loss of temporal and inferior rim, with resolving disc hemorrhage and peripapillary atrophy.

Geijssen and Greve[32] noted peripapillary atrophy in the entity of senile sclerotic glaucoma. However, Jonas and Xu[33] felt that there were similar degrees of paripapillary atrophy between normal-tension glaucoma and primary open-angle glaucoma in their study population.

It therefore becomes problematic to define what if any features of the optic disc are characteristic of

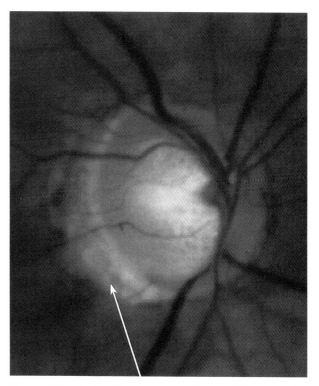

Figure 12.6 Peripapillary atrophy. Peripapillary atrophy in normal-tension glaucoma (arrow). This change is typical of what has been termed 'senile sclerotic glaucoma'.

normal-tension glaucoma. Our inability to do so undoubtedly reflects on our inability to define what are likely to be the many entities which may result in glaucomatous optic atrophy, the complexities of attempting to study and analyze the optic disc, and the tremendous physiological variability that is typical of the eye and optic nerve.

VISUAL FIELD DEFECTS

The diagnosis of normal-tension glaucoma is made on the basis of progressive visual field loss and/or optic disc changes in the absence of elevated intraocular pressure. For the most part, visual field defects in normal-tension glaucoma are similar to defects found in high-tension glaucoma[34]. Nasal steps, paracentral scotomas and arcuate defects predominate.

Subtle differences between visual fields of normal-tension glaucoma and high-tension glaucoma subjects appear to exist. Numerous studies have compared the visual fields seen in normal-tension glaucoma with those seen in high-tension glaucoma. Anderton and Hitchings[35,36] as well as Caprioli and Spaeth[37] found a higher incidence of defects near fixation, especially superonasally, in normal-tension glaucoma (Figures 12.7–12.9). Caprioli and Speath noted that visual field defects in normal-tension glaucoma had greater depth and a steeper slope than the defects of high-tension glaucoma. Other studies, however, have not supported these findings. Motolko and others[38,39], and Greve and Geijssen[40] found no significant difference in the proximity of field defects near fixation between the normal-tension and high-tension glaucoma groups. King et al.[41] even found that defects in high-tension glaucoma tended to be closer to fixation.

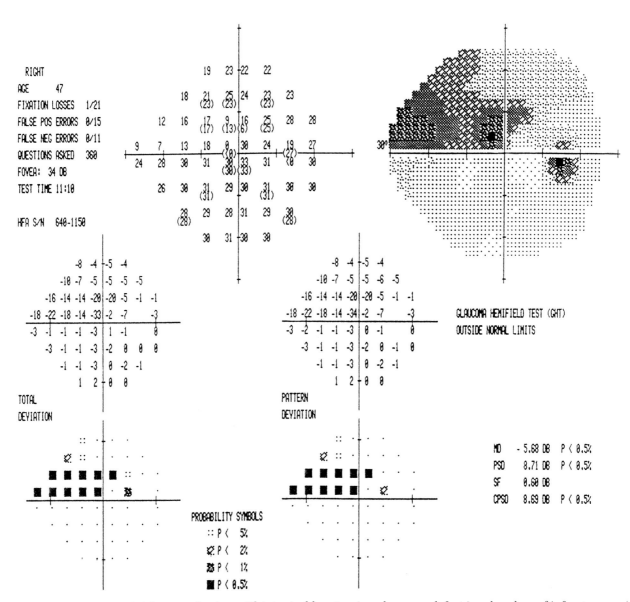

Figure 12.7 Superonasal defect near fixation. This typical low-tension glaucoma defect involves loss of inferotemporal nerve fibers. It is very dense and comes close to fixation.

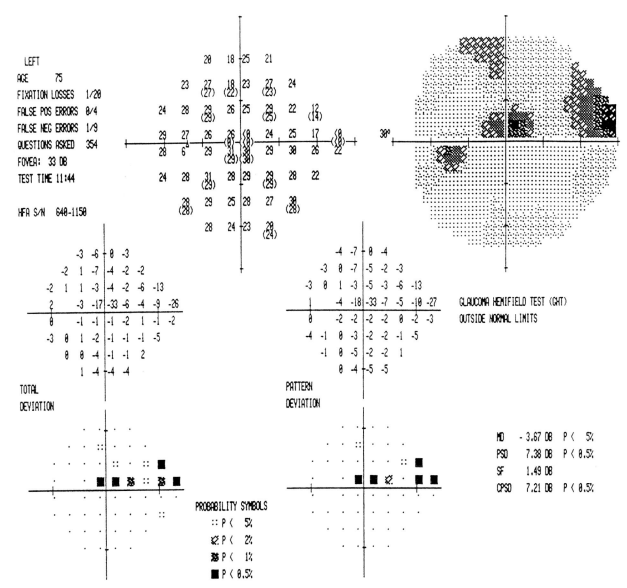

Figure 12.8 Example of a visual field defect near fixation. Note the depth of the defect and the sharp drop-off between the defect and the surrounding points.

The assertion that normal-tension glaucoma field defects are 'deep, steep, and creep' towards fixation in comparison to high-tension glaucoma fields is still being debated. Phelps et al.[42] attribute the disparate findings of the various studies to the different methodologies used.

Most studies have found that the superior hemifield and particularly the superonasal quadrant are the most frequent locations for normal-tension glaucoma defects. Furthermore, Araie et al.[43,44] reported that the inferior hemifield just below fixation might be relatively spared. Inferior defects that do occur are also typically deep with steep slopes (Figure 12.10).

Other differences between normal-tension glaucoma fields and high-tension glaucoma fields have been shown. Several groups, including Drance et al.[45], Chauhan et al.[46] and Araie et al.[43,44], have shown that diffuse visual field loss is more common

in the high-tension group. This finding is based on the decreased overall sensitivity of the 'spared' hemifield (no local defect) in high-tension glaucoma. Araie et al. concluded that, even in the late stages of disease, diffuse depression may be more common in high-tension glaucoma. Zeiter and others[47] reported that localized defects in the inferior hemifield may be more common in normal-tension glaucoma.

The difference between normal-tension and high-tension glaucoma with respect to diffuse versus local field loss may be attributable to the difference in intraocular pressure rather than some other intrinsic difference between normal-tension and high-tension glaucoma. Instead of comparing normal-tension with high-tension glaucoma groups, several studies compared glaucoma subjects (both low tension and high tension) having diffuse visual field loss with those having localized field defects.

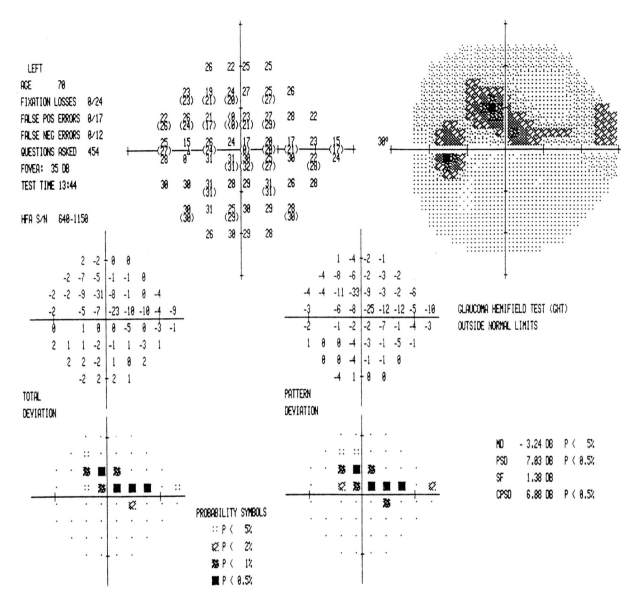

Figure 12.9 Another example of a defect near fixation.   Note that the overall pattern is that of a nerve fiber layer defect.

Glowazki and Flammer[48], Caprioli et al.[49], and Samuelson and Spaeth[50] all found significantly higher intraocular pressures in subjects with diffuse field loss than in subjects with localized field loss (Figure 12.11).

While these differences between normal-tension and high-tension glaucoma fields are no-doubt important to our scientific understanding of normal-tension glaucoma, the clinical significance is less clear. Distinguishing between normal-tension and high-tension glaucoma is obviously not based on the visual field defects. However, we should be aware that defects near fixation might be quite common in persons with normal-tension glaucoma. Defects near fixation (Figure 12.12) are clearly more worrisome than more peripheral ones. In monitoring for the progression of disease, we must realize that the existing defects may deepen rather than enlarge, so particular attention should be paid to the total deviation at each point.

Several studies have addressed the rate of progression of visual field changes in normal-tension glaucoma. Two retrospective analyses found a rather alarming rate of progression. Glicklich et al.[51] found progression in 53% at 3 years and 62% at 5 years. Noureddin et al.[52] found progression in 37% of eyes with a mean follow-up of 28 months. A very high rate of progression was initially seen in the Collaborative Normal-tension Glaucoma Study[53,54] in which a duplicate field determination was necessary to confirm a change. However, by statistical reanalysis of the field data, the study group found a very high false-positive rate for progression. The criteria for progression were revised to include two sets of duplicate fields (four total) spaced 3 months apart that showed the same change of at least 10 dB. This increased testing reduced the false-positive rate to only 2%. The estimated rate of progression by the revised criteria was only 1.3% per patient per 3-month period. In light of the findings of the

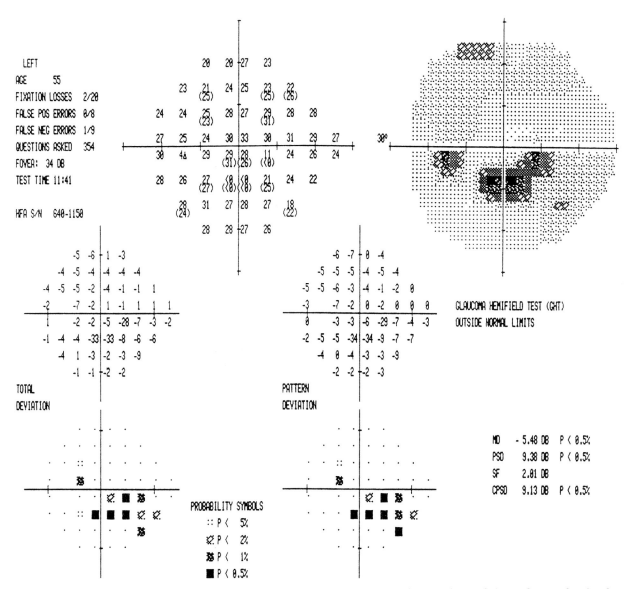

Figure 12.10 Inferior field defect. Although less common than superior defects, inferior defects also tend to be deep and steep and may be close to fixation.

Normal-tension Glaucoma Treatment Trial[55], we may need to repeat visual field testing several times before concluding that progression has occurred in a person with normal-tension glaucoma.

TREATMENT OF NORMAL-TENSION GLAUCOMA

The treatment of low-tension glaucoma remains as much an enigma as the disease itself. In general, the accepted clinical treatment of low-tension glaucoma parallels that for primary open-angle glaucoma. Individuals are usually started on medical therapy designed to lower their intraocular pressure and may undergo laser or glaucoma filtering surgery with very low pressures as the target goal. The Collaborative Normal-tension Glaucoma study provided the most convincing evidence that lowering intraocular pressure does decrease the

rate of progression in this disease. With a target pressure lowering of 30%, the study found that treatment reduced the progression rate by about two-thirds compared to untreated controls. The Early Manifest Glaucoma Trial also found that pressure-lowering treatment reduced the rate of progression in its subset of subjects with normal-tension glaucoma compared to untreated controls[56,57].

While critically important, reduction of intraocular pressure may not be the only potential treatment for normal-tension glaucoma. Therapy for low-tension glaucoma is always being critically re-evaluated and novel approaches to therapy in some individuals are being considered. Based on studies that suggest a vascular autoregulatory dysfunction or vasospasm in normal-tension glaucoma, some individuals have recommended therapy specific for these proposed pathophysiological abnormalities[58]. In addition, interest is increasing to consider agents that may have neuroprotective effects.

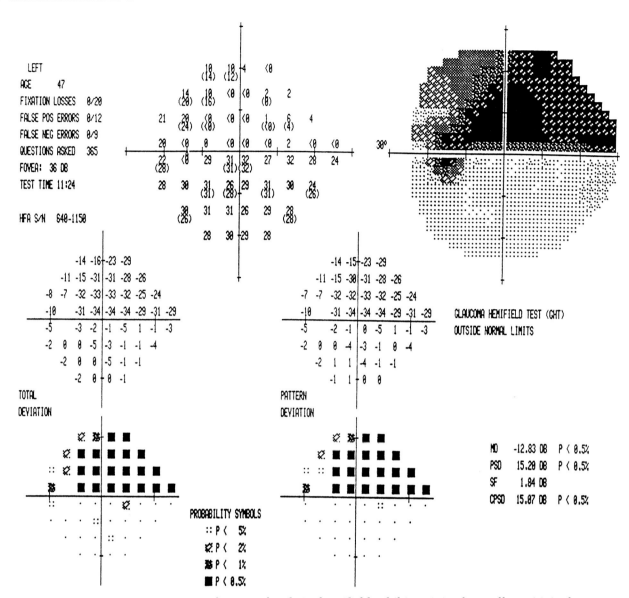

Figure 12.11 Superior hemifield loss. The 'spared' inferior hemifield exhibits minimal overall sensitivity loss.

While medical treatment for normal-tension glaucoma is generally similar to treatment for primary open-angle glaucoma, some potentially important variations should be considered. There have been some suggestions that the β_1-antagonist, betaxolol, may improve blood flow or provide neuroprotective benefits to help preserve visual function and thus may be of benefit in low-tension glaucoma. However, long-term studies addressing the efficacy of betaxolol, although suggestive, are not complete. Non-selective beta blockers generally lower pressure more than a selective beta blocker; however, there are concerns regarding potential vasoconstriction related to the pharmacological properties of these agents. In fact, the Collaborative Normal-tension Glaucoma Study avoided beta blockers for this reason. Although direct evidence of clinically significant vasospasm in low-tension glaucoma has been suggested, the evidence for such an effect is still to be defined.

The development of neuroprotective agents has been a very active area of glaucoma research and normal-tension glaucoma patients may achieve the greatest benefit from this type of therapy. The highly selective α_2-agonist, brimonidine tartrate, has shown neuroprotective effects in cell culture and in a variety of animal models. Brimonidine is also being evaluated as a neuroprotective agent in a large clinical trial[59]. Other compounds, some already available such as memantine, are being investigated as potential neuroprotective agents.

Newer therapeutic approaches directed at improving blood flow to the optic nerve have also been considered. Calcium channel blockers have received the most interest and study. Although some suggestive indirect evidence does exist that individuals on calcium channel blockers may have better visual field survival, these studies are open to criticism and there is still much work to be done. In addition, these agents can be associated with serious

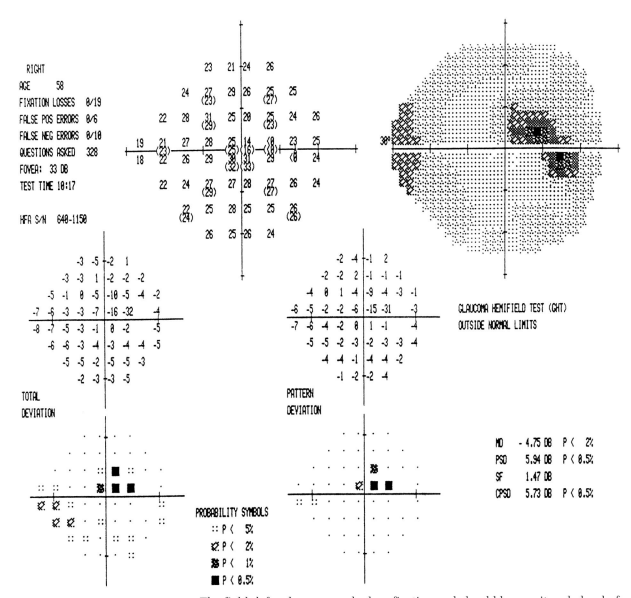

Figure 12.12 Paracentral scotoma. The field defect has encroached on fixation and should be monitored closely for further deepening of the defect.

systemic side-effects, such as hypotension and a reported increased risk of heart attack. Other novel approaches to treating low-tension glaucoma are being investigated and will hopefully lead to more satisfactory medical approaches in the future.

Most clinicians agree that, in the face of progressive low-tension glaucoma, aggressive surgical therapy should be considered. Several studies have suggested that, with aggressive surgery and intraocular pressure lowering to the low teens or below, visual field progression can be slowed or halted in many individuals. When considering glaucoma filtering surgery for low-tension glaucoma, many clinicians and glaucoma specialists will consider the use of an anti-metabolite such as 5-fluorouracil or mitomycin C. Although the use of anti-metabolites

increases the likelihood of obtaining low intraocular pressures, one must also deal with the short-term complications of hypotony, choroidal effusions, and flat anterior chamber, as well as the potential long-term complications of cataract progression, bleb leaks, and endophthalmitis.

Unfortunately, despite what might be considered as optimal therapy for an individual with low-tension glaucoma, many of these individuals seem to progress. Our lack of understanding of the etiology of low-tension glaucoma undoubtedly contributes to our therapeutic failures. Further research is necessary to define the underlying causes that predispose to low-tension glaucoma so that future therapy may be directed at specific pathophysiological abnormalities.

REFERENCES

1. von Graefe A. Uber die glaucomatose Natur die Amaurosenmit Sehnervenexcavation und uber das Weses und die Classification des Glaucomas. Archiv Ophthalmol 1861; 8: 271–97

2. von Graefe A. Amaurose mit Sehnervenexcavation. Archiv Ophthalmol 1857; 3: 484–7

3. von Graefe A. Die Iridectomie bei Amaurous mit Sehnervenexcavation. Archiv Ophthalmol 1857; 3: 546–8

4. Duke-Elder S, Jay B. Disease of the Lens and Vitreous: Glaucoma and Hypotony. London: Kimpton, 1969

5. Sjögren H. A study of pseudoglaucoma. Acta Ophthalmol 1946; 24: 239–94

6. American Academy of Ophthalmology. Primary Open-Angle Glaucoma. Preferred Practice Pattern. San Francisco: American Acad of Ophthalmology 2003: 3. Available at www.aao.org/ppp. Accessed 13 October 2006

7. Leydhecker W, Akiyama K, Neumann HG. Der intraokulare Druck gesunder menschlicher Augen. Klin Monatsbl Augenheilkd 1958; 133: 662

8. Armaly MF. Ocular pressure and visual fields: a ten year follow-up study. Arch Ophthalmol 1969; 81: 25–40

9. Bankes JLK, Perkins ES, Tsolokis S, et al. Bedford glaucoma survey. Br Med J 1968; 1: 791–6

10. Linner E, Stromberg U. The course of untreated ocular hypertension. A tonographic study. Acta Ophthalmol 1964; 42: 836–48

11. Perkins ES. The Bedford Glaucoma Survey. 1. Long term follow-up borderline cases (abstr). Br J Ophthalmol 1973; 57: 179

12. Schappert-Kimmijser J. A five-year follow-up of subjects with intraocular pressure of 22–30 mmHg without anomalies of the optic nerve and visual field typical for glaucoma at first investigation. Ophthalmologica 1971; 162: 289–95

13. Klein BEK, Klein R, Linton KLP. Intraocular pressure in an American community: the Beaver Dam Eye Study. Invest Ophthalmol 1992; 33: 2224–8

14. Tielsch JM, Sommer A, Witt K, et al. Blindness and visual impairment in an American urban population: the Baltimore Eye Survey. Arch Ophthalmol 1990; 108: 286–90

15. Spaeth GL. A new classification of glaucoma including focal glaucoma. Surv Ophthalmol (Suppl) 1994; 38: S9–S15

16. Emara BY, Tingey DP, Probst LE, Motolko MA. Central corneal thickness in low-tension glaucoma. Can J Ophthalmol 1999; 6: 319–24

17. Copt RP, Thomas R, Mermoud A. Corneal thickness in ocular hypertension, primary open-angle glaucoma, and normal tension glaucoma. Arch Ophthalmol 1999; 117: 14–16

18. Morad Y, Sharon E, Hefetz L, Nemet P. Corneal thickness and curvature in normal-tension glaucoma. Am J Ophthalmol 1998; 125: 164–8

19. Lewis RA, Hayreh SM, Phelps CD. Optic disk and visual field correlations in primary-open angle low-tension glaucoma. Am J Ophthalmol 1983; 6: 148–52

20. Miller KM, Quigley HA. Comparison of optic disc features in low-tension and typical open-angle glaucoma. Ophthalmic Surg 1987; 13: 882–9

21. Levene RZ. Low tension glaucoma: a critical review and new material. Surv Ophthalmol 1980; 19: 621–63

22. Tuulonen A, Airaksinen PJ. Optic disc size in exfoliative, primary open angle and low tension glaucoma. Arch Ophthalmol 1992; 5: 211–13

23. Jonas JB, Sturmer J, Papastathopoulos K, et al. Optic disc size in normal pressure glaucoma. Br J Ophthalmol 1995; 4: 1102–5

24. Nicolela MT, Drance SM. Various glaucomatous optic nerve appearances. Ophthalmology 1996; 103: 640–9

25. Caprioli J, Spaeth GL. Comparison of the optic nerve head in high- and low-tension glaucoma. Arch Ophthalmol 1985; 5: 1145–9

26. Fazio P, Krupin T, Feitl M, et al. Optic disc topography in patients with low-tension and primary open angle glaucoma. Arch Ophthalmol 1990; 5: 705–8

27. Javitt JC, Spaeth GL, Katz LJ, et al. Acquired pits of the optic nerve: increased prevalence in patients with low-tension glaucoma. Ophthalmology 1986; 2: 1038–44

28. Kitazawa Y, Shirato S, Yamamoto T. Optic disc hemorrhages in the glaucomas. Ophthalmology 1986; 2: 853–7

29. Drance SM. Disc hemorrhages in the glaucomas. Surv Ophthalmol 1989; 19: 331–7

30. Hendrickx KH, van den Enden A, Rasker MT, Hoyng PFJ. Cumulative incidence of patients with disc hemorrhages in glaucoma and the effect of therapy. Ophthalmology 1994; 2: 1165–72

31. Buus DR, Anderson DR. Peripapillary crescents and halos in normal-tension glaucoma and ocular hypertension. Ophthalmology 1989; 2: 16–19

32. Geijssen HC, Greve EL. The spectrum of primary open-angle glaucoma 1: senile sclerotic glaucoma versus high tension glaucoma. Ophthalmic Surg 1987; 18: 207–13

33. Jonas JB, Xu L. Parapapillary chorioretinal atrophy in normal-pressure glaucoma. Am J Ophthalmol 1993; 6: 501–5

34. Drance SM. The visual field of low-tension glaucoma and shock-induced optic neuropathy. Arch Ophthalmol 1977; 95: 1359–61

35. Anderton S, Hitchings RA. A comparative study on visual fields of patients with low-tension glaucoma and those with chronic simple glaucoma. Doc Ophthalmol Proc Series 1983; 35: 97–9

36. Hitchings RA, Anderton SA. A comparative study of visual field defects seen in patients with low-tension glaucoma and chronic simple glaucoma. Br J Ophthalmol 1983; 67: 818–21

37. Caprioli J, Spaeth GL. Comparison of visual field defects in the low-tension glaucomas with those in the high-tension glaucomas. Am J Ophthalmol 1984; 97: 730–7

38. Motolko M, Drance SM, Douglas GR. Visual field defects in low-tension glaucoma: comparison of defects in low-tension glaucoma and chronic open angle glaucoma. Arch Ophthalmol 1982; 100: 1074–7

39. Motolko M, Drance SM, Douglas GR. The visual field defects of low-tension glaucoma: a comparison of the visual field defects in low-tension glaucoma with chronic open angle glaucoma. Doc Ophthalmol Proc Series 1983; 35: 107–11

40. Greve EL, Geijssen HC. Comparison of glaucomatous visual field defects in patients with high and with low intraocular pressures. Doc Ophthalmol Proc Series 1983; 35: 101–5

41. King D, Drance SM, Gouglas G, et al. Comparison of visual field defects in normal-tension glaucoma and high-tension glaucoma. Am J Ophthalmol 1986; 101: 204–7

42. Phelps CD, Hayreh SS, Montague PR. Comparison of visual field defects in the low-tension glaucomas with those in the high-tension glaucomas. Am J Ophthalmol 1984; 98: 823–5

43. Araie M, Yamagami J, Suziki Y. Visual field defects in normal-tension and high-tension glaucoma. Ophthalmology 1993; 100: 1808–14

44. Araie M, Hori J, Koseki N. Comparison of visual field defects between normal-tension and primary open-angle glaucoma in the late stage of the disease. Graefe's Arch Clin Exp Ophthalmol 1995; 233: 610–16

45. Drance SM, Douglas GR, Airaksinen PJ, et al. Diffuse visual field loss in chronic open-angle and low-tension glaucoma. Am J Ophthalmol 1987; 104: 577–80

46. Chauhan BC, Drance SM, Douglas GR, Johnson CA. Visual field damage in normal-tension and high-tension glaucoma. Am J Ophthalmol 1989; 108: 636–42

47. Zeiter JH, Shin DH, Juzych MS, et al. Visual field defects in patients with normal-tension glaucoma and patients with high-tension glaucoma. Am J Ophthalmol 1992; 114: 758–63

48. Glowazki A, Flammer J. Is there a difference between glaucoma patients with rather localized visual field damage and patients with more diffuse visual field damage? Doc Ophthalmol Proc Series 1987; 49: 317–20

49. Caprioli J, Sears M, Miller JM. Patterns of early visual field loss in open-angle glaucoma. Am J Ophthalmol 1987; 103: 512–17

50. Samuelson TW, Spaeth GL. Focal and diffuse visual field defects: their relationship to intraocular pressure. Ophthalmic Surg 1993; 24: 519–25

51. Gliklich RE, Steinmann WC, Spaeth GL. Visual field change in low-tension glaucoma over a five-year follow-up. Ophthalmology 1989; 96: 316–20

52. Noureddin BN, Poinoosawmy D, Fietzke FW, Hitchings RA. Regression analysis of visual field progression in low tension glaucoma. Br J Ophthalmol 1991; 75: 493–5

53. Collaborative Normal-tension Glaucoma Study Group. Comparison of glaucomatous progression between untreated patients with normal-tension glaucoma and patients with therapeutically reduced intraocular pressure. Am J Ophthalmol 1998; 126: 487–97

54. Collaborative Normal-tension Glaucoma Study Group. The effectiveness of intraocular pressure reduction in the treatment of normal-tension glaucoma. Am J Ophthalmol 1998; 126: 498–505

55. Schulzer M. Normal-tension Glaucoma Study Group. Errors in the diagnosis of visual field progression in normal-tension glaucoma. Ophthalmology 1994; 101: 1589–95

56. Heijl A, Leske MC, Bengtsson B, et al. Reduction of intraocular pressure and glaucoma progression – results from the Early Manifest Glaucoma Trial. Arch Ophthalmol 2002; 120: 1268–79

57. Leske MC, Heijl A, Hussein M, et al. Factors for glaucoma progression and the effect of treatment. Arch Ophthalmol 2003; 121: 48–56

58. Chung HS, Harris A, Evans DW, et al. Vascular aspects in the pathophysiology of glaucomatous optic neuropathy. Surv Ophthalmol 1999; 43(Suppl 1): S43–S50

59. Krupin T, Liebmann JM, Greenfield DS, et al., Low-Pressure Glaucoma Study Group. The Low-pressure Glaucoma Treatment Study (LoGTS): study design and baseline characteristics of enrolled patients. Ophthalmology 2005; 112: 376–85

13 Ocular blood flow

Alon Harris, Christian P Jonescu- Cuypers

INTRODUCTION

From the most basic standpoint, the eye offers a unique opportunity to study hemodynamics. It is the only location in the body where capillary blood flow may be observed in humans non-invasively. Over 100 years ago, Wagemann and Salzmann observed vascular sclerosis in many of their glaucoma patients. Through the years, numerous other researchers have uncovered pieces of the ocular blood flow puzzle: documenting reductions in the capillary beds, sclerosis of nutritional vessels, vascular lesions and degeneration, and other circulatory pathologies in many eye diseases including glaucoma. A century of observation and circumstantial evidence suggesting a vascular component in the pathogenesis of glaucoma is now supported by direct experimental evidence. This transition from theory to fact took 100 years because the technology required to make such specialized measurements of homodynamic function have only recently become available. Now that the link has been established, there has been a focus on ocular hemodynamics in glaucoma and the effect of intraocular pressure (IOP)-reducing medications on ocular perfusion.

OCULAR VASCULATURE

The ophthalmic artery is the source for blood flow to the eye but the left and right ophthalmic arteries derive blood from the heart through slightly different routes. The left carotid artery is one of three branches of the aortic arch. The right carotid artery is a branch of the brachiocephalic artery, itself one of the three branches of the aortic arch (Figure 13.1). Both left and right common carotids split to form the internal and external carotid arteries. The only branch of the internal carotid artery outside the cranium is the ophthalmic artery (Figure 13.2). The ocular vasculature is exceedingly complex. The various layers of tissue in the retina receive nourishment from both the uveal and the retinal vasculature.

The ophthalmic artery (OA) supplies both major ocular vascular beds: the retinal and uveal systems. Its major branches include branches to the extraocular muscles, the central retinal artery and the posterior ciliary arteries (Figure 13.3). The uveal system, which supplies blood to the iris, ciliary body, and choroid, is supplied by one to five posterior ciliary arteries (PCA). They emerge from the ophthalmic artery in the posterior orbit. Short posterior ciliary arteries (SPCAs) penetrate the sclera surrounding insertion of the optic nerve (Figure 13.4). These vessels supply the peripapillary choroid, as well as the majority of the anterior

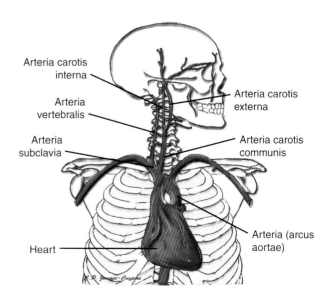

Figure 13.1   Origin and path of arteria carotis.

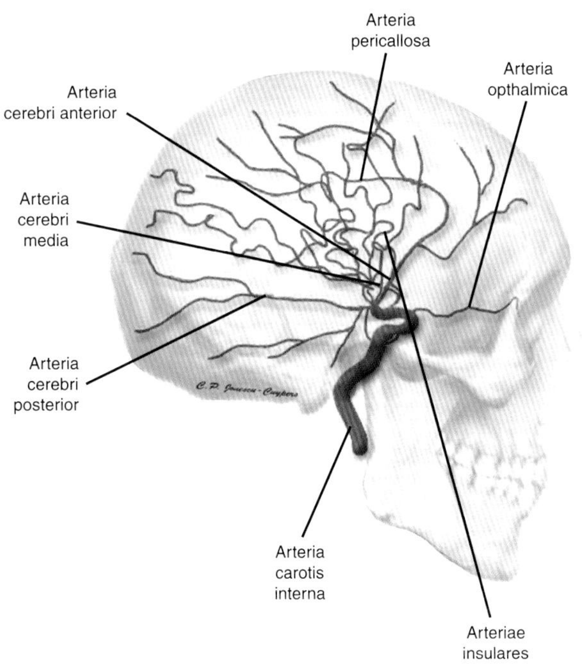

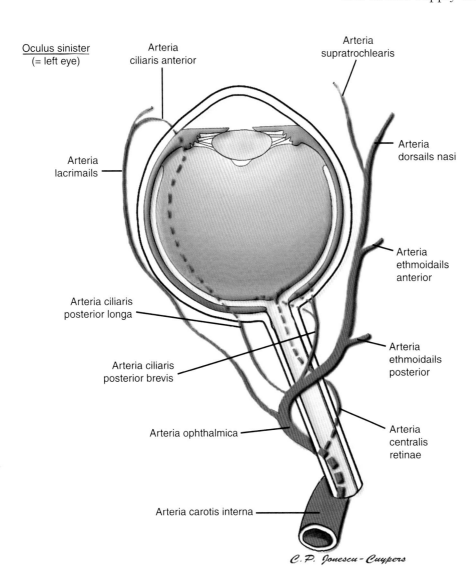

Arteria
pericallosa

Arteria
cerebri anterior

Arteria
opthalmica

Arteria
cerebri
media

Arteria
cerebri
posterior

Arteria
carotis
interna

Arteriae
insulares

Figure 13.2   Cerebral vasculature.

optic nerve. Some SPCAs course, without branching, through the sclera directly into the choroid; others divide within the sclera to provide branches to both the choroid and the optic nerve. Often, a non-continuous arterial circle exists within the perineural sclera, the circle of Zinn–Haller. This structure is formed by the convergence branches from the short posterior ciliary arteries. The circle of Zinn–Haller provides blood for various regions of the anterior optic nerve, the peripapillary choroid, and the pial arterial system.

VASCULATURE OF THE CHOROID

The outer choroid is composed of large non-fenestrated vessels, while the vessel caliber of the inner choroid is much smaller. The innermost layer of the choroid, the choriocapillaris, is composed of richly anastomotic, fenestrated capillaries beginning at the optic disc margin (Figure 13.5). The capillaries of the choriocapillaris are separate and distinct from the capillary beds of the anterior optic nerve. The SPCAs supply most of the optic nerve head

Oculus sinister
(= left eye)

Arteria
ciliaris anterior

Arteria
supratrochlearis

Arteria
lacrimails

Arteria
dorsails nasi

Arteria
ethmoidails
anterior

Arteria ciliaris
posterior longa

Arteria ciliaris
posterior brevis

Arteria
ethmoidails
posterior

Figure 13.3   Branches originating from the arteria carotis interna.

Arteria ophthalmica

Arteria
centralis
retinae

Arteria carotis interna

C. P. Jonescu-Cuypers

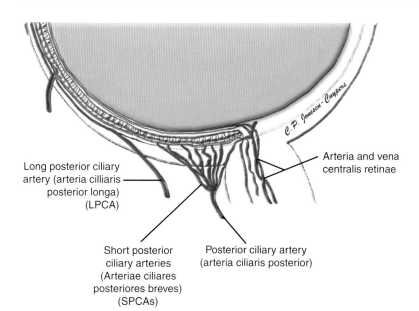

Figure 13.4 Choroidal and retinal vasculature.

Long posterior ciliary artery (arteria cilliaris posterior longa) (LPCA)

Short posterior ciliary arteries (Arteriae ciliares posteriores breves) (SPCAs)

Posterior ciliary artery (arteria ciliaris posterior)

Arteria and vena centralis retinae

Choriocapillaris

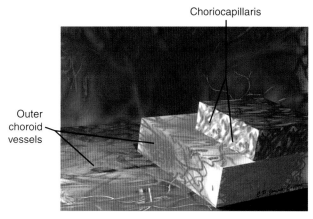

Outer choroid vessels

Figure 13.5   Cross section of choroidal vascular bed.

and the portion of the choriocapillaris posterior to the equator. The choriocapillaris anterior to the equator is supplied by the long posterior ciliary arteries (LPCAs) and the anterior ciliary arteries (ACAs). The LPCAs pierce the sclera and course anteriorly through the suprachoroidal space to branch near the ora serrata. Each LPCA then sends three to five branches posteriorly to supply the choriocapillaris anterior to the equator. The ACAs, branches of the OA, accompany the rectus muscles anteriorly to supply the major circles of the iris (Figure 13.6). Before reaching the iris, 8–12 branches pass posteriorly through the ciliary muscle to supply the anterior choriocapillaris together with the LPCAs (Figure 13.7). Functional anastomoses between the choriocapillaris anterior and posterior to the equator have not been demonstrated. This represents a peripheral choroidal watershed zone.

Venous drainage from the choriocapillaris is mainly through the vortex vein system. Minor

drainage occurs through the ciliary body via the anterior ciliary veins. The vortex veins drain into the inferior (IOV) and superior (SOV) ophthalmic veins (Figure 13.8). The SOV exits the orbit through the superior orbital fissure and drains into the cavernous sinus. The IOV sends a branch to the SOV and then exits the orbit through the inferior orbital fissure into the pterygoid plexus.

The retinal system is supplied by the central retinal artery (CRA) and sustains the inner retina. The CRA, itself a branch of the ophthalmic artery, penetrates the optic nerve approximately 12 mm behind the globe. The CRA courses adjacent to the central retinal vein through the center of the optic nerve, then emerges from the optic nerve within the globe, where it branches into four major vessels.

The anterior optic nerve may be divided into four anatomic regions: the superficial nerve fiber layer, the prelaminar region, the lamina cribrosa, and the retrolaminar region (Figure 13.9).

The superficial nerve fiber layer, the anterior-most region, is continuous with the nerve fiber layer of the retina and is the only nerve head structure visible by fundus examination (Figure 13.9, yellow shaded). It is supplied by retinal arterioles arising from the branches of retinal arteries. These small vessels originate in the surrounding nerve fiber layer and run toward the center of the optic nerve head. They have been referred to as 'epipapillary vessels'. The temporal nerve fiber layer may receive additional blood from a cilioretinal artery when it is present. No direct choroidal or choriocapillaris contribution is observed in the superficial nerve fiber layer.

Immediately posterior to the nerve fiber layer is the prelaminar region, which lies adjacent to the peripapillary choroids (Figure 13.9, red shaded). In this region, ganglionic axons group into

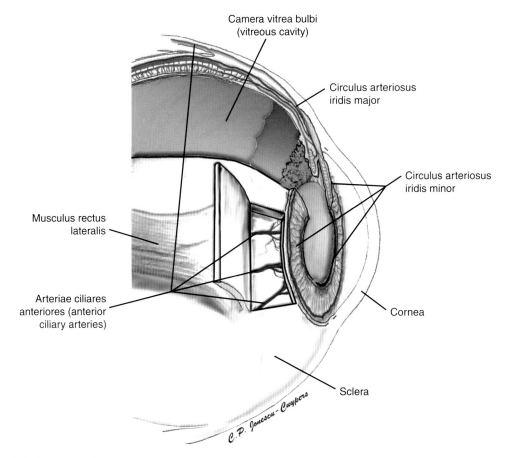

Figure 13.6   **Anterior segment.**

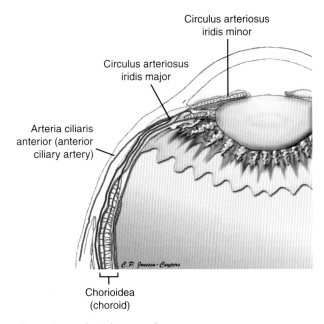

Figure 13.7   **Anterior vessels.**

bundles for passage through the lamina cribrosa. The prelaminar region is supplied primarily by branches of the SPCAs and by branches of the circle of Zinn–Haller, though some investigators have observed a vascular contribution to the prelaminar region from peripapillary choroidal arterioles. The amount of choroidal contribution may be difficult to ascertain, as there are branches from both the circle of Zinn–Haller and from the SPCAs which course through the choroid and ultimately supply the optic nerve in this region. These vessels do not originate in the choroid, but merely pass through it. The direct arterial supply to the prelaminar region arising from the choroidal vasculature is minimal. This minimal contribution from the choroidal vasculature is limited to small arterioles. There is no vascular contribution from the choriocapillaris.

More posteriorly, the laminar region is continuous with the sclera and is composed of the lamina cribrosa (Figure 13.9, green shaded). The lamina cribrosa is a structure consisting of fenestrated connective tissue which allows the passage of neural axons through the scleral coat. Like the prelaminar

Vena ophthalmica
superior

Figure 13.8 Venous drainage of the orbit and globe.

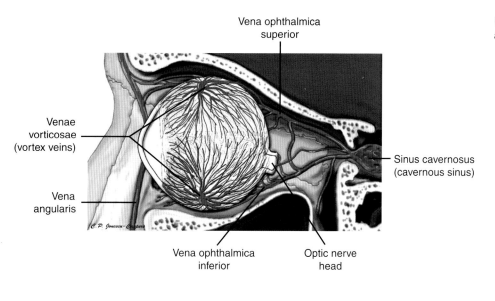

Venae
vorticosae
(vortex veins)

Vena
angularis

Sinus cavernosus
(cavernous sinus)

Vena ophthalmica
inferior

Optic nerve
head

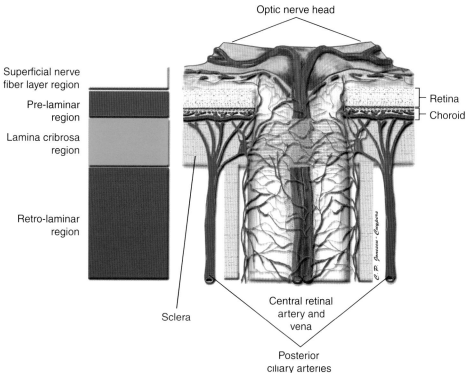

Optic nerve head

Superficial nerve
fiber layer region

Pre-laminar
region

Lamina cribrosa
region

Retro-laminar
region

Retina

Choroid

Sclera

Central retinal
artery and
vena

Posterior
ciliary arteries

Figure 13.9   Optic nerve head vasculature. (Figures 13.1–13.9 from Atlas of Ocular Blood Flow: Vascular Anatomy, Pathophysiology and Metabolism with permission from Elsevier).

region, the lamina cribrosa also receives its blood supply from branches of the SPCAs and branches of the circle of Zinn–Haller. These precapillary branches perforate the outer lamina cribrosa before branching centrally, forming a capillary network throughout the fenestrated connective tissue. Larger vessels of the peripapillary choroid may contribute occasional small arterioles to the lamina cribrosa region.

Finally, the retrolaminar region lies posterior to the lamina cribrosa and, marked by the beginning of axonal myelination, is surrounded by the meninges of the central nervous system (Figure 13.9, blue shaded). The retrolaminar region has two blood supplies – the CRA and the pial system. The pial system is an anastomosing network of capillaries located immediately within the pia mater. The pial system originates at the circle of Zinn–Haller and may also be fed directly by the SPCAs. Its branches extend into the optic nerve to nourish the axons. The CRA may provide several small intraneural branches in the retrolaminar region. Some of these branches anastomose with the pial system.

There is a marked interindividual variation in the vascular patterns of the anterior optic nerve, peripapillary retina and posterior choroid. The predominant variability observed among individuals is in the arterial supply. Varying numbers of branches have been found in the posterior ciliary arteries, the SPCAs, the number of branches from the LPCAs, and the number of branches from the ACAs.

The most recent evidence suggests that glaucoma characteristically damages the photoreceptors and the horizontal cells, as well as the retinal ganglion cells. The retinal ganglion cells are nourished by the retinal circulation, while the photoreceptors receive their blood supply from the underlying choroid. Therefore, to define how enhanced blood flow improves visual function, it is essential to evaluate blood flow to the retina and choroid, for the retinal ganglion cells and photoreceptor cells, respectively.

Several soluble vasoactive molecules mediate retinal vascular autoregulation, including endothelium-derived nitric oxide, endothelins, superoxide anions, rennin–angiotensin, and vascular endothelial growth factor (VEGF).

TECHNIQUES FOR EXAMINING OCULAR BLOOD FLOW

Technological revolutions in medical science have enabled clinicians and researchers to better visualize ocular blood flow (OBF). In the past two decades, ocular hemodynamics assessment has evolved from a subjective description of visible vessels to direct quantitative measurement of blood flow parameters. Each technique provides a different aspect of ocular hemodynamics and therefore different ones are required in order to quantify the various vascular beds comprising the ocular circulation.

PULSATILE OCULAR BLOOD FLOW

The pulsatile ocular blood flow (POBF) device (the OBF Labs (UK) Ltd unit is pictured in Figure 13.10) is a pneumotonometer that measures IOP in real time. It is based on the principle (Figure 13.11) that blood volume in the eye increases with the systolic pulse, and decreases during diastole. When the volume increases, eye pressure increases as well. If the relationship between eye pressure and eye volume is identical for everyone, then transient changes in IOP can be used to calculate absolute transient changes in ocular volume. As with a car tire that is leaking air, however, the true volume of blood entering the eye is unknown, because the rate of venous flow (the leak) is not measured, is

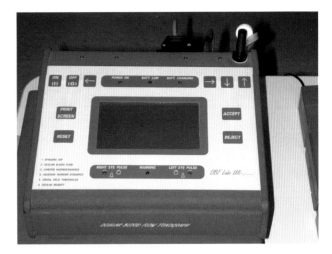

Figure 13.10 Pubsatile ocular blood flow device. (OBF Labs (UK) Ltd. Malmesbury, Wiltshire, England.)

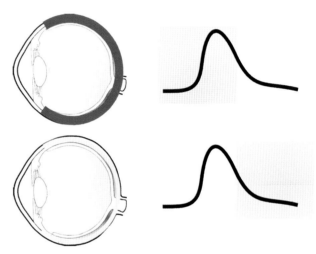

Figure 13.11 Representation of the principle of pulsatile ocular blood flow measurements. Blood volume in the eye increases with the systolic pulse and decreased during diastole.

unknown, and varies between individual eyes. The IOP pulse wave is transformed into an ocular volume wave using the presumed universal relationship. The change in volume over time is reported as the pulsatile ocular blood flow.

OCULO-OPHTHALMODYNAMAMOGRAPHY

The oculo-ophthalmodynamamograph (OODG) device is a pneumotonometer that measures IOP in real time, similar to the POBF device (Figure 13.12). The OODG differs from the POBF in that it is used in combination with a scleral suction cup. During the measurement, IOP is increased. With sufficient IOP increase, flow ceases within each of the vascular beds within the globe. When blood flow ceases within a vascular bed, its contribution to the IOP waveform measured by the pneumotonometer

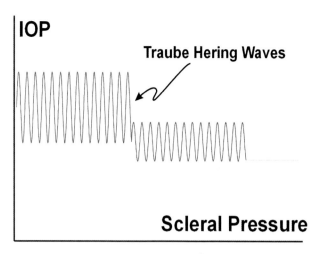

Figure 13.12 Waveform produced by the oculo-ophthalmo-dynamamograph (OODG). This measures IOP in real time.

disappears. The OODG uses this phenomenon to directly quantify the perfusion pressure within the uveal and retinal beds.

COLOR DOPPLER IMAGING

Fundamentals

Ultrasound uses sound waves to locate structures in the body. By timing the delay between sound transmission and echo, ultrasound can measure the depth and location of an anatomic structure, e.g. A-scan ultrasound measurements of axial length. The time between transmission of a sound wave into the eye and the returning echo from the back of the eye provides a precise measurement of axial length. This measurement does not require clear optical media and can be performed in the presence of many ophthalmic diseases. By sweeping the A-scan in a line through the eye, a map of structural locations through a slice is obtained. This is commonly known as B-scan ultrasound and has been used to produce gray-scale images of ophthalmic structures. Color Doppler imaging (CDI) is based on B-scan technology, with an additional processing step (Figure 13.13). The frequency of the returning B-scan sound waves is analyzed. When a wave is reflected by a moving source, such as flowing blood, it is Doppler shifted to a different frequency. The amount of the shift is described by the Doppler equation (Figure 13.14), where V_{Blood} is the blood flow velocity, Wavelength is the wavelength of the incident sound wave, and $Cos\theta$ is the cosine of the angle between the blood velocity vector and the incident sound wave vector. Doppler shifted sound is displayed using color-coded pixels within the gray-scale image. Red pixels represent movement toward the CDI probe, and blue represents movement away from the probe. Samples of Doppler shifts (or velocities as calculated using the

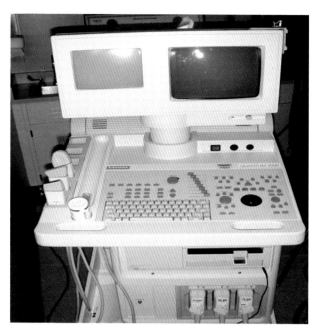

Figure 13.13 Color Doppler imaging ultrasound machine. (Siemens Quantum 2000, Siemens Ultrasound, Isaquaah, WA.)

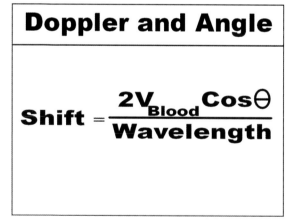

Figure 13.14 Formula for calculating blood flow velocities from Doppler shift.

equation in Figure 13.14) may be collected from specified vessels within the image. These data are collected in real time during the cardiac cycle. A number of data may be obtained from the resulting velocity waveform. The peak systolic velocity (PSV) is located by the ultrasonographer and is equal to the greatest observable flow velocity obtained by the blood during systole. The end-diastolic blood flow velocity (EDV) can also be located by the ultrasonographer (Figure 13.15). Using both of these measurements, Pourcelot's resistive index (RI) may be computed (Figure 13.16); RI is an indication of the resistance to flow in the vasculature distal to the point of measurement.

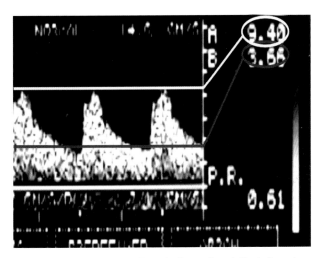

Figure 13.15   Peak systolic velocity and end diastolic velocity. These are marked by the ultrasonographer and resistive index is then calculated from these values.

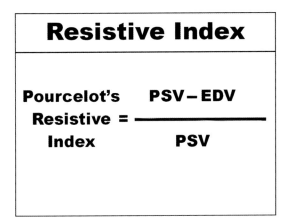

Figure 13.16 Formula for calculation of Pourcelot's Resistive Index. This uses peak systolic and end diastolic velocities.

Hemodynamic measurements

CDI is used to measure blood flow velocities in the ophthalmic, CRA and SPCAs. Due to the large difference between the ophthalmic and smaller CRA and SPCAs, the system settings are changed to appropriate ranges of depth and velocity. The waveforms of the various vessels provide additional information. The dicrotic notch is clearly evident in the ophthalmic artery waveform (Figure 13.17), while still evident yet less pronounced in the CRA and missing from the SPCA.

In glaucomatous eyes with high resistance to flow, SPCA waveforms take on the appearance of a haystack with almost no end-diastolic flow. CDI thus allows quantification of flow velocities in the retrobulbar vasculature in research and clinical settings. The appearance of waveforms may also provide insight into the condition of the patient's ocular vascular health.

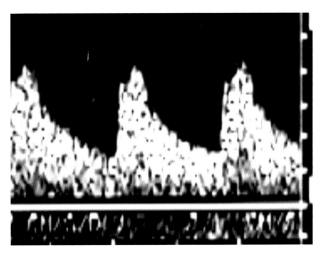

Figure 13.17   Waveform produced by the ophthalmic artery. This is distinct from the other vessels by a dicrotic notch.

ANGIOGRAPHY

Fundamentals

Ophthalmic angiography dates back to 1961 when, at the Indiana University School of Medicine, Novotny and Alvis first described a method for photographing fluorescein as it passed through the human retina. Their early technique was limited to one image every 12 seconds. Today fluorescein angiography can be performed with scanning laser ophthalmoscopes (SLO) which are capable of a wide range of imaging applications in ophthalmology. The Rodenstock SLO is an imaging device that produces fundus images (Figure 13.18). The Heidelberg retina angiography (HRA) unit is a digital imaging platform equipped with argon and infrared lasers (Figure 13.19).

Both the HRA and Rodenstock SLO utilize a confocal optical system (Figure 13.20). For each point of the image, light is focused to a point on the fundus. Light reflected from this point is quantified by a photodetector. Confocal systems create

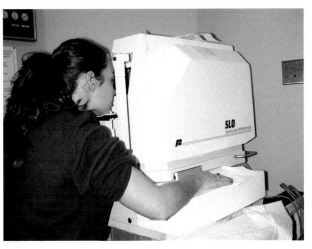

Figure 13.18   Rodenstock Scanning Laser Ophthalmoscope.

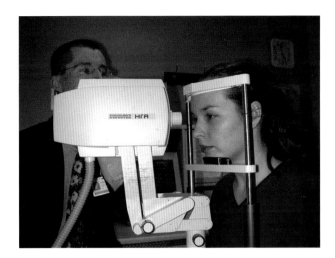

Figure 13.19   Heidelberg Retinal Angiograph.

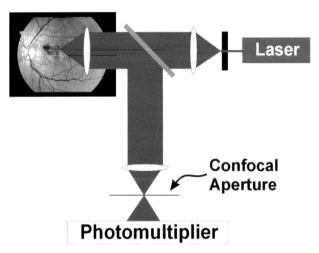

Figure 13.20 Diagrammatic representation of a confocal optical system. This is utilized in the Rodenstock Scanning Laser Ophthalmoscope and Heidelberg Retinal Angiograph.

sharp images by blocking scattered light from the image. Only light from the point of interest is focused to a point at the aperture.

The HRA and Rodenstock SLO are also used to quantify retinal hemodynamics. By recording fluorescein and indocyanine green angiograms, both of the SLO systems provide valuable data concerning the movement of blood through the retinal and choroidal vasculature; however, measurement of volumetric blood flow by angiography is currently impossible.

Equipped with argon, infrared, and helium–neon lasers, and a number of apertures and filters, the Rodenstock SLO has a large number of imaging modes. Temporal resolution has increased to 30 images per second and spatial resolution is maximized by using a scanning laser to illuminate the fundus one point at a time. Images obtained from the Rodenstock SLO are recorded on videotape because of the large amount of image data. While the

improvements in image collection are important, improvements in image interpretation and analysis continue to provide new insight into the physiology and pathophysiology of ocular hemodynamics.

Video images obtained from Rodenstock SLO angiography are analyzed using digital video analysis equipment. Each frame of a video segment of interest is digitized. This allows the brightness in specified areas to be quantified. As dye enters retinal vessels, it becomes bright. By quantifying the brightness in two locations on a retinal vessel, the amount of time for fluorescein dye to move from a proximal to a distal location may be measured (Figure 13.21). Utilizing the image-processing capabilities of the analysis system, the distance between the two brightness measurement locations may also be measured. Combining distance and time data yields the mean dye flow velocity (MDV) through retinal vessels. If the same system is used to measure vessel diameter, volumetric flow through the retinal arteries may be calculated.

Hemodynamic measurements at 40°

In order to obtain an accurate measurement, sample areas on retinal arteries are located on a length of vessel void of branches. A plot of the brightness of a vein in time may be used with the arterial plots in order to measure the arteriovenous passage (AVP) time. The AVP time is an indication of the overall status of the retinal microcirculation, requiring passage of dye from retinal arteries to retinal veins (Figure 13.22).

Hemodynamic measurements at 20°

Measurements of blood velocity in the perifoveal retina were first estimated using the blue field entoptic phenomenon. Illuminated by a bright blue light, the leukocytes cast a shadow on retinal

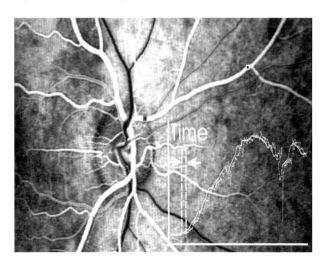

Figure 13.21   Image of fluorescein angiogram indicating the appearance of dye arrival in the arteries.

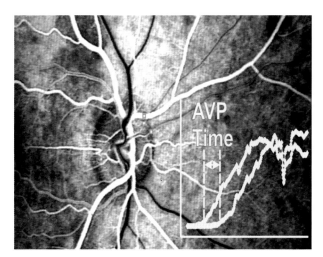

Figure 13.22 Image of fluorescein angiogram indicating arterial venous passage time.

receptors. In the perifoveal region, where the retinal capillaries thin to a single layer, these moving shadows are visible; the average subject describes their appearance as that of spermatozoa in a microscope. Using the blue field effect, Riva constructed a blue field entoptic simulator. The simulator allows a subject to adjust the density, speed, and pulsatility of simulated leukocyte shadows on a computer screen to match their own. Besides the subjectivity of this process, the problem with estimating blood velocity based on the movement of leukocytes is that leukocytes are much bigger than the retinal capillaries. Forcing their way through the capillaries, they must fold up by rubbing on the endothelial wall. Outnumbering the leukocytes by 600 to 1, the erythrocytes move more readily through the capillaries, making the forced movement of leukocytes more the exception than the rule.

Using the 20° field, the SLO's high spatial and temporal resolution makes it possible to record microdroplets of fluorescein dye passing through the perifoveal capillaries. Dark areas between the bright droplets are thought to be rouleux formations of erythrocytes. These droplets therefore represent the movement of red blood cells through the vasculature. If the intent of blood flow measurement is better understanding of the delivery of oxygen to tissue, this method, which concentrates on the movement of erythrocytes, is preferred for description of the velocity of retinal capillaries. Quantification is accomplished using the same system as that used for measurement of the mean dye velocity in 40° angiograms. The number of frames required for bolus transit across the capillary is used to determine time, and the digital video analysis system is used to measure the length of the capillary. Combined, a precise measurement of capillary transit velocity (CTV) is obtained.

Thus, retinal blood velocities can be measured in the large retinal arteries using 40° fluorescein angiography, and capillary velocities in both the perifoveal and optic disc areas can be measured using a 20° field. Either measurement requires both an SLO and a video analysis system. Currently, the software required for this analysis is not commercially available.

Indocyanine green angiography

Indocyanine green (ICG) angiography can be performed on either a Rodenstock SLO or the Heidelberg HRA digital SLO. ICG dye is excited by near-infrared light with maximum excitation at 805 nm, and maximum emission at 835 nm. These wavelengths of light are able to penetrate the retinal pigment epithelial layer and produce excellent images of choroidal structure. These structures are not visible using a 488-nm argon laser during fluorescein angiography. A technique has been developed which allows quantification of choroidal hemodynamics using ICG angiograms.

A modified injection technique is used. Twenty-five milligrams of ICG are dissolved into 2 ml of solvent. One milliliter of the solution is injected per examination. The small volume of dye allows a rapid injection time of approximately 1 second. The injection is immediately followed by a 2-ml saline flush. Like fluorescein angiography, verbal commands are used to guide subject fixation. Figure 13.23 demonstrates the appearance of dye in the choroid following intravenous injection. For ICG angiography, the nasal edge of the disc is situated at the edge of the 40° field of view. Examinations are recorded on S-VHS videotape and processed off-line. A digital image processor with customized software is used to perform the analysis. Six locations on the image are identified – two near the optic disc (located superiorly and inferiorly on the temporal side) and four around the macula (Figure 13.24). The average

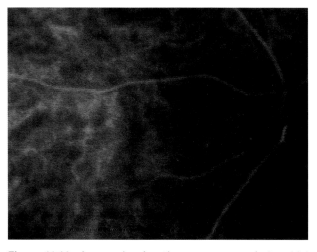

Figure 13.23 Image showing the appearance of choroidal vasculature. This is shown at the time of dye arrival following indo-cyanine green injection.

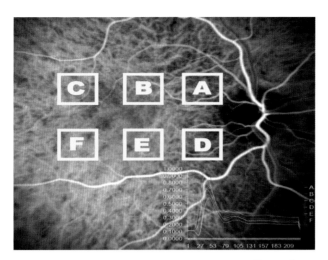

Figure 13.24   Image with six locations marked. From these the average brightness in each area is computed for each frame of the angiogram.

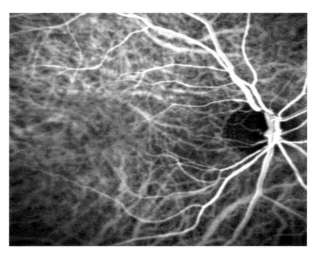

Figure 13.25   Image of the fundus acquired using the Heidelberg Retinal Angiograph.

brightness in each of the six areas is computed for each frame of the angiogram. Area brightness is graphed with time on the x-axis and brightness on the y-axis. The analysis identifies three parameters from the brightness maps: slope, time to achieve 10% of total brightness, and curve width. The slope provides information concerning the average speed of dye entry into each area. The 10% time provides a more precise but noisier look at dye velocity into each area. The width of the curve provides information on the amount of time required for dye to enter and then leave the choroid. The mean value and range for all six areas are also computed.

The Heidelberg HRA system is a completely digital SLO that is also capable of producing fundus angiograms. Instead of recording a video sequence onto super VHS tape, each frame is stored individually on the HRA hard drive. The number of frames that can be acquired is limited by the memory of the HRA computer. The total length of any individual segment is, therefore, limited to a short amount of time (1–2 minutes at full frame rates) before recording must stop and frames are saved to the hard drive. The HRA is more sensitive to small head movements than the Rodenstock SLO. At 20 frames per second, 1200 images are generated each minute. Each image contains 65 536 individual pixels, each pixel representing the fluorescence detected at a 30×30 μm area of the fundus (Figure 13.25). The greatest advantage of the HRA is that the images produced are digital.

Conversely, Rodenstock SLO data begin as a voltage level that is digitized within the SLO imaging system. This digital level is converted back to analog to form the video signal out of the machine. The signal is stored in analog format on the S-VHS tape, and converted back to digital by a frame grabber for analysis. In each of these steps, there is some small amount of signal degradation. In the case of HRA, there is no digitization required for computer analysis of angiograms. Images are, and remain, in their original pristine state. HRA images, however, are of a lower spatial and temporal resolution than Rodenstock SLO images.

INTERFEROMETRY

Interferometry is a technique used to directly measure the pulsation of the fundus relative to the cornea. As implied by its name, interferometry is based on the interference pattern formed by two sources of light: one reflected from the fundus and one reflected from the cornea. The two beams are created from a single laser beam passing through the center of the eye. The beam is partially reflected by the cornea, and also partially reflected by the retina (Figure 13.26).

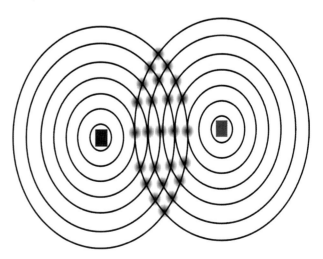

Figure 13.26   Diagrammatic representation of the principle of interferometry.

Since the source of the two reflections is a single laser, the reflected light from each source has the same frequency. The result is a stationary interference pattern. The intensity pattern is a function of the distance between the two reflective sources which vary with location but do not vary with time. As the fundus pulses with the cardiac cycle, the locations of the nodes within the interference pattern move. The magnitude of fundus pulsation can be calculated if the change in node spacing is known. This spacing is measured by the interferometer using a linear array detector. The detector quantifies the light level along its axis.

LASER DOPPLER TECHNIQUES

The Canon laser blood flowmeter

The Canon laser blood flowmeter (CLBF) is the only hemodynamic assessment device capable of measuring volumetric blood flow in absolute units. The CLBF is a Windows-based flowmeter that uses two lasers to simultaneously measure blood velocity and vessel diameter. Blood flow is calculated from these two measurements (Figure 13.27). Used in a manner similar to a fundus camera, the CLBF provides an image of the fundus, from which the technician can identify a large retinal artery or vein to be measured (Figure 13.28). The unit then performs measurements at the specified site. The velocity measurement is based on the Doppler principle. The CLBF utilizes an innovative solution that allows the unit to deduce the orientation of the blood vessel under investigation.

Laser Doppler flowmeter

Laser Doppler technology has been employed to quantify ophthalmic blood flow. The Laser Doppler Flowmeter (LDF) is a laser Doppler device consisting of a modified fundus camera and computer. Unlike the CLBF, the LDF is not designed to examine velocity in large vessels, but volumetric flow in the capillary beds of retinal tissue. Though no longer commercially available, the device is well represented in the medical literature. The operator must position an illuminating laser onto a location of interest and a detector over the illumination point. The complexity and difficulty of operation have kept the Riva LDF from gaining popularity clinically or in research.

Heidelberg Engineering GmbH of Heidelberg, Germany has produced a scanning version of the LDF. The Heidelberg Retinal Flowmeter (HRF) scans the fundus, creating a map of retinal blood flow (Figure 13.29). Three flow parameters are displayed: volume, flow, and velocity. Values are in arbitrary units, absolute values depending on the optical scattering characteristics of individual eyes. Unlike the stationary laser point of the LDF and CLBF, the HRF laser quickly scans the fundus. Each scan line is divided into 256 individual points. Doppler shifts from each point are considered independently.

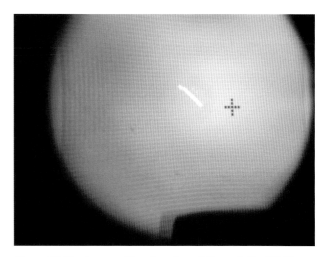

Figure 13.28   Image of fundus viewed through the CLBF.

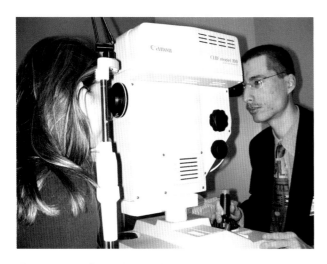

Figure 13.27   Canon Laser Blood Flow meter (CLBF).

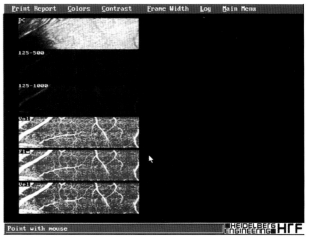

Figure 13.29   Map of retinal blood flow produced by Heidelberg Retinal Flowmeter (HRF).

Scattered light from each point is quantified as with LDF; however, only scattered light from the point of illumination is analyzed by the HRF. Since separation of the incident beam and detection point (as use: ! in the LDF) increases penetration of the measurement, HRF measurements will tend to be concentrated on surface vasculature. Further, the system is confocal, with a focal plane thickness of 400 μm, therfore eliminating the contribution of deeper tissue to the measurement.

As technology improves, the temporal and spatial resolution of hemodynamic measurements improves. When resolution surpasses the dimensions of capillaries, new problems in data interpretation occur. Previous technologies, including Riva's LDF, measure flow per volume of tissue to describe local hemodynamics. When capillaries and the areas between them can be resolved, a quantitative method is required to describe this new information. Utilizing the high spatial resolution of the HRF, an analysis technique has been developed which quantifies capillary density in concert with quantification of blood flow within those same capillaries. Using the HRF, flow measurements of living tissue are obtained at a resolution sufficient to discern capillaries and the avascular tissue between them. The percentage of tissue between capillaries is calculated as a percentage of total tissue volume. Individual flow measurements within those same capillaries are described in a histogram (Figure 13.30). Cumulative percentage landmarks

are then used to describe the distribution of capillary flow. This provides a complete assessment of the hemodynamics in a given tissue. To its advantage, the HRF measures volumetric flow, though in arbitrary units. Further, the HRF represents an important advance in hemodynamic analysis. With subcapillary resolution, the device has forced us to reconsider how we approach the description of blood flow. While the exact meaning of HRF blood flow measurements remains unclear, it has been demonstrated, through the use of *in vitro* models, that the HRF is sensitive to small changes in blood flow. The greatest disadvantage of the HRF is that flow measurements are in arbitrary units. The gold standard of ml/min/g has not been met and it is unlikely that the current instrument will ever be able to produce absolute measurements of blood flow.

Laser speckle flowmetry

Another technique called laser speckle flowmetry uses the interference pattern created by light reflected from the fundus and anterior surface of the cornea to measure the amplitude of fundus pulsation with the cardiac cycle (Figure 13.31). The laser speckle technique is a non-invasive technique capable of measuring a blood velocity parameter, albeit in arbitrary units. Further, the technique has produced reproducible measurements. The two greatest disadvantages of the technique are: (1) the technology

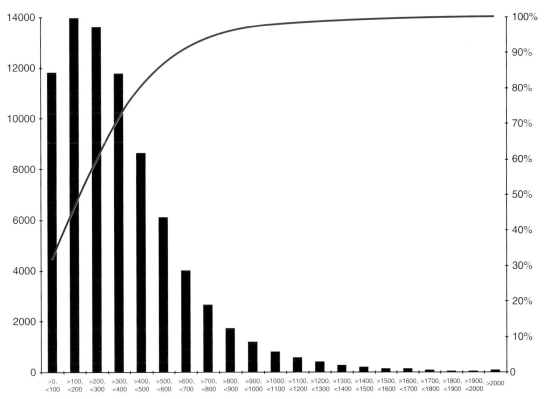

Figure 13.30   Individual flow measurements from within the capillaries as measured using the HRF.

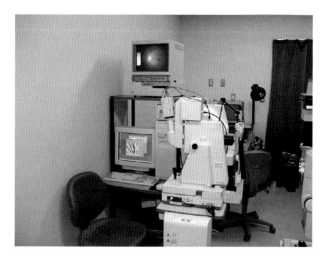

Figure 13.31   Laser speckle flowmeter.

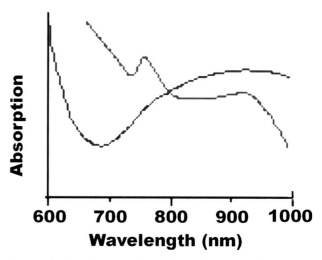

Figure 13.33   Plot showing absorption at various wavelengths.   From the digital spectral retinal oximeter.

is not commercially available; and (2) the meaning of the raw normalized blur measurement is not clearly understood. The technique is appropriate for the measurement of change over time if the optics are not significantly altered. The effect of progressive cataract on laser speckle measurements is unknown.

Digital spectral retinal oximetry

A new technique is digital spectral retinal oximetry, a non-invasive oxygen measurement based on optical methods, which detect the ratio of oxygenated (red) to deoxygenated (blue) blood (Figure 13.32). As evidenced by their different colors, oxygenated and deoxygenated hemoglobin possess different optical characteristics. Measurement involves passing two wavelengths of light through (or bouncing them off) the tissue of interest. The ratio between the resulting light intensities represents oxygen tension (Figures 13.33 and 13.34). The application of oximetry measurements in the study of basic ophthalmic disease processes as well as the pharmaceutical

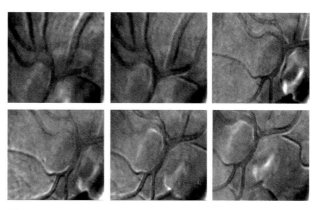

Figure 13.34   Images obtained with the digital spectral retinal oximeter at differing wavelengths.

effects of existing topical medications on retinal oxygen tension is of immense interest to both government funding agencies and pharmaceutical companies alike.

Magnetic resonance oximetry

Magnetic resonance oximetry measurements are based on the principle that oxygen is a paramagnetic compound that directly influences the spin-lattice relaxation rate (1/T1). The T1 relaxation time is a function of many factors besides local oxygen tension. To eliminate other factors that can affect the observed T1, such as flow, measurements are limited to the posterior vitreous near the retina. Oxygenation of the posterior vitreous near the retina is used as a measure of inner retinal oxygenation (Figure 13.35).

Retinal Vessel Analyzer

The Retinal Vessel Analyzer (RVA) from Jena produces real-time measurements of large retinal vessels

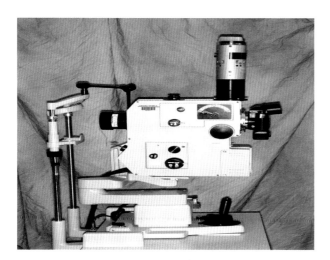

Figure 13.32   Digital spectral retinal oximeter.

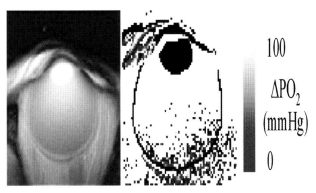

Figure 13.35 Image and digital representation of the inner retina using magnetic resonance oximetry.

with a spatial resolution less than 1 μm. This is accomplished through a statistical process. The physical resolution of the device is approximately 17 μm per pixel. By performing a rapid series of vessel diameter measurements and maintaining a floating average over time, the device has demonstrated the ability to accurately monitor the pulsation of retinal vessels throughout the cardiac cycle. The RVA provides information on vascular tone and may be useful in the examination of the effect of vasoactive compounds on the large retinal vasculature.

CONCLUSIONS

According to evidence-based medicine in 1993, the effectiveness of IOP reduction in glaucoma treatment had not yet been established. Today, the role of vascular factors in the management of glaucoma is in the same position as IOP was just over a decade ago. The only vascular factor consistently meeting the criteria required for clinical consideration is diastolic perfusion pressure. There is currently no evidence supporting the role of ischemia in the clinical management of the disease, in spite of numerous small clinical findings supporting the role of vascular deficits and ischemia in glaucoma. Existing clinical research supports the funding of a large-scale prospective ocular hemodynamic study in glaucoma. Technology for the comprehensive assessment of vascular hemodynamics exists in the clinical research environment. The technology for metabolic measurements of retinal oxygen consumption is under development and will be applied in clinical research in the near future. Using these techniques, the literature contains numerous examples of altered blood flow in ophthalmic disease. Current technologies cannot be used to determine whether altered blood flow is primary or secondary to IOP and/or optic nerve damage. Longitudinal studies may provide better insight into the role of ocular blood flow deficits in disease progression, but at a great cost in time and materials. As technology improves, more direct measurements may provide the answers to some basic questions:

- How great a blood flow deficit is necessary to cause glaucomatous damage?
- What is the threshold of perfusion deficit before nerve cell damage occurs?
- How can we identify this threshold?

Measurement of metabolism may provide the answer. Several types of measurement would be of interest. Desired measurements include retinal oximetry, quantification of metabolites, reduction/oxidation potentials, or perhaps ATP/NADH$^+$ levels. Using spectral analysis of reflected light, work is underway in the development of retinal oximetry, but a system suitable for clinical use is still years away. These measurements will allow us to fine-tune glaucoma medications as we gain understanding of how various drugs effect the environment in which neurons must survive.

Further reading

Alm A. Alder's Physiology of the Eye. St Louis: Mosby, 1992: 198

Anderson DR. Ultrastructure of human and monkey lamina cribrosa and optic nerve head. Arch Ophthalmol 1969; 82: 800–14

Anderson DR. Vascular supply to the optic nerve of primates. Am J Ophthalmol 1970; 70: 341–51

Anderson DR, Braverman S. Reevaluation of the optic disk vasculature. Am J Ophthalmol 1976; 82: 165–74

Bill A, Sperber GO. Control of retinal and choroidal blood flow. Eye 1990; 4: 319–25

Blunt MJ, Steele EJ. The blood supply of the optic nerve and chiasma in man. J Anat 1956; 90: 486–93

Bohdanecka Z, Orgul S, Prunte C, Flammer J. Influence of acquisition parameters on hemodynamic measurements with the Heidelberg Retina Flowmeter at the optic disc. J Glaucoma 1998; 7: 151–7

Burk RO, Tuulonen A, Airaksinen PJ. Laser scanning tomography of localised nerve fibre layer defects. Br J Ophthalmol 1998; 82: 1112–17

Butt Z, McKillop G, O'Brien C, et al. Measurement of ocular blood flow velocity using colour Doppler imaging in low tension glaucoma. Eye 1995; 9: 29–33

Chauhan BC, Drance SM. The relationship between intraocular pressure and visual field progression in glaucoma. Graefes Arch Clin Exp Ophthalmol 1992; 230: 521–6

Chauhan BC, Smith FM. Confocal scanning laser Doppler flowmetry: experiments in a model flow system. J Glaucoma 1997; 6: 237–45

Chung HS, Harris A, Halter PJ, et al. Regional differences in retinal vascular reactivity. Invest Ophthalmol Vis Sci 1999; 40: 2448–53

Costa VP, Harris A, Stefansson E, et al. The effects of antiglaucoma and systemic medications on ocular blood flow. Prog Retin Eye Res 2003; 22: 769–805

Cristini G. Common pathological basis of the nervous ocular symptoms in chronic glaucoma. Br J Ophthalmol 1951; 35: 11–120

Duke-Elder WS. Textbook of Ophthalmology. St Louis, MO: CV Mosby, 1940: 3354

Francois J, Neetens A. Increased Intraocular Pressure and Optic Nerve Atrophy. den Haag: DW Junk, 1966

Funk J, Muller-Velten R, Ness T. [Measuring retinal circulation with the Heidelberg retinal flowmeter: reproducibility of data and no effect of metipranolol in normal probands]. Klin Monatsbl Augenheilkd 2000; 217: 263–8

Galassi F, Sodi A, Ucci F, et al. Ocular hemodynamics and glaucoma prognosis: a color Doppler imaging study. Arch Ophthalmol 2003; 121: 1711–15

Glovinsky Y, Quigley HA, Dunkelberger GR. Retinal ganglion cell loss is size dependent in experimental glaucoma. Invest Ophthalmol Vis Sci 1991; 32: 484–91

Griesser SM, Lietz A, Orgul S, et al. Heidelberg retina flowmeter parameters at the papilla in healthy subjects. Eur J Ophthalmol 1999; 9: 32–6

Harrington DO. The pathogenesis of the glaucoma field: clinical evidence that circulatory insufficiency in the optic nerve is the primary cause of visual field loss in glaucoma. Am J Ophthalmol 1959; 47: 177–85

Harris A, Kagemann L, Evans DW, et al. A new method for evaluating ocular blood flow in glaucoma: pointwise flow analysis of HRF-images. Invest Ophthalmol Vis Sci 1997; 38: 439

Harris A, Chung HS, Ciulla TA, Kagemann L. Progress in measurement of ocular blood flow and relevance to our understanding of glaucoma and age-related macular degeneration. Prog Retin Eye Res 1999; 18: 669–87

Harris A, Jonescu-Cuypers CP, Kagemann L, Ciulla TA, Kreiglstein GK, eds. Atlas of Ocular Blood Flow: Vascular Anatomy, Pathophysiology, and Metabolism. Philadelphia: Butterworth Heinemann, 2003

Hayashi N, Tomita G, Kitazawa Y. Optic disc blood flow measured by scanning laser-Doppler flowmetry using a new analysis program. Jpn J Ophthalmol 2000; 44: 573–4

Hayashi N, Tomita G, Kitazawa Y. [Optic disc blood flow measured by scanning laser-Doppler flowmetry using a new analysis program]. Nippon Ganka Gakkai Zasshi 2000; 104: 148–53

Hayreh SS. The central artery of the retina. Its role in the blood supply of the optic nerve. Br J Ophthalmol 1963; 47: 651–63

Hayreh SS. Blood supply of the optic nerve head and its role in optic atrophy, glaucoma, and oedema of the optic disc. Br J Ophthalmol 1969; 53: 721–48

Hayreh SS. Structure and blood supply of the optic nerve. In: Heilmann K, Richardson KT, eds. Glaucoma: Conceptions of a Disease: Pathogenesis, Diagnosis, Therapy. Stuttgart: Georg Thieme, 1978: 78–96

Henkind P, Levitzky M. Angioarchitecture of the optic nerve. I. The papilla. Am J Ophthalmol 1969; 68: 979–86

Hill DW. Measurement of retinal blood flow. Transophthalmol Soc 1976; 96: 199–201

Hollo G, van den Berg TJ, Greve EL. Scanning laser Doppler flowmetry in glaucoma. Int Ophthalmol 1996; 20: 63–70

Jonas JB, Gusek GC, Naumann GO. Optic disc, cup and neuroretinal rim size, configuration and correlations in normal eyes. Invest Ophthalmol Vis Sci 1988; 29: 1151–8

Jonescu-Cuypers CP, Chung HS, Kagemann L, et al. New neuroretinal rim blood flow evaluation method combining Heidelberg retina flowmetry and tomography. Br J Ophthalmol 2001; 85: 304–9

Jonescu-Cuypers CP, Harris A, Bartz-Schmidt KU, et al. Reproducibility of circadian retinal and optic nerve head blood flow measurements by Heidelberg retina flowmetry. Br J Ophthalmol 2004; 88: 348–53

Jonescu-Cuypers CP, Harris A, Wilson R, et al. Reproducibility of the Heidelberg retinal flowmeter in determining low perfusion areas in peripapillary retina. Br J Ophthalmol 2004; 88: 1266–9

Kagemann L, Harris A, Chung H, et al. Photodetector sensitivity level and Heidelberg retina flowmeter measurements in humans. Invest Ophthalmol Vis Sci 2001; 42: 354–7

Ko MK, Kim DS, Ahn YK. Morphological variations of the peripapillary circle of Zinn–Haller by flat section. Br J Ophthalmol 1999; 83: 862–6

Lachenmayr B, Gleissner M, Rothbacher H. [Automated flicker perimetry]. Fortschr Ophthalmol 1989; 86: 695–701

Lieberman MF, Maumenee AE, Green WR. Histologic studies of the vasculature of the anterior optic nerve. Am J Ophthalmol 1976; 82: 405–23

Loewenstein A. Cavernous degeneration, necrosis and other regressive processes in optic nerve with vascular disease of eye. Arch Ophthalmol 1945; 34: 220–5

Logan JF, Rankin SJ, Jackson AJ. Retinal blood flow measurements and neuroretinal rim damage in glaucoma. Br J Ophthalmol 2004; 88: 1049–54

Michelson G, Schmauss B. Two dimensional mapping of the perfusion of the retina and optic nerve head. Br J Ophthalmol 1995; 79: 1126–32

Michelson G, Schmauss B, Langhans MJ, et al. Principle, validity, and reliability of scanning laser Doppler flowmetry. J Glaucoma 1996; 5: 99–105

Michelson G, Welzenbach J, Pal I, Harazny J. Automatic full field analysis of perfusion images gained by scanning laser Doppler flowmetry. Br J Ophthalmol 1998; 82: 1294–300

Nasemann JE, Carl T, Pamer S, Scheider A. [Perfusion time of the central retinal artery in normal pressure glaucoma. Initial results]. Ophthalmologe 1994; 91: 595–601

Nicolela MT, Hnik P, Schulzer M, Drance SM. Reproducibility of retinal and optic nerve head blood flow measurements with scanning laser Doppler flowmetry. J Glaucoma 1997; 6: 157–64

Olver JM, Spalton DJ, McCartney AC. Microvascular study of the retrolaminar optic nerve in man: the possible significance in anterior ischaemic optic neuropathy. Eye 1990; 4: 7–24

Olver JM, Spalton DJ, McCartney AC. Quantitative morphology of human retrolaminar optic nerve vasculature. Invest Ophthalmol Vis Sci 1994; 35: 3858–66

Onda E, Cioffi GA, Bacon DR, Van Buskirk EM. Microvasculature of the human optic nerve. Am J Ophthalmol 1995; 120: 92–102

Quaranta L, Manni G, Donato F, Bucci MG. The effect of increased intraocular pressure on pulsatile ocular blood flow in low tension glaucoma. Surv Ophthalmol 1994; 38 (Suppl): S177–S181

Quigley HA, Nickells RW, Kerrigan LA, et al. Retinal ganglion cell death in experimental glaucoma and after axotomy occurs by apoptosis. Invest Ophthalmol Vis Sci 1995; 36: 774–86

Ravalico G, Pastori G, Toffoli G, Croce M. Visual and blood flow responses in low-tension glaucoma. Surv Ophthalmol 1994; 38 (Suppl): S173–S176

Rhodes R, Tanner G. Medical Physiology. New York: Little Brown, 1995

Rojanapongpun P, Drance SM, Morrison BJ. Ophthalmic artery flow velocity in glaucomatous and normal subjects. Br J Ophthalmol 1993; 77: 25–9

Schumann J, Orgul S, Gugleta K, et al. Interocular difference in progression of glaucoma correlates with interocular differences in retrobulbar circulation. Am J Ophthalmol 2000; 129: 728–33

Singh S, Dass R. The central artery of the retina. II. A study of its distribution and anastomoses. Br J Ophthalmol 1960; 44: 280–99

Trew DR, Smith SE. Postural studies in pulsatile ocular blood flow: II. Chronic open angle glaucoma. Br J Ophthalmol 1991; 75: 71–5

Williamson TH, Harris A. Ocular blood flow measurement. Br J Ophthalmol 1994; 78: 939–45

Wolf S, Arend O, Sponsel WE, et al. Retinal hemodynamics using scanning laser ophthalmoscopy and hemorheology in chronic open-angle glaucoma. Ophthalmology 1993; 100: 1561–6

Zinser G. Scanning laser Doppler flowmetry: principle and technique. In: Pillunat LE, Harris A, Anderson DR, Greve EL, eds. Current Concepts on Ocular Blood Flow in Glaucoma. The Hague: Kugler Publications, 1999: 197–204

14 The developmental glaucomas

Carlo E Traverso, Fabio De Feo

INTRODUCTION

The congenital glaucomas are a broad group of entities defined as glaucoma associated with a developmental anomaly that is present at birth. Included in this group are primary congenital glaucoma as well as glaucoma associated with other developmental anomalies, both ocular or systemic. The term 'developmental glaucoma' is synonymous with congenital glaucoma.

PRIMARY CONGENITAL GLAUCOMA

Primary congenital glaucoma is characterized by an isolated trabeculodysgenesis in the absence of visible iris or corneal abnormalities. On examination, two major types of peripheral iris profiles may be seen: a flat iris insertion or a 'wrap around' configuration (Figures 14.1 and 14.2). A more severe variant of the disease exhibits peripheral iris stromal atrophy and anomalous iris vessels (Figures 14.3 and 14.4). Figure 14.5 illustrates normal iris vessels for comparison. The inheritance is sporadic with glaucoma occurring in approximately 1/12 500 live births, although a higher incidence is seen in the setting of consanguinity. Two-thirds of the patients are male with bilateral disease in approximately 75% of cases. Some clinicians further classify congenital glaucoma by age of onset: congenital (at birth), infantile (after birth, up to age 2 years), and juvenile (after age 2 years).

The treatment of primary congenital glaucoma is largely surgical (see Chapter 21), although medications may be used acutely to gain control of intraocular pressure and minimize corneal edema while awaiting surgery. Prognosis is related to the age of disease onset with a poorer prognosis associated with onset at birth. Even with successful IOP control, visual outcome may be limited by associated ocular problems such as myopia, retinal detachment,

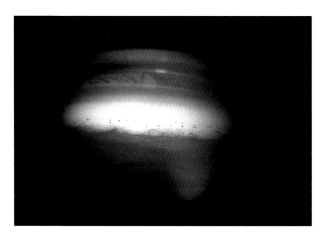

Figure 14.1 Developmental glaucoma, gonioscopic view. Note flat iris profile with anterior insertion. The iris processes extend irregularly over the ciliary band, and pigment granules are scattered up to Schwalbe's line. One anomalous vascular loop is visible over the trabecular meshwork.

and lens subluxation from pressure-induced buphthalmos (Figure 14.6), as well as corneal decompensation and amblyopia.

CONGENITAL GLAUCOMA ASSOCIATED WITH INHERITED ANOMALIES

Ocular anomalies

Corneal anomalies
Microcornea, defined as a corneal diameter of less than 10 mm, is not a specific disease but rather associated with other ocular conditions such as persistent hyperplastic primary vitreous, nanophthalmos, micro-ophthalmos, rubella, and Rieger's syndrome (Figure 14.7). Glaucoma may result from angle closure secondary to anterior segment crowding. Similarly, cornea plana and sclerocornea can be associated with angle anomalies and glaucoma (Figure 14.8).

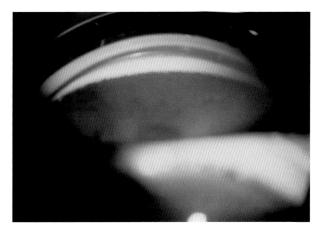

Figure 14.2   Developmental glaucoma, gonioscopic view.   Note concave peripheral iris profile with 'wrap around' configuration.

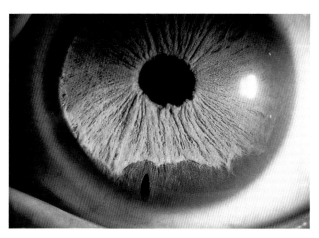

Figure 14.3   Iris hypoplasia.   The superficial stroma is thin, especially in the inferior periphery, and there is hypoplasia of the sphincter muscle.

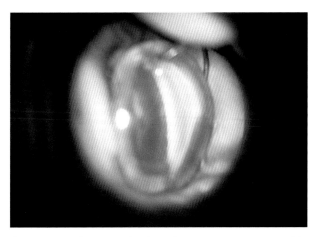

Figure 14.4   Gonioscopic view of anomalous vessels on iris surface.

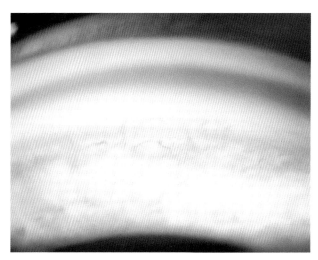

Figure 14.5   Gonioscopic view of normal iris surface vessels for comparison.   Note exposed greater iris circle vessels, which are commonly seen in patients with light-colored irides.

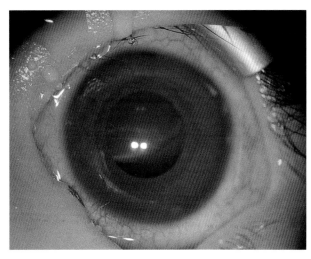

Figure 14.6   Spontaneous lens subluxation in a 12-month-old infant with primary congenital glaucoma and buphthalmos.

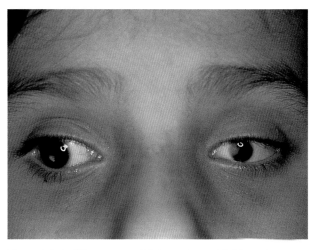

Figure 14.7   Microcornea OS in patient with Rieger's anomaly and bilateral glaucoma.

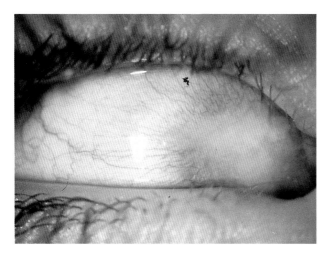

Figure 14.8 Sclerocornea.

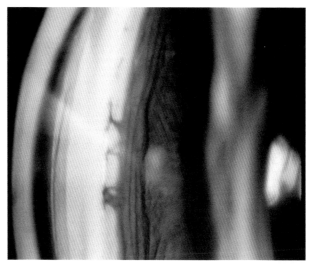

Figure 14.9 Axenfeld's anomaly, gonioscopic view. T-shaped strands of iris tissue bridge over the angle recess up to Schwalbe's line.

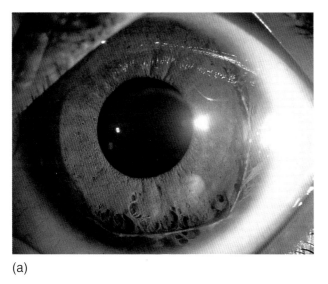

(a)

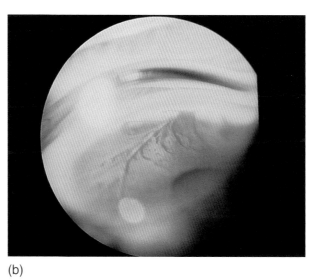

(b)

Figure 14.10 Axenfeld's anomaly with posterior embryotoxon. (a) The posterior embryotoxon seems to have been pulled from the angle wall, so that it lies over the iris surface like a clothesline. (b) Gonioscopic view shows the suspended embryotoxon as a refractile rope with multiple strands of iris attached to it.

Iris/corneal anomalies

Axenfeld/Rieger/Peter's comprise a group of conditions known as anterior segment dysgenesis syndrome to reflect their proposed etiology. Recalling that corneal endothelium, trabecular meshwork, Schlemm's canal, and the iris stroma all develop from neural crest tissue, it is hypothesized that altered embryologic development of neural crest tissue leads to the spectrum of clinical findings in this group of diseases.

Axenfeld's anomaly (Figures 14.9 and 14.10) is characterized by T-shaped iris strands drawn up to a prominent Schwalbe's line as well as anterior iris stromal atrophy. It is bilateral with an autosomal dominant inheritance pattern. Up to 50% of patients may develop glaucoma that presents in infancy or later.

Rieger's anomaly is further along this clinical spectrum and shares many of the findings of Axenfeld's with a greater degree of anterior iris stromal atrophy. Findings include polycoria, corectopia and pupillary distortion. Like Axenfeld's anomaly (and unlike iridocorneal endothelial syndrome), it is bilateral with an autosomal dominant inheritance pattern. Glaucoma is present in roughly 50% of patients with onset in infancy or later. Non-ocular anomalies may also be present and include dental (hypo- and microdentia), facial (hypotelorism, malar hypoplasia), and systemic findings (short stature, cardiac defects, empty sella, deafness, and mental deficiency) (Figures 14.11, 14.12, and 14.13). The term Rieger's syndrome is used when both ocular and systemic findings are present.

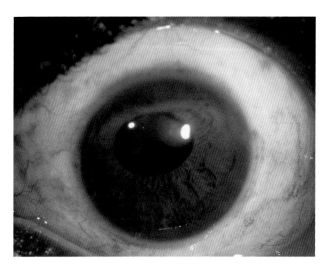

Figure 14.11 Rieger's anomaly. Note adhesions extending to the mid-periphery of the cornea. A posterior embryotoxon is prominent in the superior quadrant.

Figure 14.12 Rieger's anomaly. There are wide adhesions and the cornea is hazy in the affected areas.

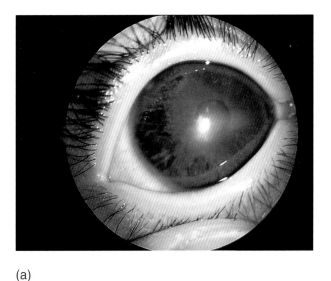

(a)

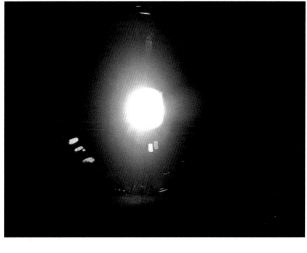

(b)

Figure 14.13 Rieger's anomaly. (a) Note marked iris hypoplasia with thinning of the peripheral anterior iris stroma allowing view of the posterior pigmented epithelium. (b) Transillumination defect of iris at 8 o'clock position.

Peter's anomaly is characterized by a central corneal opacity and adhesions between the iris collarette and corneal endothelium. Often there is absence of corneal endothelium and Descemet's membrane as well as stromal thinning underlying the central corneal opacity. Lenticular opacity may be present as well. Even in the presence of normal-appearing angle structures, 50% of patients will develop open angle glaucoma. Glaucoma may present in infancy or later (Figure 14.14).

Iris anomalies

Aniridia is a bilateral inherited ocular abnormality caused by mutations in the PAX 6 gene which may occur sporadically or with an autosomal dominant pattern. The sporadic form is associated with a 20% prevalence of Wilms' tumor (Miller syndrome).

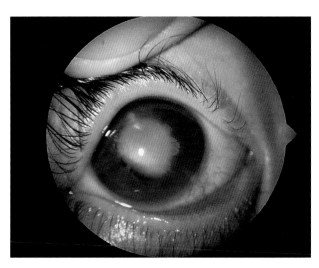

Figure 14.14 Peter's anomaly. Note the central corneal opacity and iridocorneal adhesions.

In addition to glaucoma, ocular findings include: rudimentary stump of iris, corneal pannus, cataract, ectopia lentis, optic nerve and foveal hypoplasia, and nystagmus (Figures 14.15, 14.16, and 14.17). The mechanism for intraocular pressure elevation may be adhesion of the iris stump to trabecular meshwork with progressive angle closure (late), or a primary trabeculodysgenesis (early). Glaucoma usually presents in the first three decades of life.

Iridoschisis usually occurs after the sixth decade of life, but occasionally is seen in children. There is bilateral patchy iris dissolution in which the anterior stroma separates from the posterior stroma, most often in the inferior quadrants. Iris strands from the anterior iris stroma may project into the angle, causing peripheral anterior synechiae, and leading to pressure elevation. Alternatively, pupillary block can occur with release of pigment and debris, further compromising outflow. Glaucoma occurs in about 50% of patients and is managed medically. Patients in whom pupillary block plays a significant role may benefit from laser peripheral iridotomy (Figure 14.18).

Lens

Microspherophakia may occur as an isolated finding or in association with systemic syndromes (see below). Clinically, the edges of the small spheric lens can be seen through the mid-dilated pupil. Other typical findings are high myopia and a shallow anterior chamber in a young person. Zonular laxity can lead to pupillary block with acute or chronic angle closure. Miotics make the pupillary block worse, since they result in further anterior lens displacement.

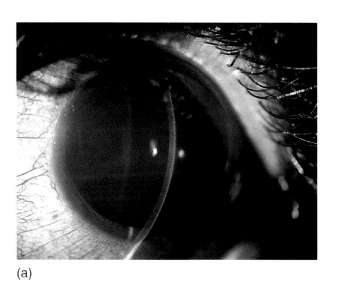

(a)

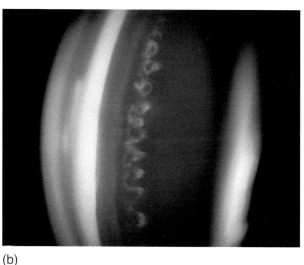

(b)

Figure 14.15 Aniridia.   (a) Slit-lamp view; (b) gonioscopic view. The angle is open.

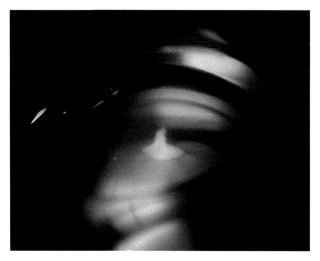

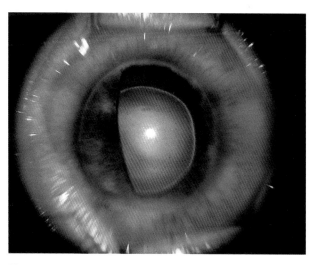

Figure 14.16 Aniridia, gonioscopic view.   There is a peripheral iris stump only. Note lens opacity with anterior pyramidal cataract.

Figure 14.17 Aniridia, partial, slit-lamp view.

Globe: nanophthalmos

The nanophthalmic eye is small but normally shaped (Figure 14.19). Small corneal diameter and short anterior–posterior length combined with a normal-sized lens leads to anterior segment crowding and angle-closure glaucoma in the fourth to sixth decades. Increased scleral thickness may lead to choroidal effusions, which can occur spontaneously or following filtering surgery.

Systemic anomalies

Lowe's syndrome

Lowe's syndrome is an X-linked recessive condition with findings of aminoaciduria and mental retardation in affected males. Characteristic ocular findings are cataracts and open-angle glaucoma in infancy.

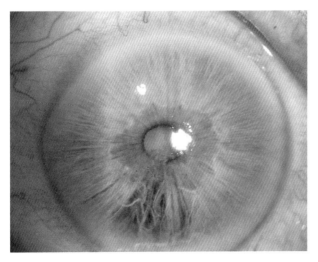

Figure 14.18 Iridoschisis in a 70-year-old patient with senile cataract.

Sturge–Weber syndrome

The hallmark of the Sturge–Weber syndrome is the hemangioma. Facial hemangiomas are most common and occur in the distribution of cranial nerve V. When cranial hemangiomas are present, there may be an associated seizure disorder. Ocular findings include lid, choroidal and episcleral hemangiomas (Figure 14.20). Glaucoma may occur due to primary angle dysgenesis (early) or increased episcleral venous pressure (late). Filtering surgery, which carries an increased risk of suprachoroidal hemorrhage, should be undertaken with great caution in patients with evidence of increased episcleral venous pressure such as blood in Schlemm's canal or dilated episcleral vessels.

Neurofibromatosis (von Recklinghausen's disease)

Neurofibromatosis is an autosomally inherited condition characterized by multiple neurofibromas, pigmented skin lesions (café au lait spots), osseous malformations and associated tumors of the brain, spinal cord, and optic nerves. The skin neurofibromas may involve the eyelids, and glaucoma occurs most commonly in this setting. The glaucoma may be due to a primary angle dysgenesis, synechial angle closure from neurofibroma tissue on the iris, or from direct infiltration of the angle by iris neurofibroma tissue.

Lens malposition syndromes

Several systemic conditions are associated with lens malposition and resulting pupillary block. Attenuated and broken zonules can lead to bilateral lens subluxation or complete dislocation into the anterior chamber (Figure 14.21). Lens subluxation is typically superior in Marfan's syndrome and inferior in homocystinuria.

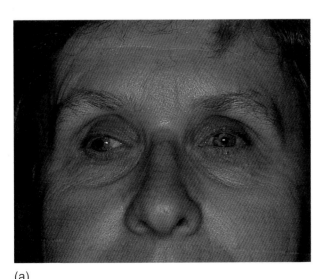

(a)

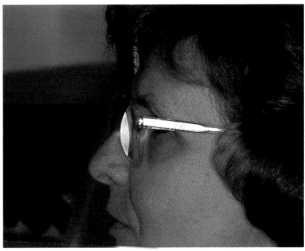

(b)

Figure 14.19 Nanophthalmos.   (a) Note small-appearing eyes. (b) The patient wearing phakic spectacles.

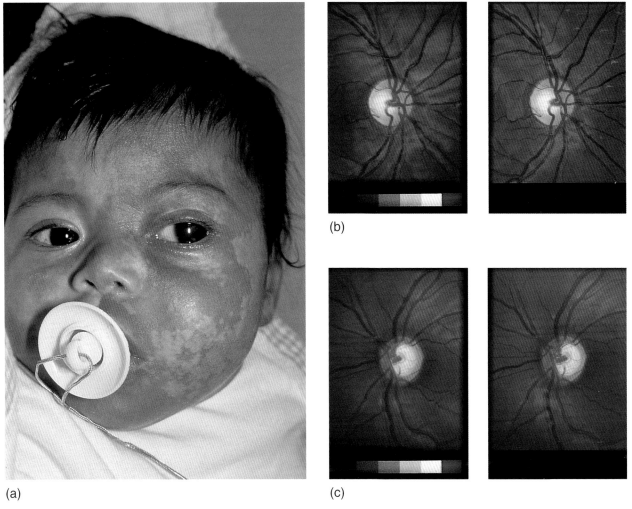

Figure 14.20 Sturge–Weber syndrome. (a) External examination. There is extensive facial hemangioma involving the first and second branches of the trigeminal nerve. Note left hemifacial hypertrophy and buphthalmos in the left eye secondary to elevated intraocular pressure. (b) Normal fundoscopic examination of the right eye. (c) Fundoscopic examination of the left eye with cupping of the optic nerve and 'tomato catsup' choroidal hemangioma.

Marfan's syndrome has an autosomal dominant inheritance and is characterized by arachnodactyly and tall stature. In addition to lens malposition and glaucoma, other ocular findings include microphakia, myopia, and retinal detachment. Systemic abnormalities include cardiac valve defects and congenital weakness of the aorta, which may lead to the development of dissecting thoracic aortic aneurysms.

Homocystinuria is a rare autosomal recessively inherited defect of the enzyme cystathione synthetase. Patients are characteristically lightly pigmented and may have osteoporosis, mental retardation, and seizures as well as tall stature. General anesthesia carries a significant risk of thrombotic vascular occlusions and should be avoided in these patients.

Patients with Weill–Marchesani syndrome exhibit short stature with short fingers and microspherophakia.

PATIENT HISTORY AND EXAMINATION

Historical information that should be obtained includes: time of symptom onset, previous medical or surgical treatment, family history of glaucoma, family history of ocular or systemic congenital abnormality, perinatal history (gestation, maternal infections, drug use, delivery), and consanguinity.

The examination of the patient is crucial for diagnosis and management, since most decisions and treatment options will be formulated solely on the basis of measured objective findings. The collection of objective findings can be performed at three levels: office evaluation, examination under sedation, and examination under anesthesia. The choice of examination level is made according to the patient's age and degree of co-operation, the ability and habits of the examining ophthalmologist as well as

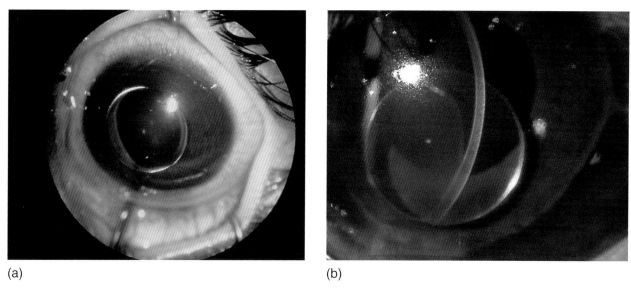

(a)   (b)

Figure 14.21   Homocystinuria with dislocation of the lens.   Homocystinuria with dislocation of the lens into the anterior chamber (a) and (b).

the anticipated amount of ocular manipulation. Below 6 months of age, a reasonably detailed examination can be carried out by pacifying the infant with feeding. After the crying triggered by administration of topical anesthetics has subsided, intraocular pressure measurement and gonioscopy are often possible without sedation. More complete examination (axial length, fundus photography, etc.) may warrant sedation or anesthesia with its attendant effects on intraocular measurement (see below).

Examination should commence with the nonocular structures to include the body, head, face, and extremities. Non-ocular findings may help make the diagnosis of a systemic syndrome associated with developmental glaucoma (see Figures 14.22 to 14.26). Attention is then directed to the ocular examination beginning with assessment of visual function (acuity, nystagmus, and amblyopia) as well as determination, if possible, of gross visual field defects.

Intraocular pressure may be measured in a number of settings and by a variety of methods. In the office, the young (less than 6 months old) infant can usually undergo accurate measurement with topical anesthetic while nursing. The Tonopen or Schiotz tonometer are most commonly used in this setting. For infants under sedation or general anesthesia, the Perkins type or the pneumotometer are additional methods (Figures 14.27, 14.28). Since most sedatives do not have a corneal anesthetic effect, use of topical anesthetic should be considered. During examination under general anesthesia, the best time for tonometry is right after induction. There are numerous factors which affect tonometry measurements regardless of the method used, including sedation and anesthesia, corneal abnormalities, and positive pressure on the periocular tissues (Figures 14.29, 14.30).

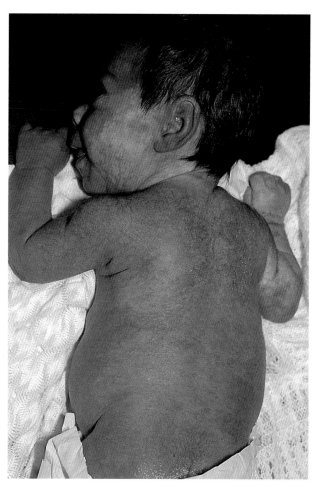

Figure 14.22 External examination of an infant with Klippel–Trenaunay Weber syndrome and bilateral developmental glaucoma.   Note hemangiomas of trunk and limbs.

The external examination often reveals the characteristic triad of photophobia, buphthalmos, and epiphora secondary to elevated intraocular

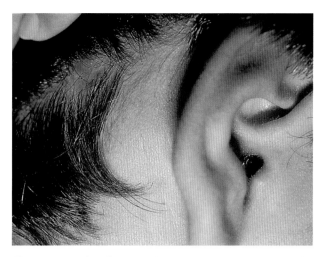

Figure 14.23 Head and neck examination of a patient with developmental glaucoma. Note earlobe malformation and scalp fibroma.

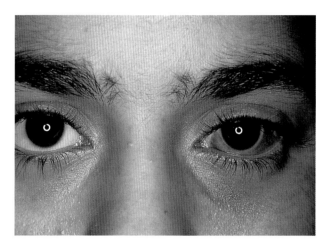

Figure 14.24 External examination in a patient with oculodermal melanocytosis involving the second branch of the trigeminal nerve and elevated intraocular pressure of the left eye. Note pigmentation of the left lower lid and sclera/episclera.

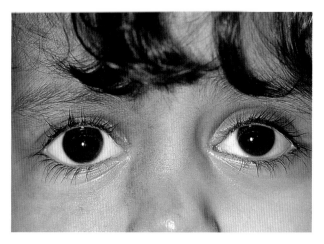

Figure 14.25 External examination of a patient with Sturge–Weber syndrome. Note the right facial hemangioma involving the second branch of the trigeminal nerve.

pressure-induced globe and corneal enlargement (Figures 14.31, 14.32). Corneal enlargement and decompensation with edema may be reversible with effective lowering of intraocular pressure (Figure 14.33). Corneal diameter is measured and monitored as an indication of long-term intraocular pressure control in young children (Figure 14.34). Beyond the age of 3–4 years, there is limited enlargement, because the sclera and cornea are less distensible. Dramatic changes may be seen in patients with advanced disease resulting in corneal ectasia or scleral thinning (Figures 14.35, 14.36). Often, a less obvious degree of scleral thinning is present in these children, posing a risk of inadvertent perforation with scleral incisions and suture passes during glaucoma filtering and shunt surgery.

Penlight examination of the cornea may reveal gross abnormalities such as an opacity or an irregular light reflex indicative of corneal edema. Slit-lamp examination (Figure 14.37) permits a more detailed examination of the cornea and other anterior segment structures. Corneal findings include epithelial and stromal edema and breaks in Descemet's membrane. When Descemet's membrane is overstretched by pressure-induced corneal enlargement, linear breaks may occur. These breaks can result in acute stromal edema with accompanying photophobia (Figure 14.38). Since both edges of the ruptured membrane roll up when the cornea eventually clears, a typical pattern of rail-like defect is evident at the level of Descemet's membrane. Breaks occurring in congenital glaucoma are known as Haab's striae and are characterized by a horizontal orientation or a location parallel to the limbus (Figure 14.39). They are usually seen in the setting of elevated intraocular pressure and enlarged corneal diameter (greater than 10.5 mm in the horizontal meridian in the newborn infant). On the other hand, breaks due to birth trauma tend to run in any direction and are accompanied by normal intraocular pressure and normal corneal diameters (Figure 14.40). Iris abnormalities such as atrophy and abnormal vessels are noted and the anterior chamber depth is assessed (Figure 14.41). Lens clarity and position are noted as well as any evidence of phakodinesis.

Gonioscopy can be performed with an indirect gonioprism or a direct goniolens (see Chapter 5). The Zeiss four-mirror gonioprism or a direct goniolens (Koeppe or Layman) is preferred over the Goldman lens since no contact gel is required. Impaired visibility from contact gel may hinder posterior pole examination or anterior segment trabecular incisional surgery. Advantages of the direct goniolens include a magnified, 360°, distortion-free view of the angle in addition to a view of the posterior pole through the undilated pupil. The lens also stabilizes the globe in the awake (co-operative) patient with nystagmus or acts as a lid speculum in the sedated/anesthetized infant (Figure 14.43a). Light and magnification are

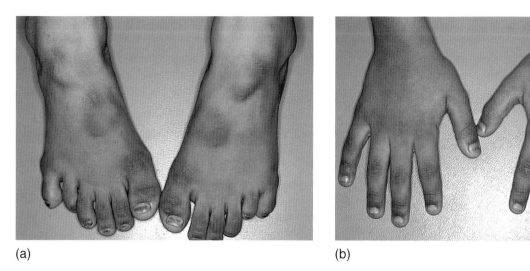

(a)   (b)

Figure 14.26   External examination of patient with developmental glaucoma and polydactyly.   (a) Of feet, and (b) of hands.

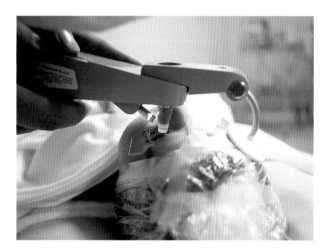

Figure 14.27   Perkins applanation tonometer.   The counterbalance modification to the Goldmann applanation tonometer allows measurement of intraocular pressure in the supine position during examination under anesthesia.

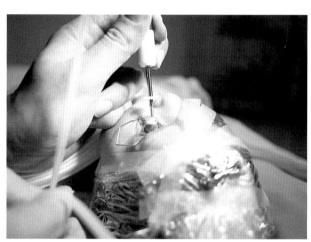

Figure 14.28   Pneumotonometer in use to measure intraocular pressure during examination under anesthesia.

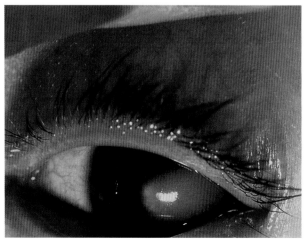

(a)   (b)

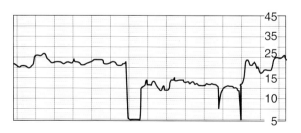

Figure 14.29   Tonometry artifacts, corneal abnormalities.   In this eye, differing tonometry tracings were obtained over normal and abnormal cornea. (a) External corneal examination. (b) Tonometry tracings. (Photographs courtesy of M Jaafar, MD, Washington, DC.)

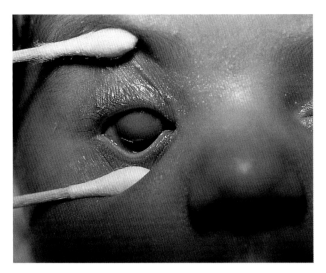

Figure 14.30   Tonometry artifacts, tight lids.   When the lid fissure is very small, one might artificially increase intraocular pressure by applying pressure to the lids. This illustrates a method of opening the fissures by placing cotton-tipped applicators over the bony orbits to minimize this artifact.

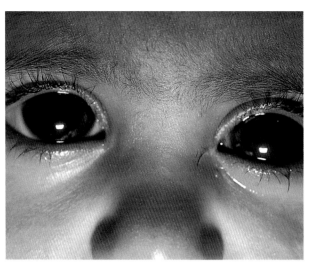

Figure 14.31   Epiphora and corneal diameter enlargement in a child with congenital glaucoma.

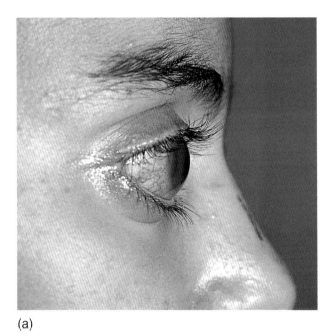

(a)

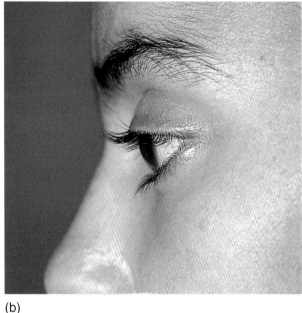

(b)

Figure 14.32   Buphthalmos in right eye of child with congenital glaucoma.   (a) Right eye. (b) Normal left eye.

obtained by means of either a portable slit lamp, the operating microscope or a light source coupled with binoculars (Figure 14.43). In normal infants, the trabecular meshwork has a pinkish, moist, transparent appearance. In trabeculodysgenesis, the color is more white/gray. However, since the normal infant angle features are often indistinguishable from primary trabeculodysgenesis, the diagnosis of developmental glaucoma cannot be ruled out solely on the basis of a 'normal' angle. Noteworthy angle features include the profile of the peripheral

iris, the true level of the iris insertion, visibility of the scleral spur and ciliary body band, presence of a prominent Swalbe's line (posterior embryotoxin), presence of a membrane over the angle, iris strands or adhesions, and angle vessels (Figures 14.44 to 14.51).

A dilated fundus examination is recommended unless goniotomy/trabeculotomy is planned during the same anesthesia. In eyes with small pupils, hazy cornea or nystagmus, a reasonable view of the posterior pole may be obtained by using a direct

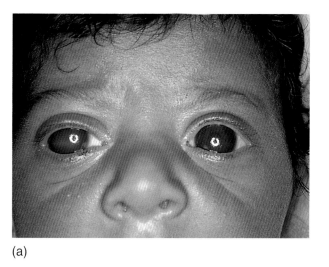

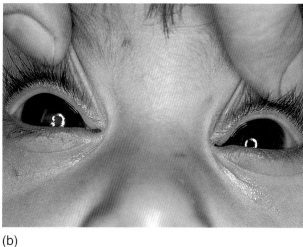

(a)   (b)

Figure 14.33   Reversible corneal edema in congenital glaucoma.   (a) Bilateral corneal edema at pressures of 40 mmHg. (b) Resolution of edema following trabeculotomy (pressure less than 20 mmHg).

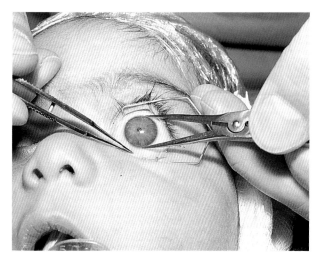

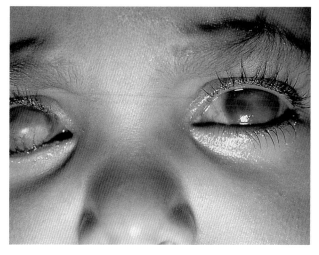

Figure 14.34   Measurement of corneal diameter during examination under anesthesia.   Diameters are measured in the vertical and horizontal meridians with calipers.

Figure 14.35   Corneal ectasia.

goniolens such as the Koeppe lens with magnification and a light source (see above). A direct ophthalmoscope may be used, but three-dimensional anatomy is not appreciated with this method and is especially important when evaluating the optic nerve head. Examination and documentation of the disc is of paramount importance for the diagnosis and management of developmental glaucomas. Disc asymmetry and enlarged (greater than 0.3) cup are rare in normal infants and children (Figure 14.52). Reversal of cupping with normalization of intraocular pressure is typically seen in infants and young children due to the distensibility of the scleral canal and lamina cribrosa (Figure 14.53). On the other hand, disc hemorrhage and venous occlusion with elevated pressure is unusual in this age group (Figures 14.54, 14.55).

DIFFERENTIAL DIAGNOSIS

Epiphora, blepharospasm, and photophobia in the infant or young child comprise the classical triad of congenital glaucoma (Figures 14.56, 14.57). Together or isolated, they are a sign of irritation due to the corneal edema secondary to elevated intraocular pressure and rupture of Descemet's membrane. However, they are not pathognomonic and other cases must be considered, as summarized in Table 14.1.

Elevated intraocular pressure can be due to topical steroid use, traumatic angle recession (Figure 14.58), or traumatic globe perforation with pupillary block. Acquired optic atrophy can be seen in retinitis pigmentosa or after trauma, as in the battered child syndrome (Figure 14.59).

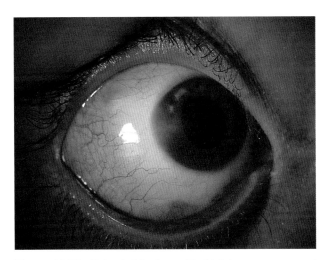

Figure 14.36 Scleral thinning with bluish appearance of underlying choroid.

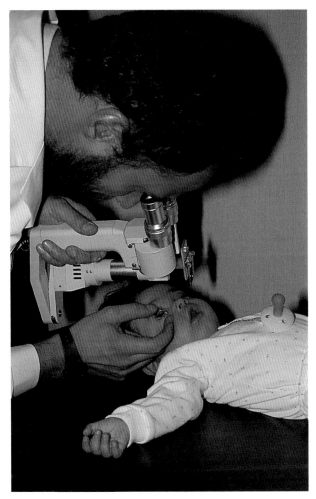

Figure 14.37 Examination under sedation. Portable slit-lamp examination of anterior segment.

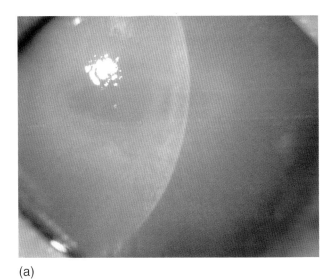

(a)

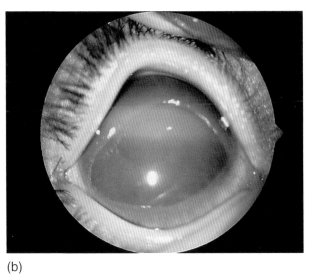

(b)

Figure 14.38 Acute corneal stromal edema secondary to breaks in Descemet's membrane. (a) Diffuse stromal edema. (b) Clearing with scar over site of rupture.

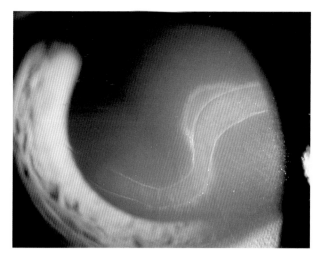

Figure 14.39 Haab's striae in congenital glaucoma. Note the typical pattern of rail-like refractile material at the level of Descemet's membrane.

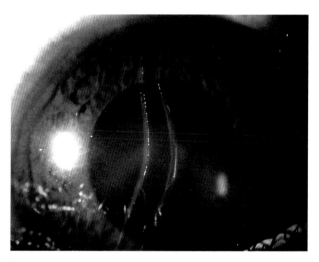

Figure 14.40 Birth trauma and breaks in Descemet's membrane. This child underwent a difficult forceps delivery. Note the vertical orientation of the corneal defect.

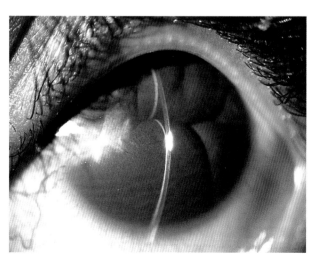

Figure 14.41 Shallow anterior chamber secondary to occluded pupil with complete pupillary block. This child had suffered a perforating injury in the past.

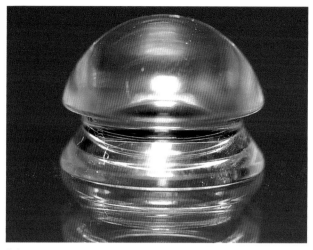

(a)

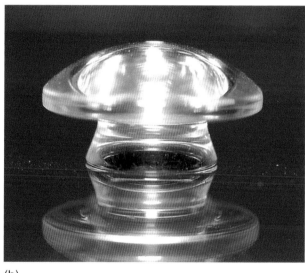

(b)

Figure 14.42 Direct goniolenses. (a) Koeppe lens. (b) Layden lens.

GENETICS OF DEVELOPMENTAL GLAUCOMAS

The most common forms of congenital glaucomas are characterized by genetic heterogenicity. Recessive forms are more evident in communities where marriages within the family are common. Abnormalities that involve a number of different chromosomes have been described and suggest that many different genes may be responsible for developmental glaucomas. Some of the genes involved in glaucomas associated with other anomalies, such as aniridia, iridodysgenesis, Peter's anomaly and Rieger's syndrome, have been identified.

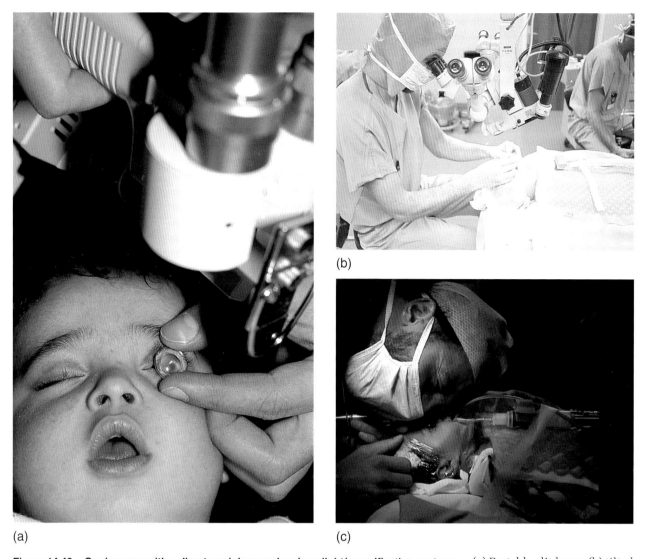

(a)

(b)

(c)

Figure 14.43   Gonioscopy with a direct goniolens and various light/magnification systems.   (a) Portable slit lamp; (b) tilted surgical microscope; (c) direct ophthalmoscope with high plus lens dialed in through a direct gonioscopy lens.

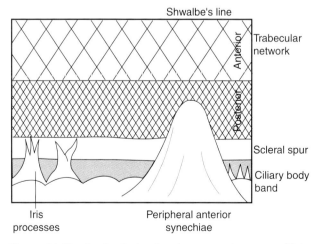

Figure 14.44   Anatomic landmarks on gonioscopy.   Note the difference between peripheral iris processes and peripheral anterior synechiae.

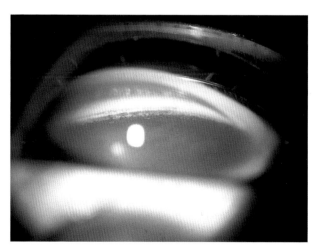

Figure 14.45   Primary congenital glaucoma, gonioscopic view.   The iris insertion is posterior and flat. The ciliary body band is covered by iris processes and is barely visible. Grayish pigment is visible just anterior to Schwalbe's line.

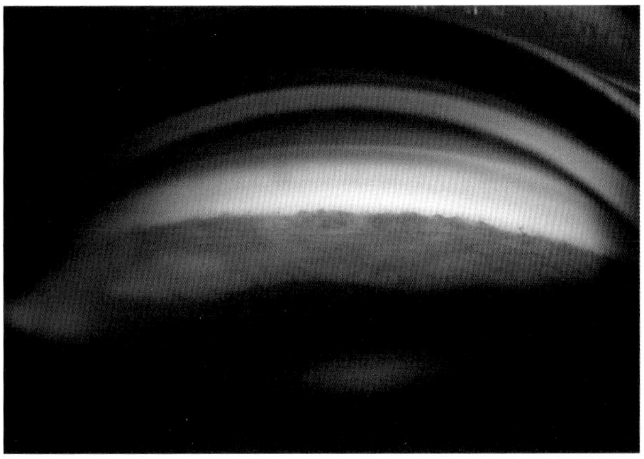

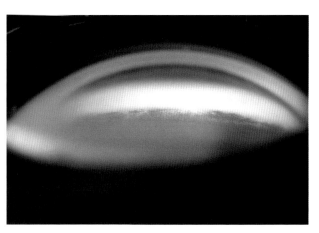

Figure 14.46 Primary congenital glaucoma, gonioscopic view. The iris insertion is anterior and flat. The tissue of the iris base extends to cover the scleral spur and most of the trabecular meshwork.

Figure 14.47 Primary congenital glaucoma, gonioscopic view. Pigmented granules of iris-like tissue appear to be enmeshed in a grayish membrane covering the trabecular meshwork.

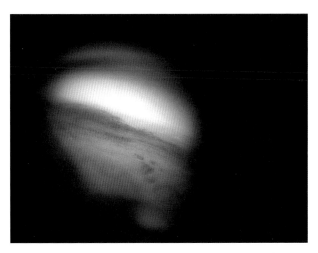

Figure 14.48 Primary congenital glaucoma, gonioscopic view. A grayish membrane covers the angle from the iris root to Schwalbe's line. Strands of irregular uveal meshwork are extended forward on the left side of the picture.

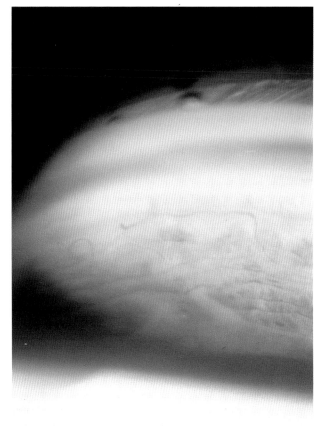

Figure 14.49 Juvenile glaucoma, gonioscopic view. Anomalous iris vessels loop in the periphery of the iris bridging over Schwalbe's line.

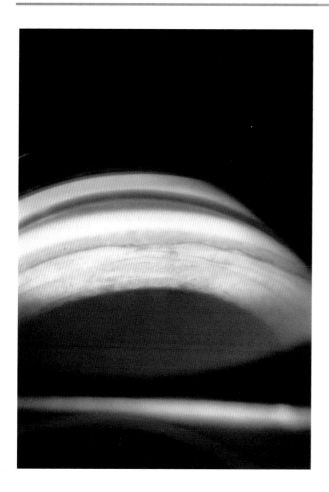

Figure 14.50 Sturge–Weber syndrome, gonioscopic view. In this patent the uveal meshwork is covering the angle structures up to Schwalbe's line.

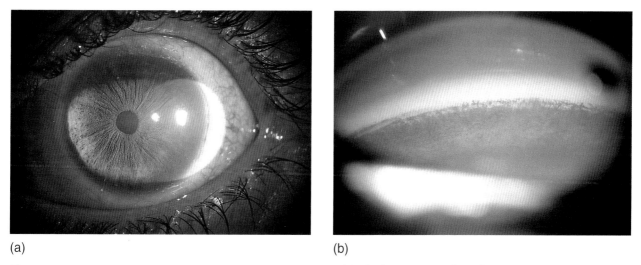

(a) (b)

Figure 14.51 Primary congenital glaucoma with iris hypoplasia. (a) Slit-lamp view. The sphincter is not visible. Radial spokes are the only iris feature. (b) Gonioscopic view. There is concavity of the peripheral iris. Strands of iris tissue extend to form a band over the trabecular meshwork. In the bottom part of the picture, darker pigment outlines Schwalbe's line.

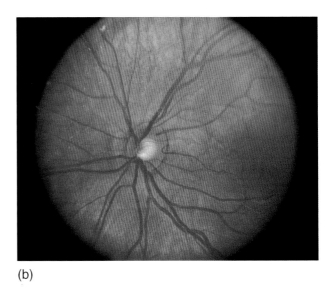

(a)   (b)

Figure 14.52   Disc rim asymmetry.   In this 11-month-old infant, the difference between (a) OD and (b) OS is striking, indicating more severe glaucomatous damage in OS.

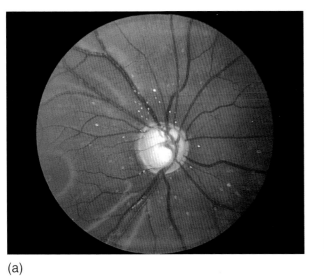
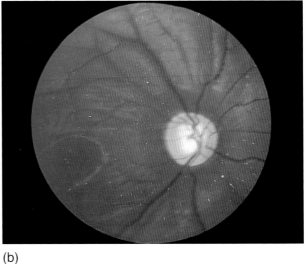

(a)   (b)

Figure 14.53   Change in optic nerve cupping with IOP changes.   (a) Before surgery with IOP levels approximately 40 mmHg. (b) After surgery with IOP of 14 mmHg.

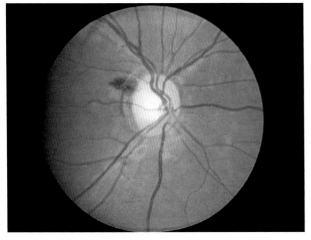
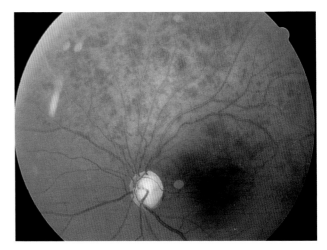

Figure 14.54   Disc hemorrhage in a case of childhood glaucoma.

Figure 14.55   Branch retinal vein occlusion in a case of advanced juvenile glaucoma.

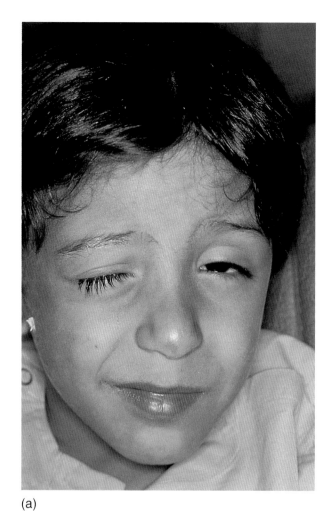

(a)

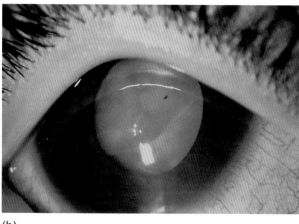

(b)

Figure 14.56 Differential diagnosis of epiphora and photophobia: trauma. This patient complained of epiphora and photophobia (a) but had a history of penetrating trauma (b) with corneal laceration and perforation of the lens.

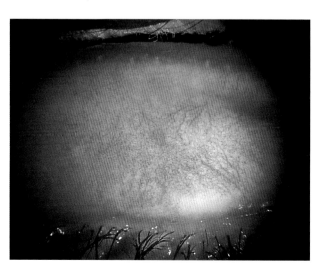

Figure 14.57 Conjunctivitis is a cause of epiphora and photophobia.

Table 14.1 Differential diagnosis of the signs of developmental glaucoma

Epiphora	Blepharospasm	Photophobia
Lacrimal duct obstruction	Corneal abrasion	Corneal abrasion
Acute dacryocystitis	Keratitis	Keratitis
Conjunctivitis	Trauma	Trauma
Trauma		Aniridia
		Albinism

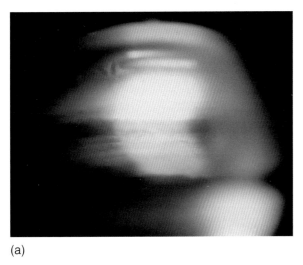
(a)

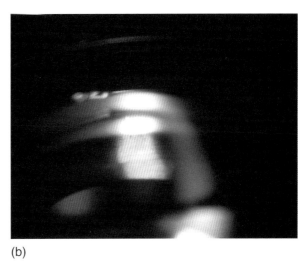
(b)

Figure 14.58 Traumatic angle recession. (a) This can be differentiated from a naturally occurring posterior iris insertion by examining the fellow eye (b).

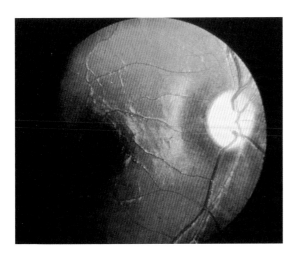

Figure 14.59 Optic nerve atrophy in a patient who suffered child abuse.

Further reading

Chang B, Smoth RS, Peters M, et al. Haploinsufficient Bmp4 ocular phenotypes include anterior segment dysgenesis with elevated intraocular pressure. BMC Genet 2001; 2: 18

Cross HE, Maumanee AE. Progressive dissolution of the iris. Surv Ophthalmol 1973; 18: 186–92

De Luise VP, Anderson DR. Primary infantile glaucoma. Surv Ophthalmol 1983; 28: 1–19

Grant WM, Walton DS. Progressive changes in the angle in congenital aniridia, with development of glaucoma. Am J Ophthalmol 1974; 78: 842–6

Hanson IM, Seawright A, Hardman K, et al. PAX6 mutations in aniridia. Hum Mol Genet 1993; 2: 915–20

Hoskins HD Jr, Shaffer RN, Heterington J Jr. Anatomical classification of the developmental glaucomas. Arch Ophthalmol 1984; 102: 1331–8

Mintz-Hittner HA. Aniridia. In: Ritch R, Shields MB, Krupin T, eds. The Glaucomas. St Louis, MO: Mosby, 1996: 859–71

Ozeki H, Shirai S, Nozaki M, et al. Ocular and systemic features of Peters' anomaly. Graefes Arch Clin Exp Ophthalmol 2000; 238: 833–9

Perveen R, Lloyd IC, Clayton-Smith J, et al. Phenotypic variability and asymmetry of Rieger syndrome associated with

PITX2 mutations. Invest Ophthalmol Vis Sci 2000; 41(9): 2456–60

Polansky JR, Nguyen TD. The TIGR gene, pathogenic mechanisms, and other recent advances in glaucoma genetics. Curr Opin Ophthalmol 1999; 10: 15–23

Quigley HA. Childhood glaucoma: results with trabeculotomy and study of reversible cupping. Ophthalmology 1982; 89: 219–23

Rabiah PK. Frequency and predictors of glaucoma after pediatric cataract surgery. Am J Ophthalmol 2004; 137: 30–7

Richardson KT. Optic cup symmetry in normal newborn infants. Invest Ophthalmol 1968; 7: 137–41

Shaffer RN, Weiss DI. Congenital and Pediatric Glaucomas. St Louis, MO: Mosby, 1970

Steinle NI, Tomey KF, Senft S, et al. Nutritional status and development of congenital glaucoma patients. Preliminary observations. In: Moyal MF, ed. Dietetics in the 90s. Role of the dietitian/nutritionist. John Libbey Eurotext, 1988: 87–90

Weatherill JR, Hart CT. Familial hypoplasia of the iris stroma associated with glaucoma. Br J Ophthalmol 1969; 53: 433–7

Wiggs JL. Molecular genetics of selected ocular disorders. In: Yanoff M, Duker JS, eds. Ophthalmology, 2nd edn. St Louis, MO: Mosby, 2004: 12–21

15 Medical therapy for glaucoma

Paul S Lee, Donna J Gagliuso, Janet B Serle

INTRODUCTION

At the present time, reduction of intraocular pressure IOP is the only proven effective therapy for reducing the risk of glaucoma development or its progression. Several large, randomized, multicenter clinical trials supported by the National Eye Institute, discussed in Chapter 9, have clearly demonstrated the benefit of reducing IOP. These trials, which include the Advanced Glaucoma Intervention Study (AGIS), the Collaborative Initial Glaucoma Study (CIGTS), the Ocular Hypertension Treatment Study (OHTS), and the Early Manifest Glaucoma Trial (EMGT), suggest that chronic differences of just a few millimeters of mercury may be significant in stabilizing glaucoma (Table 15.1). As in other disciplines of medicine, the decision on when to initiate treatment and the selection of therapy is based on the individual patient. In addition to carefully assessing the expense, inconvenience, and potential ocular and systemic side-effects of treatment, the patient's overall health and life expectancy are also considered. These factors will help to determine how aggressively an individual patient should be treated, since the goal of therapy is the preservation of useful vision for the patient's lifetime.

Table 15.1 Summary of NEI-sponsored clinical trials in patients with open-angle glaucoma or ocular hypertension

Study	Stage of glaucoma (mean db)[1]	Treatment groups	Treated IOP (mmHg)	% IOP reduction from baseline	Rate of progression (%)	Duration (years)
AGIS	'Advanced' (−10.4)	ATT TAT[2]	12.3[3]	50	'0'[4]	10
CIGTS	Newly diagnosed (−5.5)	Surgery versus medication	14–15 17–18	48 37	14 11	5
OHTS	Preperimetric (0.24)	Medications versus untreated	19.3	22.5	4.4 9.5	6.5
EMGT	Newly diagnosed (−4.7)	ALT + betaxolol versus untreated	15.5	25	45 62	4

1. For each of the studies mean decibel measured on baseline HVF 24-2 or 30-2 Full Threshold (OHTS) was included in this table in order to compare the studies and define the relative similarities and differences in stage of glaucoma.

2. Patients in the AGIS trial were randomized to two treatment regimens ATT (trabeculoplasty-trabeculectomy-trabeculectomy) or TAT (trabeculectomy-trabeculoplasty-trabeculectomy). Black patients had less progression with ATT, white patients with TAT, but antimetabolites were not used during filtration surgery.

3. Only patients in the AGIS trial with a mean IOP of 12.3 mmHg were included in this table.

4. These patients when evaluated as a group did not progress, although some individuals improved and others progressed during the AGIS trial.

TARGET INTRAOCULAR PRESSURE

AGIS, CIGTS, OHTS, and EMGTS have provided guidelines for establishing target IOP in glaucoma patients (Table 15.1). Each of these clinical trials evaluated patients with different stages of glaucoma. Patients in the AGIS study, who had a mean IOP of 12.3 mmHg and IOP of less than 18 mmHg at all visits, on average, had no progression in visual fields over 8 years of treatment. Higher IOP during the study was correlated with greater visual field progression. Patients with newly diagnosed early OAG in the treated arm of the EMGTS had IOP reduced by 25% from baseline, from 20.6 to 15.5 mmHg, and the rate of progression reduced from 62 to 45%. In the OHTS the rate of progression to glaucoma was 4.4% in the treated patients compared to 9.5% in the untreated group. The IOP of the treated group was reduced by 22.5% to a mean of 19.3 mmHg. The newly diagnosed glaucoma patients in the CIGTS trial had similar rates of progression, whether in the surgical treatment arm with IOP ranging from 14 to 15 mmHg, or in the medical treatment arm with IOP ranging from 17 to 18 mmHg.

Different rates of progression in these studies are explained by the various ways visual field progression was determined, patients at different stages of glaucoma and with different types of glaucoma, and possibly the variety of treatments used to lower the IOP. What we have gleaned from these studies is that the lower the IOP the slower the rate of progression of the disease. Currently, the accepted thinking is that the more advanced the disease, the lower the target IOP. As these studies represent a relatively short time period in the course of disease in a glaucoma patient, it may be that achieving lower IOP earlier in the disease will prove to be more beneficial. Fortunately for our patients, lower target IOP is more easily achievable due to the more effective and better tolerated ocular hypotensive medications that became available in the mid-1990s.

When initiating therapy for a newly diagnosed glaucoma patient, consideration must be given to starting with medical therapy or going straight to surgery. The CIGTS has suggested that at 5 years from initial treatment there is no real difference in progression rates between patients initially treated medically versus those treated surgically. Certainly, surgery carries more risk compared to medical therapy, but perhaps lower cost over the course of a patient's lifetime. At present, the standard of care in the United States remains initial medical therapy in most cases of newly diagnosed open-angle glaucoma, with an individualized target in mind, periodically reassessing the patient for control and progression. The medical regimen is adjusted accordingly, with surgery remaining an option should it be necessary.

PRINCIPLES OF MEDICAL THERAPY FOR GLAUCOMA

Six different classes of topical ocular hypotensive medications (Table 15.2) are available for the treatment of glaucoma: prostaglandin analogs, selective and non-selective β-adrenergic antagonists, selective α_2-adrenergic agonists, carbonic anhydrase inhibitors, direct and indirect-acting cholinergic agonists, and non-selective α and β adrenergic agonists (Figure 15.1). The mechanism by which each class reduces IOP, either by decreasing aqueous inflow or increasing outflow is described in Table 15.2. Each class includes several different compounds and formulations, increasing the number of potential therapeutic options.

Various factors must be considered when determining initial treatment for an individual patient. These factors include medical history, history of prior adverse reactions to ocular medications, cost of therapy, frequency of dosing, and anticipated compliance with therapy. Ultimately, the physician must weigh which medication has the highest benefit/risk ratio and take into consideration which medication will result in the highest compliance.

COMPLIANCE

Since glaucoma is usually an asymptomatic disease, patients may have difficulty accepting the diagnosis and the need for life-long medication, particularly when vision is unaffected and they are asymptomatic. The lack of symptoms and preservation of central vision until late in the course of the disease hinders compliance since the patient does not realize the potential gravity of the situation. In addition, the medications may burn or sting and may be expensive, which poses additional barriers to compliance. It is important to take the time to explain the disease process, demonstrate the potential for (or the presence of) visual field loss, and emphasize the benefit of the prescribed treatment plan on reduction of visual field loss.

Even 'convinced and committed' patients have limits on what they can successfully manage, especially when multiple medications are prescribed. Compliance studies demonstrate reduced compliance with a higher number of medications and increased dosing of medications. Several other factors have been identified which lead to reduced compliance, and these are listed in Table 15.3.

The medications currently available are extremely effective and, in many patients, when dosed as recommended, do stabilize glaucoma. It is anticipated that medications that will be developed in the future will be even more effective and may be able to be administered less frequently, thereby

Table 15.2 Topical ocular hypotensive medications: class, mechanism of action, and reductions in IOP

Class	Primary mechanism of action	Secondary mechanism of action	Trough and peak IOP reduction (%)[1]
Prostaglandin analogs	Increase uveoscleral outflow	Increase trabecular outflow	25, 35
Non-selective and selective β-adrenergic antagonists	Decrease aqueous flow		17, 29
Carbonic anhydrase inhibitors	Decrease aqueous flow		15, 24
Selective α_2-adrenergic agonists	Decrease aqueous flow	Increase uveoscleral outflow[2]	14, 28
Cholinergic agonists and anticholinesterase inhibitors	Increase trabecular outflow		27
Non-selective adrenergic agonists	Increase uveoscleral outflow		14

1. The range in reduction of IOP is from investigations of these drugs as single agent therapy. If an agent is used in combination with other drugs, less of a reduction in IOP is achieved.

2. Of the two available selective α_2-agonists, only brimonidine increases uveoscleral outflow.

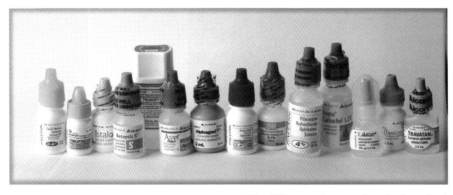

Figure 15.1 Classes of topical ocular hypotensive medications. Six different classes of topical ocular hypotensive medications are available for the treatment of glaucoma: prostaglandin analogs, selective and non-selective β-adrenergic antagonists, selective α2-adrenergic agonists, carbonic anhydrase inhibitors, direct and indirect-acting cholinergic agonists, and non-selective α and β adrenergic agonists.

potentially improving patient compliance. Currently, devices that may assist with instillation of the drops and act as dosing reminders are under evaluation. These devices include Xalease which is a delivery aid specifically for use with Xalatan, the Lumigan Compliance Aid for Lumigan which is a reminder device having a flashing light and optional alarm, and the Travatan dosing aid specifically for use with Travatan. The Travatan dosing aid has an audible alarm, a flashing light, and a one-drop dispenser mechanism, and it records when the drop is dispensed (Figure 15.2). These devices may be beneficial for some patients, but additional methods to enhance compliance that are tailored to the individual patient may need to be developed. Additionally it is important to educate our patients as to what is meant by q.d., or b.i.d, or t.i.d. dosing. Preferable terminology is every 24 hours and every 12 hours for q.d. and b.i.d. dosing respectively. In order to devise a reasonable three-times-a-day dosing regimen, a discussion with the patient as to the typical times they awaken and retire is helpful. The waking hours can be evenly divided so that the medication administration will be every 5–6 hours. If a patient is taking two or more topical medications, they need to be instructed to wait at least 5 minutes between dosing.

Table 15.3 Barriers to compliance with glaucoma therapy
Financial limitations
Education
Physical inability to instill drops
Other medical conditions
Life events (death, celebrations)
Forgetfulness
Travel
Side-effects
Understanding of the disease
Complexity of medical regimen
Daily schedule (regular or variable routine)

GAUGING EFFICACY

Ongoing assessment of the ocular hypotensive efficacy of a glaucoma regimen involves multiple IOP measurements at different times of the day, and occasionally diurnal IOP measurements. Diurnal measurements should be considered in patients whose IOP appears well-controlled on single office measurements, but are demonstrating progressive optic nerve or visual field change. Diurnal evaluation of IOP is most commonly performed in the office during the day, every one and one-half to two hours for several hours. Diurnal variation in IOP is greater in glaucoma patients than in individuals without glaucoma, and large variability in IOP throughout the day is a risk factor for progression. Thus it is important, particularly when a new medication is added, to determine that the IOP reduction is consistent throughout the day and is due to the treatment instituted and not the patient's baseline diurnal variation. Overnight diurnal IOP measurements are conducted very infrequently, in part because of the inconvenience and the uncertainty of the effect on IOP of awakening a patient. Recent studies have suggested that IOP is higher in the supine position than in the sitting position, and that IOP increases during the nighttime in some patients. These nocturnal elevations may explain progression in patients in whom IOP appears to be adequately controlled throughout the day.

Initiation of therapy or the addition of a new medication to a patient's regimen is typically done by adding one medication at a time. The new topical therapy is added to one eye and the untreated contralateral eye serves as a control. This has been called the one-eye therapeutic trial and has been recommended and used by glaucoma specialists for several decades. In addition to assessing therapeutic efficacy, unilateral instillation can also be used to gauge ocular side-effects. Although the one-eye therapeutic trial has been used for decades, recently acquired evidence questions the usefulness of the one-eye trial in predicting the efficacy of the therapy in the second eye. The difference in efficacy between the two eyes may be explained in part by asymmetric diurnal variation, asymmetric untreated IOP, and a cross-over effect from the first eye treated. Therefore, IOP should be reassessed in both eyes several weeks after adding the medication to the second eye.

Two to four weeks after initiation of therapy the IOP is again measured, sooner in patients with very high intraocular pressure or advanced glaucomatous damage. IOP reductions may be observed in both the treated and the contralateral control eye. The reduction in the control eye has been explained by diurnal variation, by a cross-over effect of the topical therapy, or by improved compliance in patients taking medication in the control eye. Reduction in the treated eye is due to the IOP-lowering effect of the medication in addition to diurnal variation. The therapeutic effect of the medication in an individual patient is estimated by assessing the difference in IOP before and after instituting therapy, between the treated and untreated eyes. The estimated efficacy in an individual patient can be compared to the anticipated efficacy of the therapy based on the documented responses to the drug in published clinical trials. If the IOP reduction is much less than anticipated and does not achieve the target, another class of compounds should be substituted. Addition of a second class of compounds should be considered when the efficacy of the first agent is similar to the anticipated efficacy, but the target IOP has not been obtained.

Large multicenter randomized clinical trials have determined the IOP reduction that can be anticipated from each of the glaucoma medications

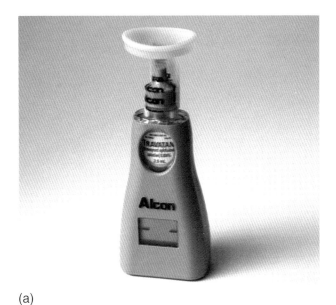

(a)

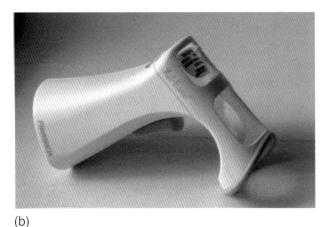

(b)

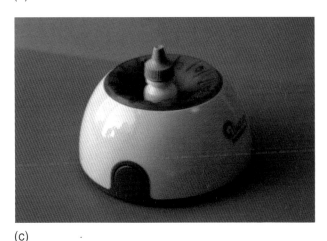

(c)

Figure 15.2 Dosing and compliance aids. Several dosing aids and compliance aids (a–c) are under evaluation for enhancing compliance with topical therapy. Each aid can be used only with the compounds manufactured by one company, due to the differences in the design of the bottles.

prescribed (Table 15.2). Responses in an individual patient may be similar to what has been defined in the large populations enrolled in these studies or may range from no response to occasionally a greater reduction in IOP. Each class of medication has been demonstrated in patients that are 'non-responders'. One explanation for a reduced response to topical ocular hypotensive therapy includes central corneal thickness. Patients with thicker central corneas may have smaller intraocular pressure reductions to topical therapy compared to patients with thinner central corneas. Measurement of central corneal thickness has become an important component of the assessment of patients with glaucoma. Thin central corneas were one of the variables associated with the development of glaucoma in the OHTS, and patients with thinner central corneas have been shown to have more advanced disease at baseline evaluation.

Additionally, medications may lose their efficacy over time. When a patient is on multiple medications, it is conceivable that one or more of the agents may be minimally effective. If it is not too inconvenient for the patient, consideration should be given to stopping a medication in one eye and performing a reverse therapeutic trial, especially when a patient has been on multiple medications for a long time without progression of the disease.

REDUCING SYSTEMIC ABSORPTION

Topically applied medications leave the eye via the nasolacrimal drainage system and are systemically absorbed when they come into contact with the mucosa in the oral and nasal pharynx. Reducing the amount of drug exiting the eye through the nasolacrimal canal will increase ocular contact time and reduce the probability of systemic side-effects.

Two fairly simple techniques may be used to decrease passage of topically applied medication into the nasolacrimal duct. The first technique is simply to close the eyelids for one to two minutes after instillation of the eye drop. This inhibits action of the 'lacrimal pump' associated with blinking that is responsible for the movement of tears across the cornea from the temporal side (where the lacrimal gland is located) to the nasal side (where the drain is located).

The second technique is punctal occlusion, in which pressure is applied to the area of the puncta and nasolacrimal sac, for one to two minutes following drop instillation, as illustrated in Figure 15.3. Both techniques, especially in combination, prolong ocular contact time with the drug, enhancing absorption while minimizing systemic absorption via the nasolacrimal duct. Decreased serum levels of topically applied medications have been demonstrated following the use of these techniques.

AVAILABLE AGENTS

Introduction of the prostaglandin analogs in 1996, the topically active carbonic anhydrase inhibitors

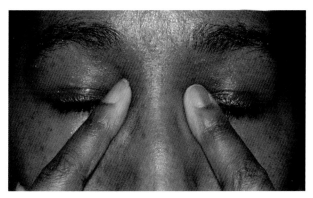

Figure 15.3 Nasolacrimal occlusion and eyelid closure. Nasolacrimal occlusion and eyelid closure should be performed for 1 to 2 minutes following instillation of topical medications to increase the amount of drug available for ocular absorption and decrease the amount of drug absorbed systemically through the nasolacrimal apparatus.

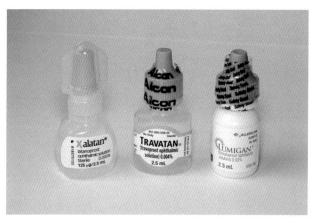

Figure 15.4 Prostaglandin $F_{2\alpha}$ derivatives. Currently, there are three prostaglandin $F_{2\alpha}$ derivatives commercially available in the USA: latanoprost (Xalatan 0.005%), bimatoprost (Lumigan 0.03%), and travoprost (Travatan 0.004%).

in 1994, and the chronic use of selective α_2-adrenergic agonists in 1993 has markedly changed the medical management of glaucoma. In addition to these three classes of compounds, β-adrenergic antagonists have been in use since 1978, parasympathomimetics since 1877, and non-selective adrenergic agonists since the 1950s. The relative efficacy, side-effects, cost, additivity, and probable compliance with each of these agents allows the physician to determine which of these medications should be prescribed for first, second, third and, if necessary, fourth line use. There are several different agents available in each class of compounds. Agents in the same class of compounds act at the same receptor and usually have similar effects on IOP. Thus, using two agents from the same class or substituting agents from the same class will typically not cause greater reductions in IOP. Side-effects of the agents in the same class may vary, due to different formulations, different preservatives and different receptor binding. Thus, medications in the same class may be substituted in an attempt to improve tolerability. A medical regimen should be designed to attain a target IOP, with the fewest associated side-effects, which the patient can administer on a regular basis.

Prostaglandin analogs

In recent years, a major shift has occurred in glaucoma management. Prostaglandin analogs have become the most common class of agents prescribed as first-line therapy in the treatment of glaucoma. This class of compounds is the most efficacious and is associated with the fewest systemic side-effects. Enhanced compliance is anticipated with the once-a-day dosing regimen.

Currently, there are three prostaglandin $F_{2\alpha}$ derivatives commercially available in the USA:

latanoprost (Xalatan 0.005%), bimatoprost (Lumigan 0.03%), and travoprost (Travatan 0.004%) (Figure 15.4). Lantanoprost, bimatoprost, and travoprost have been shown to be more effective than once or twice daily administration of timolol. Solo administration of these prostaglandins reduces intraocular pressure between 25% and 35%. The recommended dosing regimen is once-daily in the evening. Studies have concluded that dosing more frequently than once daily and that dosing in the morning rather than in the evening is less efficacious. There is no clear explanation for these findings regarding the optimal dosing regimen. These three FP receptor agonists reduce IOP primarily by increasing aqueous outflow through the uveoscleral pathways. They also secondarily increase traditional, pressure-dependent outflow, but do not reduce aqueous humor flow rates. The increase in outflow is due to the effect of the prostaglandins on the extracellular matrix in the uveoscleral pathway. Chronic administration of prostaglandins stimulates secretion of matrix metalloproteinases which initiate degradation of the extracellular matrix between bundles of the ciliary muscle, allowing for increased aqueous egress from the eye. The parent compounds of these three prostaglandins are prodrugs. They are cleaved by corneal esterases and enter the anterior chamber as free acids (Figure 15.5). The free acids have potent agonist activity at the FP receptor, while bimatoprost itself is also an FP receptor agonist.

These three prostaglandin analogs have been shown to be similarly efficacious in a number of studies. A few studies have suggested IOP reductions of 0.5–1.0 mmHg greater with bimatoprost compared to latanoprost. These IOP differences have occasionally been statistically significant and the clinical significance of these small differences remains to be determined. Data gathered from the

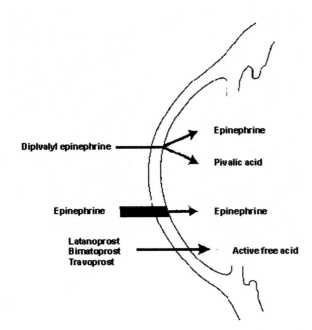

Figure 15.5 Prodrug metabolism. Prodrugs are designed to have enhanced penetration by varying the lipid and aqueous solubility characteristics, allowing for lower concentrations of active drug to be topically applied. The lower concentration of administered drug reduces ocular and systemic side-effects. Dipivalyl-epinephrine is a prodrug of epinephrine. In this case pivalyl acid is substituted for hydroxyl groups on the epinephrine molecule creating a more lipid-soluble compound that has 17 times greater penetration through the cornea. Esterases cleave the substituted pivalyl during transit through the cornea, producing pivalic acid and epinephrine. The three commercially available prostaglandins are also lipophilic prodrugs. Lantanoprost and travoprost are isopropyl esters, while bimatoprost is an ethyl amide. All three compounds are hydrolyzed within the eye to their corresponding free acids. The free acids are potent stimulators of the FP-receptor, which is responsible for the hypotensive effect of this class of drugs.

phase III clinical trials suggest that travoprost may be more effective in lowering intraocular pressure in black patients than in non-black patients. A rigorously designed study to address this question directly needs to be performed.

Ocular side-effects that may be annoying to patients include hyperemia and foreign-body sensation. The degree of conjunctival hyperemia associated with these three agents is generally mild and rarely a cause for discontinuation of therapy. Bimatoprost has been reported to cause the greatest degree of conjunctival hyperemia, and latanoprost the least degree of hyperemia. Individual patients may have enhanced responses or improved tolerability to one of these three compounds. Thus, in individual patients experiencing side-effects or in patients having less than expected IOP reductions, substitution of a different prostaglandin may occasionally lead to enhanced IOP control and/or to a reduction in side-effects such as hyperemia and foreign-body sensation.

Numerous ocular side-effects that are primarily of cosmetic significance have been reported. These include darkening of the iris, hypertrichosis, hyperpigmentation and occasional poliosis of eyelashes, increased pigmentation of the periocular tissues, and increased hair growth on the periocular tissues (Figure 15.6). The iris hyperpigmentation is most commonly observed in eyes that are not uniform in color, such as green-brown, yellow-brown and blue/gray-brown. The percentage of patients exhibiting iris hyperpigmentation varies depending upon the methodology used to measure pigment, the retrospective or prospective nature of the study, and possibly the ethnicity of the patients studied. Typically iris hyperpigmentation has been reported in 10–30% of patients, although one study in Japanese patients with homogeneous brown eyes reported an increase in iris pigmentation in 52% of patients at 12 months. Another study reported that up to 90% of patients with iris colors susceptible to color change had increased pigmentation after 2 years of close follow-up. Increased iris pigmentation is usually observed after a minimum of 3 months of treatment, and there is little information available about the reversibility of iris pigmentation following discontinuation of these agents. Periocular hyperpigmentation has been reported in Caucasian patients and in African-American patients, and reverses within weeks to months of discontinuing the prostaglandin analog. Hyperpigmentation of the iris and periocular tissues is due to an increase in the quantity of pigment within the melanocytes, and is not due to a proliferation of these pigmented cells.

Other ocular side-effects which have been associated with the use of topical prostaglandins include cystoid macular edema (CME), uveitis, and herpetic keratitis. CME has been observed in both pseudophakic and phakic patients with predisposing factors, such as a compromised blood–aqueous barrier or prior episodes of CME. Anterior uveitis has been observed in patients with prior episodes of inflammation or intraocular surgery, but very rarely in patients without these predisposing factors. Recurrences of herpes simplex keratitis have been observed during treatment with prostaglandins, and in some cases have not resolved until the prostaglandins have been discontinued. Prostaglandins should be used cautiously in patients potentially predisposed to or having a history of these adverse ocular effects. In contrast to ocular side-effects, the incidence of systemic side-effects is rare and includes upper respiratory tract infections, flu-like syndrome and headaches.

Distribution of a fourth prostaglandin analog, unoprostone isopropyl (Rescula), was discontinued in the United States in 2004. This drug was developed and initially marketed in Japan. It is a less potent prostaglandin analog and has less of an

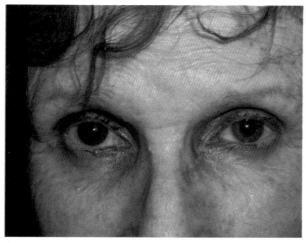

(a)

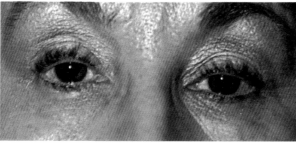

(b)

Figure 15.6   Ocular side-effects of prostaglandin analogs. Ocular side-effects that have been described with prostaglandin analogs include ocular hyperemia and foreign body sensation. Depicted is a patient (a) with unilateral pseudoexfoliative glaucoma treated with bimatoprost for several years in the right eye only. There is marked asymmetry in iris color, lash length and thickness, and inferior periorbital pigmentation. (b) This patient has been treated bilaterally for several years with topical latanoprost and has notable thickening and lengthening of the eyelashes. Other ocular side-effects of prostaglandin analogs that are primarily of cosmetic significance include occasional poliosis of eyelashes and increased hair growth on the periocular tissues.

effect on uveoscleral outflow than latanoprost, bimatoprost or travoprost. In contrast to these three agents, when used clinically, unoprostone isopropyl was dosed twice daily, was less efficacious than timolol dosed twice daily, and thus was less efficacious than latanoprost, bimatoprost or travoprost dosed once daily. The side-effect profile of unoprostone isopropyl was similar to that of the other three prostaglandin drugs. The smaller ocular hypotensive effect of this agent may be due to the lower potency of unoprostone isopropyl at the FP receptor.

Beta-adrenoreceptor antagonists

There are two types of topical ocular beta blocker: non-selective β1 and β2 adrenergic antagonists,

and selective β1 adrenergic antagonists. Non-selective β-adrenergic receptor antagonists are used as first- or second-line agents in the management of glaucoma. They are the second most efficacious class of compounds, following prostaglandins, can be prescribed once or twice daily, and are relatively well tolerated. Beta adrenergic receptors are found in many different tissues (vascular, cardiac, pulmonary and ocular). The receptors in the heart and blood vessels are primarily β1, while those in the lung are primarily β2. Agents that block both β1 and β2 receptors are classified as non-selective, while agents that primarily block β1 receptors are classified as cardioselective or simply as selective. Systemic blockade of β receptors decreases cardiac rate and blood pressure, and, in susceptible patients, can lead to bronchospasm. Blockade of the β receptors within the eye decreases aqueous humor production, thus decreasing intraocular pressure. Non-selective β-adrenoreceptor antagonists are highly effective intraocular pressure-lowering agents, typically lowering IOP by 25–30%. Selective β1 adrenergic antagonists are less effective than non-selective β-adrenoreceptor antagonists, typically lowering IOP by 20–25%. Both non-selective and selective β-adrenergic antagonists reduce IOP by reducing aqueous humor flow rates and do not alter pressure-independent or pressure-dependent outflow.

Several different formulations of non-selective β-adrenergic antagonists are available, including various solutions and gel-forming suspensions (Table 15.4). The efficacy of the various formulations is comparable when administered once or twice daily. Dosing of once-daily beta blockers is typically recommended in the morning, as beta blockers do not reduce aqueous humor formation or IOP during sleep. Patients should be instructed to administer once-daily beta blockers every 24 hours, as the maximum efficacy may wane in some patients after 24 hours. Thus, in patients taking non-selective beta blockers once daily, they should be reminded to instill the drops at the same time each morning. There may be differences in tolerability in individual patients due to the different preservatives and formulations, and some patients may express a preference for a specific product. Allergic reactions to all of these solutions and suspensions have been reported (Figure 15.7). The preservative-free unit dose formulation of timolol maleate (Ocudose) which is available at 0.25 and 0.5% concentrations can be prescribed in patients who have ocular allergies to preservatives. Some investigators have reported a lower incidence of systemic side-effects with gel formulations than with solutions. This may be due to less passage of drug into the nasolacrimal duct, which is attributed to the longer residence of the gels within the conjunctival fornices.

Table 15.4	Non-selective and selective β-adrenergic antagonists			
Generic	**Tradename**	**Concentration**	**Formulation**	**Preservative**
Timolol maleate	Timoptic XE	0.25, 0.5%	Gel	BDB 0.012%
	Timoptic	0.25, 0.5%	Solution	BAK 0.01%
	Timoptic Ocudose	0.25, 0.5%	Solution	None
	Istalol	0.5%	Solution	BAK 0.005%
	Timolol GFS	0.25, 0.5%	Gel	BDB 0.012%
Timolol hemihydrate	Betimol	0.25, 0.5%	Solution	BAK 0.01%
Levobunolol	Betagan	0.25, 0.5%	Solution	BAK 0.004%
Metipranolol	OptiPranolol	0.3%	Solution	BAK 0.004%
Carteolol	Ocupress*	1.0%	Solution	BAK 0.005%
Betaxolol	Betoptic S	0.25%	Suspension	BAK 0.01%
	Generic	0.5%	Solution	BAK 0.01%

BDB, benzododecinium bromide; BAK benzalkonium chloride

*Carteolol is no longer available as a branded product; only the generic is manufactured

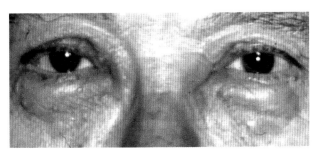

Figure 15.7 Allergic reaction to Timoptic XE. This patient used Timoptic solution without ocular side-effects for years, but developed an allergy to Timoptic XE following the initial instillation. Presumably the allergic response to Timoptic XE was due to the different preservative and vehicle. Recommended dosing of Timoptic XE is once daily, and is comparable in efficacy to once- or twice-daily dosing of solutions of non-selective β-adrenergic antagonists. Once-daily dosing of Timoptic XE may be associated with fewer systemic side-effects than once- or twice-daily dosing with solutions of non-selective β-adrenergic antagonists due to prolonged ocular contact and less passage of the drug through the naso-lacrimal system.

Carteolol (Ocupress; no longer available as a branded product), 1.0% solution is comparable in efficacy to 0.5% timolol maleate. Carteolol possesses a quality known as intrinsic sympathomimetic activity (ISA). Carteolol, while acting as a β-adrenergic competitive antagonist, also causes mild stimulation of the β receptors. Thus, it may have less of an effect on the cardiovascular and respiratory systems. Although studies have shown that carteolol causes a smaller reduction of serum high-density lipoprotein-cholesterol (HDL-C) compared to timolol, topical β-adrenoreceptor antagonist

therapy has not been associated with an increased risk of myocardial infarction, despite the association of reduced serum HDL-C with an increased risk of myocardial infarction.

Metipranolol (Optipranolol) 0.3% solution is also comparable in efficacy to timolol 0.5% solution. Initial formulations outside the USA caused granulomatous uveitis. The drug was reformulated and this side-effect has not subsequently been reported.

Betaxolol (Figure 15.8) is the only commercially available topical β1 selective intraocular pressure-lowering medication. It is available as a 0.25% suspension (Betoptic-S) and a 0.5% solution. The suspension is more comfortable than the solution for most patients, but the two are equally efficacious. Both formulations lower intraocular pressure between 20% and 25% from baseline. This agent can be considered in patients with mild to moderate pulmonary disease without other contraindications to this class of compounds. All β-adrenoreceptor antagonists must be used with caution in any patient with a history of reactive airway disease. It is advisable to consult with a patient's internist or pulmonologist prior to prescribing these agents in patients with pulmonary disease. Betaxolol has intrinsic calcium channel blocking activity, which may increase ocular blood flow. Additional investigations of this property and the potential clinical benefit need to be conducted.

Ocular side-effects with topical beta blocker therapy rarely are a cause for discontinuation and include transient blurring of vision, punctate keratopathy, and ocular dryness. Topical beta blockers are extremely well tolerated, although numerous systemic side-effects have been reported to be

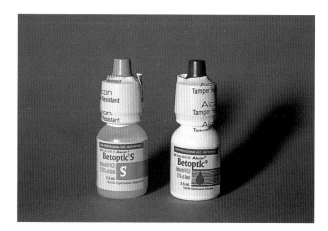

Figure 15.8 Betaxolol: a selective β1-adrenergic antagonist. Betaxolol is the only selective β1 adrenergic antagonist available. It is available as a suspension of 0.25% (Betoptic S) and as a generic solution (betaxolol) formulated as 0.5%. The suspension is generally more comfortable and causes less burning and stinging upon instillation. Twice daily dosing with these two formulations causes similar reductions in IOP.

associated with their use. An extensive review has demonstrated no support for many of the accepted associations, such as worsening of claudication, depression, hypoglycemic unawareness, or prolonged hypoglycemia in non-insulin-dependent diabetes, sexual dysfunction, or impaired neuromuscular transmission. Systemically administered beta blockers are used to treat mild, moderate, and even severe congestive heart failure. Topical beta blockers do cause mild reductions in heart rate which are most commonly asymptomatic. Patients who develop symptomatic bradycardia while administering systemic or ophthalmic β-adrenergic blockers may have underlying cardiac conduction disturbances, and in these patients a cardiac work-up should be considered. β2-Adrenergic blockade, regardless of route of administration, may exacerbate or trigger bronchospasm in patients with asthma or pulmonary disease associated with hyper-reactive airways. Therefore, these agents must be prescribed cautiously if at all in patients predisposed to pulmonary disease.

Carbonic anhydrase inhibitors

Carbonic anhydrase is an enzyme found predominantly in the ciliary epithelium, the kidney, the central nervous system, and red blood cells. It catalyzes the combination of water and carbon dioxide to form bicarbonate and hydrogen ions. Within the ciliary epithelium hydrogen ions are exchanged for sodium ions, some bicarbonate is exchanged for chloride, and bicarbonate and/or chloride are actively transported into the aqueous, with sodium and water passively following. The enzyme carbonic anhydrase must be inhibited at least 99% in

order to decrease aqueous formation. This degree of inhibition results in reductions in aqueous humor formation of up to 30% with maximum doses of oral carbonic anhydrase inhibitors (CAI) and up to 19% with maximum doses of topical CAIs.

The first clinically active orally administered CAI, acetazolamide, was introduced in the 1950s. Soon after its introduction, the numerous and substantial side-effects caused by CAIs became apparent. Therefore, in the 1950s the search began for a topically active CAI. Three orally administered CAIs are currently available. Acetazolamide is available in 125 and 250-mg tablets which are administered four times daily, and 500-mg time-release capsules (Diamox Sequals, which are large, oval orange pills) for twice-daily use. Methazolamide is available in 25 and 50-mg tablets which are administered two to three times daily, and dichlorphenamide (Daranide) is available in 50-mg tablets administered two to three times daily. Methazolamide has a theoretical advantage over acetazolamide in that it is less bound to plasma proteins, and thus may elicit less systemic toxicity than acetazolamide.

Clinical use of the orally administered CAIs, especially in the long term, is limited by the potential for systemic side-effects. Since all CAIs are sulfa derivatives, they must be used with caution, if at all, in patients with sulfa allergies. Frequently encountered side-effects include anorexia, weight loss, fatigue and drowsiness, general malaise, tingling and numbness in the hands and feet, metallic taste in the mouth after ingestion of carbonated beverages, gastrointestinal upset (including diarrhea and nausea), potassium loss with the attendant complications of hypokalemia (which could be fatal in patients taking digitalis), kidney stones (less common with methazolamide), systemic acidosis, and shortness of breath. Idiosyncratic reactions may result in fatal aplastic anemia, estimated to occur in 1 in 18 000 patient-years. Indications for oral CAIs include short-term adjunctive therapy, particularly for acute pressure elevations or to temporize prior to planned surgical intervention, and if necessary for chronic use in patients who are unwilling or unable to administer topical medications or are unable to undergo glaucoma surgery.

The numerous side-effects of oral CAIs resulted in five decades of research which culminated in the development and release of the first topically active CAI, dorzolamide 2% (Trusopt). Used three times daily, the drug is approximately equal in efficacy to betaxolol, and slightly less effective than timolol. It is an excellent additive drug to topical β-adrenoreceptor antagonists, resulting in reductions in intraocular pressure reaching 35% from baseline. Many glaucoma specialists are of the opinion that twice-daily dosing of dorzolamide is sufficient when the drug is used as additive therapy, although the effectiveness of twice-daily dosing when used in combination with other drugs for 24-hour pressure control is unproven. The drug is fairly well tolerated with minimal or no systemic side-effects. The most common side-effects are stinging and burning upon instillation, reported in up to 33% of patients, and bitter taste, which has been reported in up to 25% of patients. Allergic blepharoconjunctivitis (Figure 15.9) occurs in a small number of patients. Since dorzolamide is a sulfa derivative, it should be used cautiously in patients with known allergy to sulfa drugs.

Subsequently in 1998 brinzolamide 1% (Azopt), a second topical CAI, was approved for clinical use. Brinzolamide is similar in efficacy to dorzolamide and is also administered two or three times daily. The most common ocular side-effects of these two agents differ, however. Because brinzolamide is a suspension, it may cause blurring upon instillation, while the most common ocular side-effect with use of dorzolamide is stinging upon instillation.

α2-Adrenergic agonists

Two α2 adrenergic receptor agonists, brimonidine tartrate (Alphagan) and apraclonidine (Iopidine) are used for the acute and chronic management of elevated IOP. Apraclonidine 1% solution was the first of these two agents to be approved, in 1987, to treat acute elevations in IOP and to prevent postoperative pressure rises following ophthalmic laser procedures and cataract surgery. Subsequently, in 1992, the 0.5% concentration was approved for

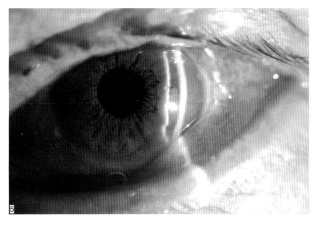

Figure 15.9   Allergic blepharoconjunctivitis and dorzolamide. Topical carbonic anhydrase inhibitors cause allergic blepharoconjunctivitis in a small percentage of patients. The allergic response is indistinguishable from that caused by other topical agents and preservatives, and includes hyperemia, chemosis, and follicles. This patient administered dorzolamide to one eye and developed this allergic response within 2 weeks of beginning instillation. Allergic responses can occur soon after beginning dosing with a medication or after months, or in some patients after years of therapy.

chronic use in treating elevated IOP. Brimonidine tartrate, approved for clinical use in 1993, is a more selective α2-adrenergic agonist than apraclonidine, and thus has fewer α1-related side-effects, including lid retraction, conjunctival blanching, and pupil dilatation. Apraclonidine and brimonidine both lower IOP by decreasing aqueous flow. Additionally, brimonidine also lowers pressure by increasing uveoscleral outflow. Brimonidine is available as a generic 0.2% solution and as 0.15% and 0.1% (Alphagan P) concentrations in a carboxymethylcellulose vehicle (Purite). Twice daily administration of brimonidine 0.2% is similar in efficacy to twice daily administration of 0.5% timolol at peak (2 hours after administration), although brimonidine is less efficacious than timolol at trough (12 hours after administration). Twice daily administration of brimonidine 0.2% is more efficacious than twice daily administration of 0.5% betaxolol at peak (2 hours after administration), and comparable in efficacy to 0.5% betaxolol at trough (12 hours after administration).

Apraclonidine 0.5% administered three times daily, similar to brimonidine, is less efficacious at trough than timolol 0.5% administered twice daily. Both apraclonidine and brimonidine have been approved by the US FDA for use three times daily. These agents are commonly prescribed twice daily due to the poor compliance with t.i.d dosing. IOP should be evaluated in the afternoon to determine whether t.i.d dosing would be beneficial in an individual patient. Side-effects include dry mouth, fatigue, drowsiness, systemic hypotension, and ocular allergy, which occurs in about 12% of patients receiving brimonidine and up to 35% of patients receiving apraclonidine (Figure 15.10). An allergic response to apraclonidine does not preclude the use of brimonidine. Between 10% and 20% of patients with a documented ocular allergic response to apraclonidine developed an allergy to brimonidine. Brimonidine was formulated in concentrations of 0.15% and 0.1% to reduce the rate of allergy. Release of and use of the generic brimonidine 0.2% has been associated with an increased rate of allergy.

If one of these selective α-adrenergic agonists is used chronically, use of the other agent will not block acute IOP elevations, such as following laser therapy. Another class of compounds that the patient is not using chronically should be administered to treat acute IOP elevations.

Brimonidine should be used with extreme caution in children, as in young patients the drug has been associated with bradycardia, hypotension, hypothermia, hypotonia, apnea, dyspnea, hypoventilation. cyanosis, and lethargy, resulting in hospitalization Although the CNS side-effects are significant, no deaths have been reported in children receiving topical brimonidine. The incidence of side-effects

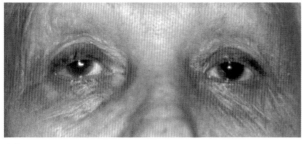

(a)

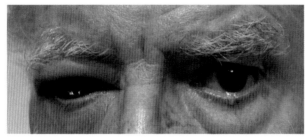

(b)

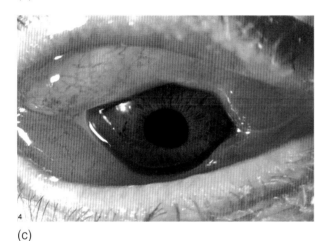

(c)

Figure 15.10 Allergic blepharoconjunctivitis with apraclonidine and brimonidine. (a) A patient with bilateral allergic blepharoconjunctivitis and marked erythema of the lids following administration of apraclonidine 0.5% b.i.d. for several months. (b and c) A patient with unilateral conjunctivitis, marked chemosis and periorbital edema following 2 weeks of unilateral treatment with generic brimonidine 0.2%. Brimonidine 0.15% (Alphagan P) has a lower incidence of ocular allergy than the 0.2% formulation, which may be due to the lower concentration of brimonidine as well as the different vehicles. The relative incidence of allergy with the newest formulation of brimonidine, 0.1%, is under evaluation. Allergic conjunctivitis can be seen with application of any and all of the topical ocular hypotensive medications in clinical use. This allergic response can be due to the drugs or the preservatives or the vehicle. Typically the allergic reaction will resolve within weeks after discontinuation of the medication. If the response is particularly severe, topical steroids can be used if not otherwise contraindicated.

increases with younger age and lower weight. The FDA-approved package insert cautions that the drug is not for use in pediatric patients less than 2

years of age. Brimonidine should be used cautiously, if at all, in patients younger than age 6 and in patients who weigh less than 20 kg.

Cholinergic agonists (miotics)

Cholinergic agonists are the oldest class of compounds that have been used to treat glaucoma, with initial reports of their use in 1877. This class of compounds is currently used infrequently because of the numerous ocular side-effects and the need for frequent instillation. Cholinergic agonists lower IOP by increasing pressure-dependent trabecular outflow facility. Stimulation of the longitudinal muscle of the ciliary body (via the parasympathetic pathways mediated by acetylcholine) increases traction on the scleral spur, which in turn increases the tension on the trabecular meshwork, resulting in increased outflow facility. This effect on IOP may be achieved by direct stimulation of the cholinergic receptors by drugs which mimic naturally occurring acetylcholine (directly applied acetylcholine is ineffective, because it is broken down by esterases in the cornea) or by indirect stimulation with drugs that inhibit the enzymatic breakdown of naturally occurring acetylcholine. Pilocarpine is a direct-acting cholinergic agonist. Carbachol, a direct-acting agent, is also a mild indirect-acting cholinesterase inhibitor. The stronger indirect-acting cholinesterase inhibitors include phospholine iodide and eserine.

The cholinergic agonists, due to their effects on pupil size and ciliary muscle tone, can markedly affect vision. Stimulation of ocular cholinergic receptors causes accommodative spasm with induced myopia due to stimulation of the circular muscle of the ciliary body, and miosis (Figure 15.11a) with decreased vision (especially in patients with early cataracts) due to stimulation of the iris sphincter. Prolonged use of miotics may result in conjunctival hyperemia, pigment epithelial cysts of the iris sphincter (Figure 15.11b), inability to dilate the pupil due to fibrosis and posterior synechiae, and uveitis due to breakdown of the blood–aqueous barrier (miotics are relatively contraindicated in inflammatory glaucoma and neovascular glaucoma). Strong miotics such as carbachol or phospholine iodide may cause cataract formation. Phospholine iodide should best be used in aphakic or pseudophakic patients, in whom it is generally well tolerated and highly effective. Miotic agents may cause retinal detachment through traction on the vitreous base, and a thorough retinal examination should be conducted prior to prescribing these agents. Systemic side-effects associated with the use of cholinergic agonists include salivation, tearing, urinary frequency, diarrhea, and excessive sweating. Additionally, anesthesiologists must be told when patients are using phospholine

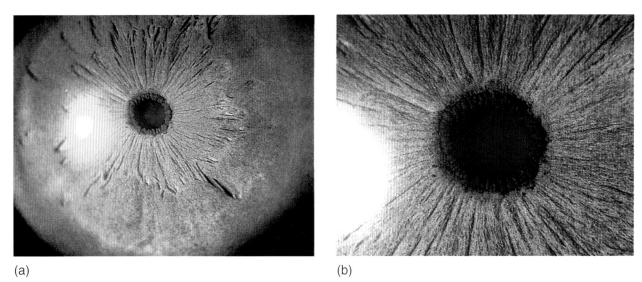

(a)   (b)

Figure 15.11 Ocular side-effects of cholinergic agents. (a) Marked miosis may cause blurring of vision and dimming of vision, or the perception that the world appears 'darker'. (b) Pigment epithelial cysts at the pupillary margin are related to chronic use of cholingerics.

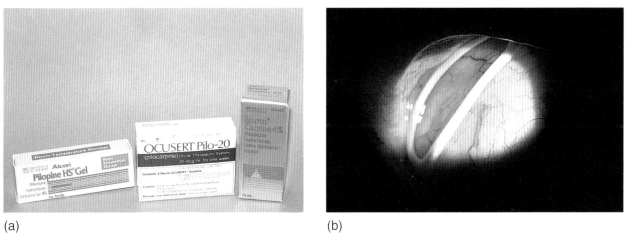

(a)   (b)

Figure 15.12 Pilocarpine formulations. (a) Numerous formulations and preparations of miotic agents have been used clinically. The options available continue to decrease, owing to the limited use of this class of compounds that has side-effects which include reductions in vision due to miosis, and accommodative spasm. (b) Ocuserts, slow-release preparations that lowered IOP for 5 to 7 days after instillation, and are shown here, have been discontinued. Pilocarpine, which had been available in concentrations of up to 10%, is currently manufactured only in concentrations of up to 4%. Pilocarpine gel is effective for up to 18–24 hours. If this preparation is used, IOP must be checked 18–20 hours after dosing to assess the duration of effect in an individual patient. If the efficacy is waning 18–20 hours following dosing, a drop of a miotic can be added 16–18 hours following instillation of the pilocarpine gel.

iodide, since inhibition of systemic cholinesterase may prolong the action of succinylcholine (used for paralysis during induction of general anesthesia), resulting in difficulty taking the patient off a ventilator. Headache or brow ache are common complaints when starting patients on miotic therapy due to ciliary spasm. Treatment should start with very low concentrations, with increase in the concentration based upon the response observed. The patients should be advised that the headache will ease up over an 'adjustment' period lasting a few days.

Pilocarpine 0.5%, 1%, 2%, 3%, and 4%, in various formulations (Figure 15.12) is the most

commonly used cholinergic and one of the least expensive glaucoma medications. It has been available for over 100 years and is the only agent derived from naturally occurring substances. In drop form, pilocarpine must be administered four times daily, due to its limited duration of action. More darkly pigmented eyes usually require higher concentrations of the drug. Alternative delivery systems have been developed in an attempt to decrease the required frequency of application and the associated side-effects. These include a 4% pilocarpine gel preparation for use once daily at bedtime. The miotic side-effects diminish during sleep, while the pressure-lowering effect lasts for

18–24 hours. If this gel formulation is used, IOP should be checked 18 hours after dosing, as some patients will require an additional drop of a miotic agent in the late afternoon for adequate 24-hour IOP control. Patients should be advised to wash off residual gel after awakening to prevent recurrences of cholinergic ocular side-effects during the day. No longer available are time-release discs (Ocuserts; Figure 15.12b), which were placed in the conjunctival fornix and released pilocarpine over a 5–7-day period. Among the other miotics still available for clinical use, carbachol 1.5% and 3% may have a longer duration of action and are administered two to three times daily, and phospholine iodide 0.125% is administered once or twice daily.

Non-selective adrenergic agonists

Epinephrine and dipivalyl-epinephrine

The nonselective adrenergic agonist compounds which include epinephrine and the prodrug dipivalyl-epinephrine are used very infrequently. This is because of the high incidence of tachyphylaxis and side-effects, the high rate of allergy, and the relatively poor efficacy compared to the other agents available to manage IOP. Non-selective adrenergic agonists can be considered in patients intolerant to other topical ocular hypotensive therapy, keeping in mind the limitations of this class of compounds. Additivity to β-adrenoreceptor antagonists is variable. One study comparing the additivity of epinephrine to a non-selective β-adrenoreceptor antagonist (timolol) or a selective β-adrenoreceptor antagonist (betaxolol) suggested better additivity to the selective β-adrenoreceptor antagonist. This suggests that the action of epinephrine may be mediated through β2 receptors, which are blocked by timolol and not by betaxolol.

Topical epinephrine applied to the glaucomatous eye lowers the IOP between 10 and 30%. Several formulations of epinephrine including bitartrate, hydrochloride, or borate salt solutions, have been in use since the early 1950s. Maximum pressure lowering occurs within 2–4 hours of administration, with duration of action between 12 and 24 hours; hence administration is usually twice daily. As epinephrine is an α1 agonist, it can cause pupil dilatation, and thus it should be used with caution (if at all) in angle-closure glaucoma or in patients with narrow angles. There is some controversy over the mechanism of action of topically applied epinephrine. It is believed to cause a short-lived increase in aqueous production, with sustained increased outflow, believed to be mostly through non-conventional, i.e. uveoscleral, pathways.

Systemic side-effects include headaches, elevated blood pressure, tachyarrythmias, and strokes. Ocular side-effects include conjunctival hyperemia, adrenochrome deposits, and, commonly, allergic blepharoconjunctivitis (Figure 5.13). Intraocular side-effects include pupillary dilatation, corneal endothelial effects, reduction in ocular blood flow due to vasospasm, rebound hyperemia, and, in aphakic and some pseudophakic patients, cystoid macular edema (Figure 15.13b).

Attempts to reduce the side-effects of epinephrine therapy while increasing absorption into the eye resulted in the development of an epinephrine 'pro-drug', dipivalylepinephrine, also known as dipivefrin or DPE. The substitution of pivalyl acid for each of the hydroxyl groups on the epinephrine molecule results in (1) a compound that is inactive as it comes out of the bottle, thus having a lower potential for systemic side-effects; and (2) a compound with markedly increased lipid solubility over the epinephrine molecule with greater penetrability into the eye, allowing for a lower concentration of the drug presented to the eye. As the drug penetrates the cornea, esterases cleave the pivalyl moieties, thus activating the drug to epinephrine (Figure 15.5). DPE has approximately 17 times more penetrability into the eye than epinephrine, and a 0.1% concentration has the pressure-lowering ability equivalent to about 1.5% epinephrine. Although the systemic side-effects have been reduced with DPE, local reactions, particularly allergy, remain a problem.

COMBINATION THERAPY

More than 50% of glaucoma patients require two or more ocular hypotensive medications for adequate IOP control. If a second or third agent is required to achieve target IOP, a different class of medication is selected. Adding a second agent in the same class already being chronically administered will not be additive. This is also true for acute dosing of medications to prevent postoperative laser or other acute IOP elevations. Optimal combinations of medications will vary in individual patients and often depend upon the factors already discussed, including tolerability, side-effects, dosing regimen and efficacy.

Compliance is one of the major obstacles to medical management of diseases. Numerous studies demonstrate that less frequent dosing of therapy leads to enhanced compliance. Unique to topical ophthalmic drugs is the washout phenomenon. Rapid instillation of successive drugs leads to reduced efficacy, as the second drug markedly decreases the concentration of the first agent in the tear film, leading to decreased absorption of the first medication instilled. Fixed combination therapy (more than one agent in the same bottle) addresses both the issues of compliance and wash-out. The goals of combination therapy are to provide efficacy and side-effect profiles that are similar to concomitant administration of the individual drugs. Combination products such

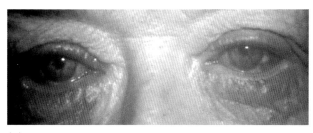

(a)

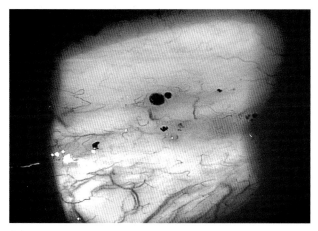

(b)

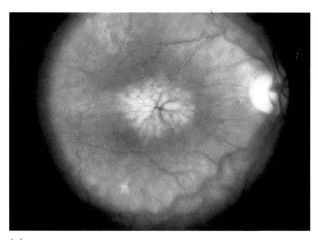

(c)

Figure 15.13 Ocular side-effects with topical epinephrine. (a) Bilateral blepharoconjunctivitis in a patient secondary to treatment with topical epinephrine. Allergic responses and tachyphylaxis appear to be more common with this class of compounds, which explain their limited use. (Photograph courtesy of Steven M Podos, MD.) (b) Chronic administration of epinephrine may result in adrenochrome deposits in the conjunctiva. These are black oxidation products of the drug which are usually asymptomatic. Occasionally these deposits cause ocular irritation. (c) Cystoid macular edema is more common in aphakic and pseudophakic patients instilling topical epinephrine agents. Higher concentrations of the drug are achieved in the posterior segment in these patients, due to absence of the lens as a barrier to diffusion, which explains the increased incidence of CME. Discontinuation of the drug typically leads to resolution of the CME.

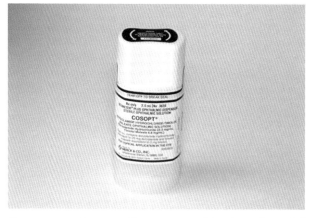

Figure 15.14 Cosopt. Cosopt, a combination of timolol 0.5% and dorzolamide 2%, is administered twice daily, every 12 hours. It is as efficacious as administering timolol 0.5% twice daily and dorzolamide 2% two or three times daily, reducing IOP up to 30–40% from untreated baseline.

as epinephrine/pilocarpine, timolol/pilocarpine, and betaxolol/pilocarpine have been available for many years but are used infrequently today. This is due to the unfavorable side-effects of pilocarpine and epinephrine, and the smaller effects on IOP compared to the other classes of ocular hypotensive compounds currently available.

Newer combination products are available and are being prescribed, but at the present time only one combination product is approved for clinical use in the USA. Cosopt, which is a combination of timolol 0.5% and dorzolamide 2%, is administered twice daily, every 12 hours (Figure 15.14). It is as efficacious as administering timolol 0.5% twice daily and dorzolamide 2% two or three times daily, reducing IOP up to 30% to 40% from untreated baseline. Studies have suggested similar efficacy with Cosopt administered b.i.d. and latanoprost administered q.h.s. Some studies have suggested enhanced efficacy with Cosopt compared to concomitant dosing with its two components, presumably due to enhanced compliance and reduced wash-out. No new side-effects have been identified with this combination therapy.

Other combination products that have been approved internationally, and are in clinical trials but not yet available in the USA, include latanoprost/timolol (Xalcom), timolol/brimonidine (Combigan) and travoprost/timolol (DuoTrav).

THE FUTURE OF MEDICAL THERAPY FOR GLAUCOMA

New drugs

Many avenues are being explored in the search for newer, more effective agents, with fewer side-effects, and that will hopefully be dosed less frequently.

It is possible that additional receptors will be identified that mediate ocular outflow and aqueous flow, leading to development of new drugs that act at these receptors. In addition to ocular hypotensive agents, drugs that regulate blood flow, drugs that are neuroprotective, agents that mediate immunological responses, and drugs that stimulate regeneration of retinal ganglion cells, may be discovered. Genetic manipulation of ocular disease may be a treatment of the future. Treatment of glaucoma will probably evolve to a combination of therapies that act on many different components of the disease and will not be limited to reducing intraocular pressure.

Neuroprotection

Although we focus on IOP in managing glaucoma, the goal of glaucoma therapy is to preserve vision. Loss of ganglion cells, manifest by changes in the optic nerve, leads to loss of vision. Therapies that directly protect the optic nerve, used in conjunction with ocular hypotensive agents, may be beneficial in managing glaucoma. There is a large and accumulating body of literature on neuroprotection. Many agents have been investigated in laboratory and clinical trials of patients with neurological disorders. Thus far, agents that definitively protect the optic nerve have not been identified. There is an ongoing international, multicentered clinical trial in glaucoma patients of one drug that has been demonstrated to be of benefit in patients with Alzheimer's disease. The drug, which is called memantine, is a glutamate antagonist. Excess levels of glutamate, which may or may not occur in glaucoma patients, are neurodestructive. Glutamate stimulates the NMDA receptor, allowing for increased calcium entry into cells. Elevated levels of calcium set off a cascade of intracellular events, leading to apoptosis, or preprogrammed cell death (Figure 15.15). Memantine is an uncompetitive blocker of the NMDA receptor. Memantine allows for normal levels of activity at the NMDA receptor while blocking excess activation and opening of this calcium channel. Side-effects of memantine, which include headache and insomnia,

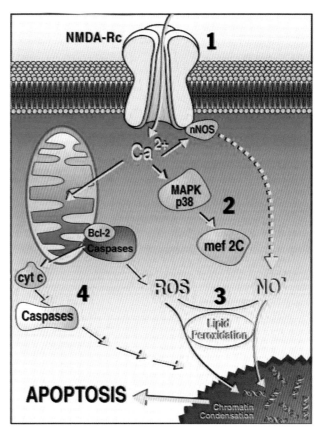

Figure 15.15 NMDA receptor. The NMDA receptor is a major glutamate receptor in the central nervous system and the eye. Overstimulation of the NMDA receptor may be a factor leading to cell injury, as overstimulation increases ingress of calcium into the cell. Elevated intracellular calcium leads to excess enzyme activity, free-radical formation, and the turn on of downstream signaling pathways, which lead to apoptosis. Apoptosis is pre-programmed cell death without surrounding inflammation. NMDA-Rc, NMDA receptor; MAPK-mef 2C, p38 mitogen-activated kinase transcription factor pathway; NO, nitrous oxide; nNOS, nitrous oxide synthetase; ROS, reactive oxygen species; cyt c, cytochrome c; Bcl 2, proteins involved in apoptosis.

are rare and very infrequently lead to discontinuation of the drug. This ongoing clinical trial may determine whether this agent is beneficial and indicated in the treatment of glaucoma.

Further reading

Advanced Glaucoma Intervention Study (AGIS): 7. The relationship between control of intraocular pressure and visual field deterioration. The AGIS Investigators. Am J Ophthalmol 2000; 130: 429–40

Alm A, Schoenfelder J, McDermott J. A 5-year, multicenter, open-label, safety study of adjunctive latanoprost therapy for glaucoma. Arch Ophthalmol 2004; 122: 957–65

Al-Shahwan S, Al-Torbak AA, Turkmani S, et al. Side-effect profile of brimonidine tartrate in children. Ophthalmology 2005; 112: 2143

Asrani S, Zeimer R, Wilensky J, et al. Large diurnal fluctuations in intraocular pressure are an independent risk factor in patients with glaucoma. J Glaucoma 2000; 9: 134–42

Bartlett JD, Olivier M, Richardson T, et al. Central nervous system and plasma lipid profiles associated with carteolol and timolol in postmenopausal black women. J Glaucoma 1999; 8: 388–95

Brandt JD, Beiser JA, Gordon MO, Kass MA, Ocular Hypertension Treatment Study (OHTS) Group. Central corneal thickness and measured IOP response to topical ocular hypotensive medication in the Ocular Hypertension Treatment Study. Am J Ophthalmol 2004; 138: 717–22

Brubaker RF. Targeting outflow facility in glaucoma management. Surv Ophthalmol 2003; 48 (Suppl 1): S17–20

Chauhan BC, Hutchison DM, LeBlanc RP, Artes PH, Nicolela MT. Central corneal thickness and progression of the visual field and optic disc in glaucoma. Br J Ophthalmol 2005; 89: 1008–12

Chiba T, Kashiwagi K, Chiba N, et al. Comparison of iridial pigmentation between latanoprost and isopropyl unoprostone: a long-term prospective comparative study. Br J Ophthalmol 2003; 87: 956–9

Costa VP, Harris A, Stefansson E, et al. The effects of antiglaucoma and systemic medications on ocular blood flow. Prog Retin Eye Res 2003; 22: 769–805

Eisenberg DL, Toris CB, Camras CB. Bimatoprost and travoprost: a review of recent studies of two new glaucoma drugs. Surv Ophthalmol 2002; 47 (Suppl 1): S105–15

Ekatomatis P. Herpes simplex dendritic keratitis after treatment with latanoprost for primary open-angle glaucoma. Br J Ophthalmol 2001; 85: 1008–9

Fechtner RD, McCarroll KA, Lines CR, Adamsons IA. Efficacy of the dorzolamide/timolol fixed combination versus latanoprost in the treatment of ocular hypertension or glaucoma: combined analysis of pooled data from two large randomized observer and patient-masked studies. J Ocul Pharmacol Ther 2005; 21: 242–9

Francis BA, Du LT, Berke S, Ehrenhaus M, Minckler DS, Cosopt Study Group. Comparing the fixed combination dorzolamide-timolol (Cosopt) to concomitant administration of 2% dorzolamide (Trusopt) and 0.5% timolol a randomized controlled trial and a replacement study. J Clin Pharm Ther 2004; 29: 375–80

Gandolfi S, Simmons ST, Sturm R, Chen K, VanDenburgh AM, Bimatoprost Study Group 3. Three-month comparison of bimatoprost and latanoprost in patients with glaucoma and ocular hypertension. Adv Ther 2001; 18: 110–21

Gordon MO, Beiser JA, Brandt JD, et al. The Ocular Hypertension Treatment Study: baseline factors that predict the onset of primary open-angle glaucoma. Arch Ophthalmol 2002; 120: 714–20; discussion 829–30

Halper LK, Johnson-Pratt L, Dobbins T, Hartenbaum D. A comparison of the efficacy and tolerability of 0.5% timolol maleate ophthalmic gel-forming solution QD and 0.5% levobunolol hydrochloride BID in patients with ocular hypertension or open-angle glaucoma. J Ocul Pharmacol Ther 2002; 18: 105–13

Henderer JD, Wilson RP, Moster MR, et al. Timolol/dorzolamide combination therapy as initial treatment for intraocular pressure over 30 mm Hg. J Glaucoma 2005; 14: 267–70

Herndon LW, Robert DW, Wand M, Asrani S. Increased periocular pigmontation with ocular hypotensive lipid use in African Americans. Am J Ophthalmol 2003; 135: 713–15

Holmstrom S, Buchholz P, Walt J, Wickstrom J, Aagren M. Analytic review of bimatoprost, latanoprost and travoprost in primary open-angle glaucoma. Curr Med Res Opin 2005; 21: 1875–83

Johnstone MA, Albert DM. Prostaglandin-induced hair growth. Surv Ophthalmol 2002; 47 (Suppl 1): S185–202

Keisu M, Wiholm BE, Ost A, Mortimer O. Acetazolamide-associated aplastic anaemia. J Intern Med 1990; 228: 627–32

Konstas AG, Katsimbris JM, Lallos N, et al. Latanoprost 0.005% versus bimatoprost 0.03% in primary open-angle glaucoma patients. Ophthalmology 2005; 112: 262–6

Law SK, Song BJ, Fang E, Caprioli J. Feasibility and efficacy of a mass switch from latanoprost to bimatoprost in glaucoma patients in a prepaid Health Maintenance Organization. Ophthalmology 2005; 112: 2123–30

Lipton SA. The molecular basis of memantine action in Alzheimer's disease and other neurologic disorders:

low-affinity, uncompetitive antagonism. Curr Alzheimer Res 2005; 2: 155–65

Liu JH, Kripke DF, Weinreb RN. Comparison of the nocturnal effects of once-daily timolol and latanoprost on intraocular pressure. Am J Ophthalmol 2004; 138: 389–95

McCarey BE, Kapik BM, Kane FE, Unoprostone Monotherapy Study Group. Low incidence of iris pigmentation and eyelash changes in 2 randomized clinical trials with unoprostone isopropyl 0.15%. Ophthalmology 2004; 111: 1480–8

Maus TL, Larsson LI, McLaren JW, Brubaker RF. Comparison of dorzolamide and acetazolamide as suppressors of aqueous humor flow in humans. Arch Ophthalmol 1997; 115: 45–9

Melles RB, Wong IG. Metipranolol-associated granulomatous iritis. Am J Ophthalmol 1994 15; 118: 712–15

Michaud JE, Friren B, International Brinzolamide Adjunctive Study Group. Comparison of topical brinzolamide 1% and dorzolamide 2% eye drops given twice-daily in addition to timolol 0.5% in patients with primary open-angle glaucoma or ocular hypertension. Am J Ophthalmol 2001; 132: 235–43

Mietz H, Esser JM, Welsandt G, et al. Latanoprost stimulates secretion of matrix metalloproteinases in tenon fibroblasts both in vitro and in vivo. Invest Ophthalmol Vis Sci 2003; 44: 5182–8

Mundorf TK, Ogawa T, Naka H, Novack GD, Crockett RS, US Istalol Study Group. A 12-month, multicenter, randomized, double-masked, parallel-group comparison of timolol-LA once-daily and timolol maleate ophthalmic solution twice-daily in the treatment of adults with glaucoma or ocular hypertension. Clin Ther 2004; 26: 541–51

Netland PA, Robertson SM, Sullivan EK, et al. Response to travoprost in black and nonblack patients with open-angle glaucoma or ocular hypertension. Adv Ther 2003; 20: 149–63

Nordmann JP, Mertz B, Yannoulis NC, et al. A double-masked randomized comparison of the efficacy and safety of unoprostone with timolol and betaxolol in patients with primary open-angle glaucoma including pseudoexfoliation glaucoma or ocular hypertension. 6 month data. Am J Ophthalmol 2002; 133: 1–10

Parrish RK, Palmberg P, Sheu WP, XLT Study Group. A comparison of latanoprost, bimatoprost, and travoprost in patients with elevated intraocular pressure: a 12-week, randomized, masked-evaluator multicenter study. Am J Ophthalmol 2003; 135: 688–703

Realini T, Vickers WR. Symmetry of fellow-eye intraocular pressure responses to topical glaucoma medications. Ophthalmology 2005; 112: 599–602

Reisberg B, Doody R, Stoffler A, et al. A 24-week open-label extension study of memantine in moderate to severe Alzheimer disease. Arch Neurol 2006; 63: 49–54

Schumer RA, Camras CB, Mandahl AK. Putative side effects of prostaglandin analogs. Surv Ophthalmol 2002; 47 (Suppl 1): S219

Schwartz M. Lessons for glaucoma from other neurodegenerative diseases: can one treatment suit them all? J Glaucoma 2005; 14: 321–3

Sharif NA, Kelly CR, Crider JY, Williams GW, Xu SX. Ocular hypotensive FP prostaglandin (PG) analogs: PG receptor subtype binding affinities and selectivities, and agonist potencies at FP and other PG receptors in cultured cells. J Ocul Pharmacol Ther 2003; 19: 501–15

Shin DH, Glover BK, Cha SC, et al. Long-term brimonidine therapy in glaucoma patients with apraclonidine allergy. Am J Ophthalmol 1999; 127: 511–15

Smith J, Wandel T. Rationale for the one-eye therapeutic trial. Ann Ophthalmol 1986; 18: 8

Stewart WC, Laibovitz R, Horwitz B, et al. A 90-day study of the efficacy and side effects of 0.25% and 0.5% apraclonidine vs 0.5% timolol. Apraclonidine Primary Therapy Study Group. Arch Ophthalmol 1996; 114: 938–42

Stjernschantz JW, Albert DM, Hu DN, Drago F, Wistrand PJ. Mechanism and clinical significance of prostaglandin-induced iris pigmentation. Surv Ophthalmol 2002; 47 (Suppl 1): S162–75

Topper JE, Brubaker RF. Effects of timolol, epinephrine, and acetazolamide on aqueous flow during sleep. Invest Ophthalmol Vis Sci 1985; 26: 1315–19

Tsai JC, McClure CA, Ramos SE, Schlundt DG, Pichert JW. Compliance barriers in glaucoma: a systematic classification. J Glaucoma 2003; 12: 393–8

Tsukamoto H, Mishima HK, Kitazawa Y, et al. A comparative clinical study of latanoprost and isopropyl unoprostone in Japanese patients with primary open-angle glaucoma and ocular hypertension. J Glaucoma 2002; 11: 497–501

van der Valk R, Webers CA, Schouten JS, et al. Intraocular pressure-lowering effects of all commonly used glaucoma drugs: a meta-analysis of randomized clinical trials. Ophthalmology 2005; 112: 1177–85

Walters TR, DuBiner HB, Carpenter SP, Khan B, VanDenburgh AM, Bimatoprost Circadian IOP Study Group. 24-Hour IOP control with once-daily bimatoprost, timolol gel-forming solution, or latanoprost: a 1-month, randomized, comparative clinical trial. Surv Ophthalmol 2004; 49 (Suppl 1): S26–35

Wand M, Gaudio AR, Shields MB. Latanoprost and cystoid macular edema in high-risk aphakic or pseudophakic eyes. J Cataract Refract Surg 2001; 27: 1397–401

Wand M, Gilbert CM, Liesegang TJ. Latanoprost and herpes simplex keratitis. Am J Ophthalmol 1999; 127: 602–4

Williams GC, Orengo-Nania S, Gross RL. Incidence of brimonidine allergy in patients previously allergic to apraclonidine. J Glaucoma 2000; 9: 235–8

Yuksel N, Karabas L, Altintas O, Yildirim Y, Caglar Y. A comparison of the short-term hypotensive effects and side effects of unilateral brimonidine and apraclonidine in patients with elevated intraocular pressure. Ophthalmologica 2002; 216: 45–9

16 Laser surgery in the treatment of glaucoma

Richard A Hill

INTRODUCTION

The development of the laser and its application in clinical medicine has been particularly important in ophthalmology. This chapter discusses the use of the laser in the treatment of glaucoma. Conditions for which lasers have proved to be useful include angle-closure glaucoma (iridotomy), plateau iris (iridoplasty), open-angle glaucoma (trabeculoplasty, laser sclerostomy), postoperative regulation of intraocular pressure following trabeculectomy (suture lysis), 'refractory' glaucomas (ciliodestructive procedures), and other miscellaneous conditions.

In 1960 Maiman first demonstrated stimulated emission of radiation using a ruby crystal and a flashlamp. The device used light amplification for the stimulated emission of radiation and is now known by the acronym 'laser'. Light produced by a laser is monochromatic (one wave length, determined by the 'lasing' medium), spatially coherent (phase correlation across beam) and temporally coherent (wavelength is stable). When laser light interacts with ocular tissue, it is either reflected, scattered, transmitted or absorbed (Figure 16.1). Clinically useful laser–tissue interactions can be classified as photochemical, thermal (photocoagulation and photothermoablation) or ionizing (Figure 16.2). Light in the range of 400–1100 nm will easily pass through cornea, aqueous, lens, and vitreous.

In current glaucoma therapy, intraocular laser effects are achieved by two main mechanisms. In the first mechanism, spatial confinement of photons occurs by absorption of photons by the ocular chromophores: melanin, hemoglobin, and xanthophyll or water (Figures 16.3 and 16.4). The deposition of energy at first causes denaturation of proteins as the tissue temperature rises. This is clinically useful for iridoplasty or coagulation of bleeding vessels. If irradiance is greatly increased (continuous wave power/area) thermally induced focal destruction of the target

Laser–Tissue Interactions

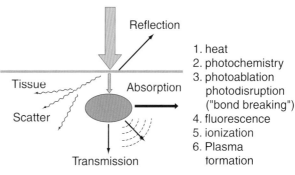

Figure 16.1 Laser–tissue interactions. Laser light may be reflected, scattered, absorbed, or transmitted, or create plasma. (Courtesy of M Berns, Beckman Laser Institute and Medical Clinic, University of California, Irvine.)

tissue occurs (photocoagulation). If the temperature rises above the boiling point of water, a steam bubble is seen to form, which contains water vapor and gaseous by-products of the tissue destroyed. This produces a typical laser ablation (Figure 16.5) in which both the surrounding edema zone of thermally altered tissues decreases and energy needed decreases (Figure 16.6) as spatial confinement of energy increases. In addition to chromophore selection, thermal damage may be limited or extended by altering the exposure time relative to the thermal relaxation time (approximately 1 μs) for biological tissues (Figure 16.7). In glaucoma therapy by continuous wave lasers (argon laser trabeculoplasty, iridectomy, cyclophotocoagulation, and iridoplasty), melanin is the major chromophore. Its absorption decreases over the 400–1000 nm range (Figure 16.3), decreasing spatial confinement of laser energy for longer wavelength lasers. In addition, longer wavelengths will exhibit less scatter, further increasing penetration into tissues. Although this facilitates some procedures such as transscleral Nd:YAG

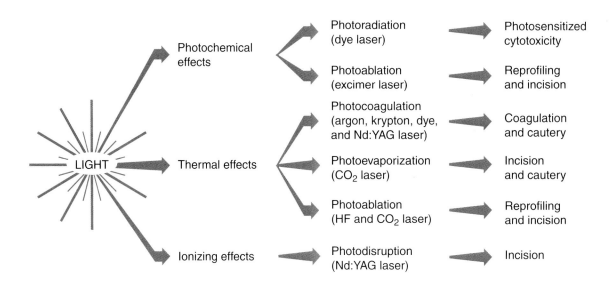

Laser Light, Interactions, and Clinical Systems

Laser–tissue interactions may be divided into photochemical, thermal, or ionizing

Figure 16.2 Clinically useful laser–tissue interactions. (Adapted from L'Esperance FA Jr. Ophthalmic Lasers. St Louis, MO: CV Mosby, 1989: 65; and from Nelson JS, Berns MW. Basic laser physics and tissue interactions. Contemp Dermatol 1988; 2: 2.)

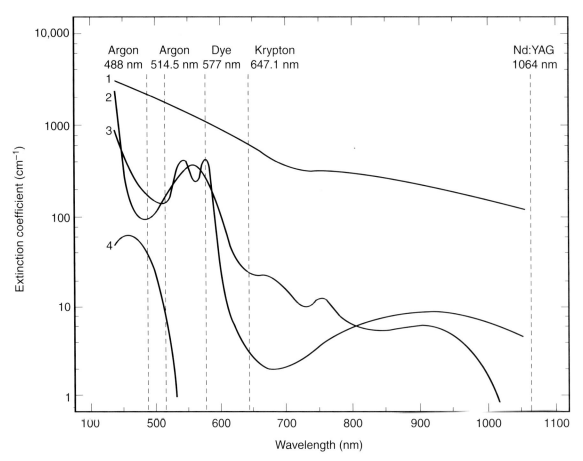

Figure 16.3 Extinction coefficient versus wavelength for ocular chromophores. Curve 1 = melanin; curve 2 = reduced hemoglobin; curve 3 = oxygenated hemoglobin; curve 4 = macular xanthophyll. (Adapted from L'Esperance FA Jr. Ophthalmic Lasers. St Louis, MO: CV Mosby, 1989: 68.)

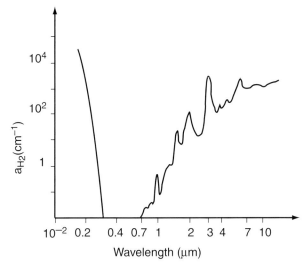

Figure 16.4 **Absorption of photons by water.** Water, as a chromophore has intense absorption in the ultraviolet and usable peaks in the infrared at 2.1 μm (holmiun lasers) and 2.94 μm (erbium lasers).

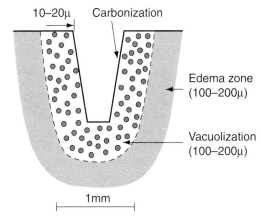

Figure 16.5 **Typical effects of a pulsed laser on biological tissues.** The edema zone represents tissue thermally denatured and is of variable thickness depending on spatial confinement of the laser light and laser pulse duration. (Adapted from Nelson JS, Berns MW. Basic laser physics and tissue interactions. Contemp Dermatol 1988; 2: 2.)

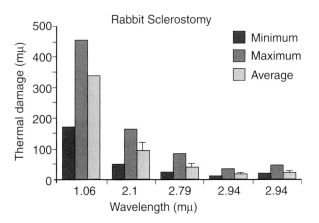

Figure 16.6 **Energy required for tissue ablation decreases as spatial confinement increases.** This results in maximum efficiency for lasers operating near absorption peaks (Figure 16.4). (Reprinted with permission from Invest Ophthalmol Vis Sci 1991; 32: 58–63.)

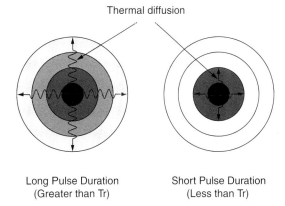

Figure 16.7 **Tissue thermal damage.** Tissue thermal damage increases by diffusion when laser pulses are longer than the thermal relaxation time for biological tissues. (Courtesy of S Nelson, Beckman Laser Institute and Medical Clinic, University of California, Irvine.)

cyclophotocoagulation, it tends to create less of a surface effect (which provides clinical feedback) in other procedures such as trabeculoplasty.

The second major mechanism by which laser affects ocular tissue occurs at the focal point of short-pulse, high-power lasers (Nd:YAG), which create optical breakdown or plasma formation. The individual laser pulses are delivered over extremely short intervals, which results in an extraordinarily high irradiance at the focal point of the laser. This irradiance is sufficient to strip electrons from atoms of molecules, creating a cloud of ions and electrons (plasma). This plasma cloud can initially absorb photons and later scatters them, providing some protection for underlying tissues. After the initial plasma cloud forms, it expands rapidly, creating

stresses that exceed the structural limits of the target tissue. This ablation mechanism is chromophore independent, and useful for iridectomy formation in light-colored irides.

LASER PERIPHERAL IRIDECTOMY

Early attempts at iridectomy formation with coherent light sources were not successful, because of poor spatial confinement of the laser energy. The longer wavelength photons traveled deeper into the iris and were less well absorbed by melanin. The application of lasers with shorter wavelengths and better spatial confinement of applied energy (such as ruby and argon) led to the reproducible

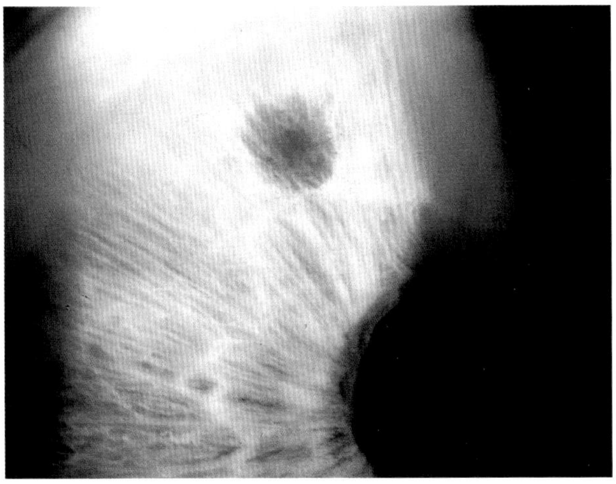

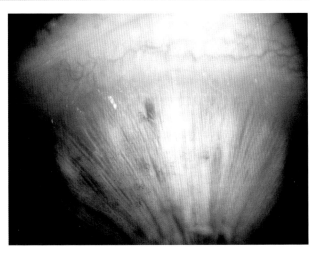

Figure 16.8 Argon laser iridectomies. Argon laser iridectomies are typically rounded with zones of thermal damage extending beyond the opening (see also Figure 16.5).

Figure 16.9 Nd:YAG laser iridectomy. Typical slit-like iridectomy produced by a short-pulse Nd:YAG laser.

creation of laser iridectomies. The argon laser was widely embraced and strategies for dealing with situations of excessive chromophore (dark irides) or insufficient chromophore (light irides) were developed by Ritch (contraction burn) and Hoskins and Migliazzo (bubble formation). In the early 1980s the argon laser iridectomy (Figure 16.8) largely replaced incisional iridectomy as initial therapy for angle closure with pupillary block. In the mid-1980s short pulsed Nd:YAG lasers became widely available for iridectomies. The mechanism of action is chromophore independent and works well in all iris colors. The radial orientation of iris fibers yields slit-like iridectomies (Figure 16.9). The simplicity of the procedure and lower iridectomy closure rates has led to rapid and widespread acceptance. In addition, the use of apraclonidine prophylaxis has decreased the incidence and severity of post-laser intraocular pressure elevations. There are, however, a number of situations where the argon laser has retained utility. For example, in the angle closure patient on anticoagulants or in an eye with chronic inflammation, the argon laser creates a zone of thermally induced tissue coagulation (Figure 16.5) which can also be used to prevent bleeding or stop bleeding resistant to contact lens pressure (Figure 16.10). Other uses of the argon laser include pretreating a spongy, thick, brown iris to minimize shredding with subsequent application of Nd:YAG energy, and in iridoplasty to break an attack of angle closure when the surgeon is unable to initially create a laser iridectomy or the angle remains occluded or occludable after laser peripheral iridectomy.

Patient evaluation

The patient examination with a Zeiss four-mirror or similarly shaped gonioscope should show occludable

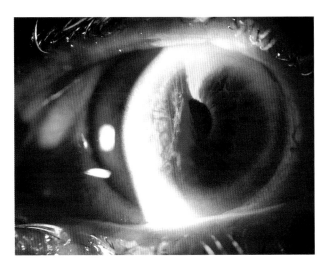

Figure 16.10 Bleeding in a patient after Nd:YAG iridectomy requiring argon laser coagulation to stop. On questioning of the patient, NSAIDs were found to be taken for arthritis but not declared as a current medication.

or occluded angles which open with compression. In patients with pigment dispersion (Figure 16.11a), laser iridectomy reverses iris concavity and iridozonular contact, although additional pilocarpine therapy may be necessary for residual iridociliary contact (Figure 16.11b). Lastly, an iridectomy may be useful in treating postoperative complications such as iris bombé, caused by posterior synechiae formed in eyes with chronic inflammation (Figure 16.12).

Contact lens selection

An Abraham or Wise (Figure 16.13) iridectomy lens will increase safety and facilitate the laser iridectomy. The use of a viscous artificial tear solution to place the contact lens (such as Celluvisc®) increases patient comfort postoperatively.

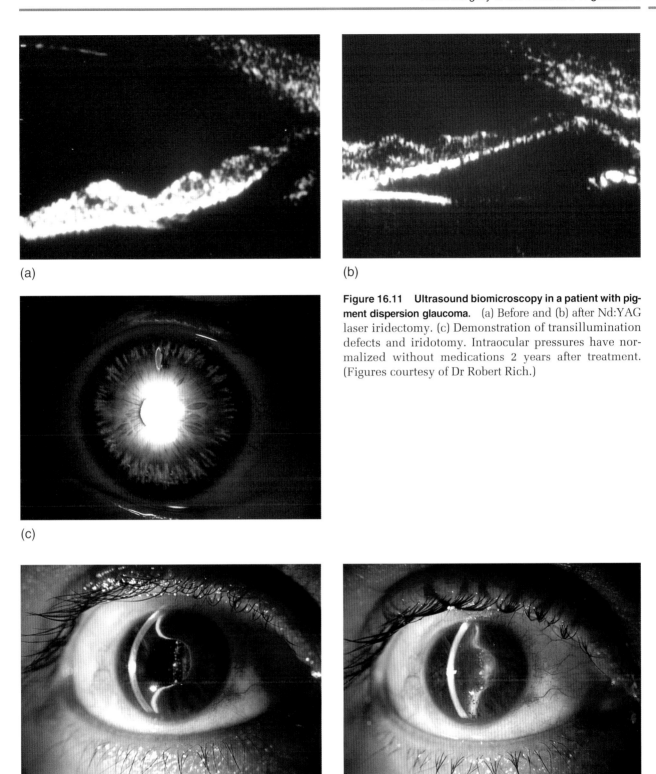

(a)

(b)

Figure 16.11 Ultrasound biomicroscopy in a patient with pigment dispersion glaucoma. (a) Before and (b) after Nd:YAG laser iridectomy. (c) Demonstration of transillumination defects and iridotomy. Intraocular pressures have normalized without medications 2 years after treatment. (Figures courtesy of Dr Robert Rich.)

(c)

(a)

(b)

Figure 16.12 Iris bombé. Chronic inflammation has produced an iris bombé configuration, in a pseudophakic eye before (a) and after (b) Ahmed Valve implantation.

Patient preparation

Apraclonidine (Iopidine®) or brimonidine (Alphagan®-P) preoperatively and postoperatively will limit pressure spikes and bleeding with iridectomies. The use of pilocarpine will tighten the iris and allow for more peripheral placement of the iridectomy, which will decrease the possibility of postoperative glare symptoms. The operation should be performed in an area of iris normally covered by eyelid. Thin areas of iris such as crypts or transillumination defects in pigment dispersion (after pilocarpine use) are preferable locations.

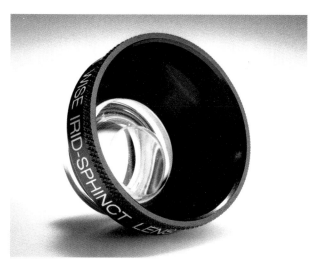

Figure 16.13 The Wise iridectomy lens. Using the Wise iridectomy lens as an example, corneal irradiance is decreased 91%, spot size on the iris is decreased 62% (increasing irradiance 7×), and potential fundus irradiance minimized by causing a 230% increase in beam diameter. (Courtesy of Ocular Instruments.)

Technique

Continuous or quasi-continuous wave laser iridectomy

Continuous wave lasers include argon, krypton, frequency doubled Nd:YAG, and diode. Historically, the 'hump,' 'drumhead,' and 'chipping away' techniques have been described for argon laser iridectomy. The chipping away technique is most commonly used. This technique is simple and straightforward. The patient must be instructed not to look at the laser light; a slight upward or inward orientation of the eye will further decrease the chances of a posterior pole laser burn. A high-power (+) lens will minimize fundus irradiance should an errant laser pulse go through a patent iridectomy. Laser spots of 50 μm size are placed at exactly the same site until the anterior lens capsule can be visualized. The surgeon adjusts the continuous-wave power and exposure times based on observed laser–tissue interactions. Darker irides that absorb laser energy well may char at 0.1 s exposure time and consideration should be given to shorter exposures. Conversely, lighter irides with poorer absorption must first be heated to denature tissue, decreasing transmission which increases focal scatter and heating. In practical practice applications, the argon laser is useful for medium brown irides. It is also useful for pretreating thick spongy irides to minimize shredding with the application of Nd:YAG energy, coagulating vessels in patients on anticoagulants and stopping hemorrhage unresponsive to contact lens pressure (Figure 16.10). If continuous-wave power needs to be above 1.0 W or exposure times above 0.1 s, consideration should be given to the use of an Nd:YAG laser. In most situations this is the laser of choice for this procedure.

Nd:YAG laser iridectomy

The Nd:YAG laser is the laser of choice for the creation of laser iridectomies. In general, multiple pulses at 1.8–3.0 millijoules/pulse and 1–2 pulses per burst are usually sufficient to create Nd:YAG laser iridectomies. The use of a high plus power lens also helps creates a shallow cutting effect. A coated, high-power Abraham or Wise lens (Figure 16.13) is placed with the aid of topical anesthesia. The patient is asked to look slightly down and a thinner area of superior iris is sought out. The aiming beam is placed directly on the surface of the iris. Lighter-colored, thinner irides will yield to a few laser pulses, while darker, thicker irides may require multiple pulses. As the stroma thins, pulses per burst and energy per burst may be decreased to minimize danger to the crystalline lens. The risk to the lens may further be reduced by iridectomy placement in the far periphery, adjusting the oculars of the slit-lamp delivery system to make the operator's retina conjugate with the focal point of the laser and careful focusing. Regardless of the laser used, the anterior lens capsule must be visualized; transillumination defects are not adequate to establish patency of an iridectomy. Nd:YAG laser iridectomies tend to be slit-like because of the radial orientation of iris fibers (Figure 16.9). A small amount of bleeding is common with this technique. It may be stopped by increasing pressure on the contact lens. Rarely, this is not sufficient (Figure 16.10) and an argon laser may be used with a large spot (200–500 μm), longer duration (0.2 s) and low power burn (200–350 mW). The post-laser pressure check should be at slightly over an hour in order to detect the majority of post-laser pressure spikes. Corticosteroids are used at q.i.d. frequency and the patient seen in 1 week for gonioscopy and to confirm discontinuation of steroids. Patients with narrow occludable angles and concurrent secondary glaucomas such as exfoliation glaucoma have low outflow states and the physician may wish to consider a 1-hour postoperative intraocular pressure check. In other patients with narrow occulable angles alone, the risk of postoperative IOP elevation is rare after apraclonidine (Iopidine®) or brimonidine (Alphagan®-P) prophylaxis.

CENTRAL AND PERIPHERAL IRIDOPLASTY

Central iridoplasty, or photomydriasis, is useful on rare occasions. Typically, a glaucoma patient who is controlled on medical therapy which includes miotics, and who has a pupillary diameter less than 2 mm, may complain of poor vision and dimness, especially if an early cataract is present. Such a patient may experience an improved quality of vision if the pupil can be enlarged to greater than 2 mm by laser pupilloplasty. Long (0.2 s), large (200 μm), and low continuous-wave power are used to shrink

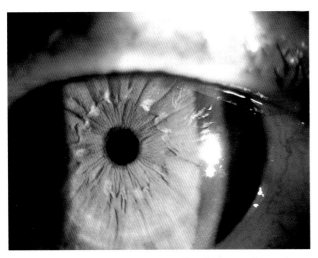

Figure 16.14 Pupilloplasty. Pupilloplasty performed at a continuous-wave power too high and a duration too short. There has been pigment release and a partial, superficial effect.

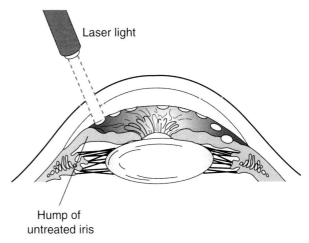

Laser light

Hump of untreated iris

Figure 16.15 The mechanical effect of low continuous-wave power, long exposure laser treatments on peripheral iris contour.

iris tissue. Spots are placed in a circular fashion every 30° around the pupil and only the minimum number of spots needed to increase pupillary size over 2 mm are used. Lenticular opacities can occur. These tend to be more common in lighter-colored irides with poorer spatial confinement of the laser energy. The operator should be vigilant for eye motion as the laser energy is applied close to the pupil. If the duration of the burn is shortened and continuous-wave power increased, pigment release and a superficial partial effect will result (Figure 16.14).

Selected narrow angles may be widened by peripheral iridoplasty, particularly if the configuration is one of plateau iris and the narrowing is not due to pupillary block. In current practice, iridoplasty is performed by inducing a deep thermal contraction burn in iris stroma, causing mechanical retraction from the filtering angle by flattening of the peripheral iris contour (Figure 16.15). The laser parameters chosen to facilitate this type of laser–tissue interaction are long burns (0.5 s), large spot size (500 μm), and low power (200–350 mW). If bubble formation occurs, the operator should stop energy application in mid-pulse and decrease continuous-wave power. The laser energy can be delivered through an Abraham contact lens to the most peripheral portion of the iris that is accessible. Six spots are placed per quadrant with 1000 μm (two laser spot) spacing. In cases of plateau iris or nanophthalmos, the laser light may need to be delivered even more peripherally and a goniolens will facilitate this. In this case the spot size should be reduced to 200 μm. In general, eyes with more chromophore (dark irides) will require less continuous-wave power than lighter irides. Iridoplasty is also a useful adjunct for cases that retain an appositional closure of the filtering angle after iridectomy or in cases where an iridectomy

cannot be initially created. Iridoplasty may also be useful to facilitate the performance of laser trabeculoplasty in eyes with a plateau iris configuration.

ARGON LASER TRABECULOPLASTY

Introduced originally by Wise and Witter, argon laser trabeculoplasty (ALT) is a frequently performed glaucoma procedure with good long-term follow-up. A variety of lasers have been used to perform trabeculoplasty. The most commonly used is the argon laser. In using this laser, operator macular photic stress may be reduced by using the argon green only rather than both the blue and green. In addition, the use of a contact lens with a metal halide coating will reduce the hazards of reflected light. The Ritch trabeculoplasty lens (Figure 16.16), has two different angles on its mirrors: 64° for the superior angle and 59° for the inferior angle. In addition, a planoconvex button is positioned over each mirror, which provides 1.4 × magnification. This reduces a 50 μm spot to 35 μm and doubles irradiance. A standard one- or two-mirror lens without a planoconvex condensing lens has an angle of 62° and produces a 54 μm spot from the original 50 μm beam, which also slightly decreases irradiance (Figure 16.17). If a one-mirror lens is used, the patient is asked to move the eye in the direction of the treating mirror to accommodate the slight variance in filtering angle anatomy. Tilting the lens will introduce astigmatic error, creating an oval beam and altered irradiance (energy per surface area).

ALT is generally indicated for the reduction of intraocular pressure in patients with primary open-angle glaucoma, although it is also used to very good effect in patients with glaucoma associated with the pigment dispersion syndrome and

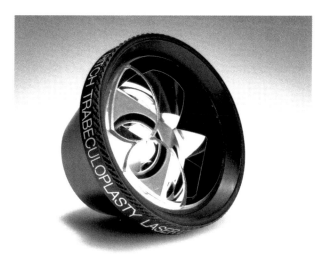

Figure 16.16 The Ritch lens. The Ritch lens has two different angles on its mirrors: 64° for the superior angle and 59° for the inferior angle. In addition, a planoconvex button is positioned over each mirror, which provides 1.4 × magnification. This reduces a 50 μm spot to 35 μm and doubles irradiance. (Courtesy of Ocular Instruments.)

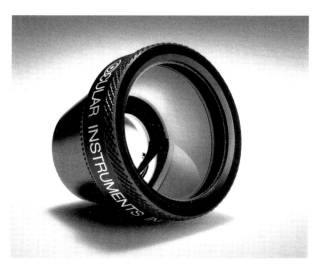

Figure 16.17 A standard one- or two-mirror lens. A standard one- or two-mirror lens without a planoconvex condensing lens has an angle of 62° and produces a 54 μm spot from the original 50 μm beam (magnification = 0.93) which also slightly decreases irradiance. (Courtesy of Ocular Instruments.)

the exfoliation syndrome. It may also work in patients with steroid-induced glaucoma. Traditionally, it is used when the patient has reached maximum tolerated medical therapy, and in such cases usually does not allow the discontinuation of any of the medications being used. Recently, economic pressures have caused a renewed interest in laser trabeculoplasty as an alternative to increasing or allowing for a decrease in topical therapy. The procedure carries an initial success rate of 70–80%, but patients should be advised

that the effect may decrease over time; approximately 10% per year of eyes will return to pretreatment pressures. Re-treatment (after 360° of the angle has already been treated) carries only about a 30% chance of success, and consideration should be given to filtering surgery once AL has failed.

Preparation

Preoperatively and postoperatively, the patient is given apraclonidine (Iopidine®) or brimonidine (Alphagan®-P), unless an allergy dictates the use of another ocular hypotensive agent. Anesthesia is achieved with topical proparacaine. Viscous artificial tears solution such as Celluvisc® may be used with the laser lens to maximize patient comfort postoperatively.

Procedure

Standard parameters of a 50 μm spot size and an exposure time of 0.1 s are usually employed. The suggested application site is the junction of the pigmented and non-pigmented trabecular meshwork. Application of laser energy at this position, easily found except in non-pigmented filtering angles, will further reduce the incidence of pressure spikes and peripheral anterior synechiae formation. This site can be found immediately below the termination of the parallel piped of light in a long thin slit beam under high magnification (Figure 16.18). The degree of pigmentation found in the trabecular meshwork and whether or not the treating lens increases irradiance will suggest to the operator what continuous-wave power to select initially. In most filtering angles, 700 mW is sufficient. A general rule of thumb is to subtract 100 mW of power for each stepwise increase in trabecular pigmentation. Continuous-wave power should be sufficient to produce blanching or small bubble formation (Figure 16.19) at 0.1 s exposure time. Laser power meters may not be accurate and the surgeon should always believe the observed laser–tissue interaction over the power meter. The surgeon should also vary the power output for variations in angle pigmentation encountered intraoperatively. Treatment at too high an irradiance or posterior placement may lead to small focal peripheral anterior synechiae formation (Figure 16.20). Standard one- and two-mirror lenses as well as specialty lenses have been used for this procedure (Figures 16.16, 16.17). Before the treating lens is rotated, the operator should note angle landmarks to avoid overlapping a treated area. Finally, careful focusing is important for a uniform treatment. Focusing starts with adjusting the oculars of the laser to make the operator's retina conjugate with the focal point of the laser. If the lens is tilted, irradiance is decreased and a larger area is irradiated.

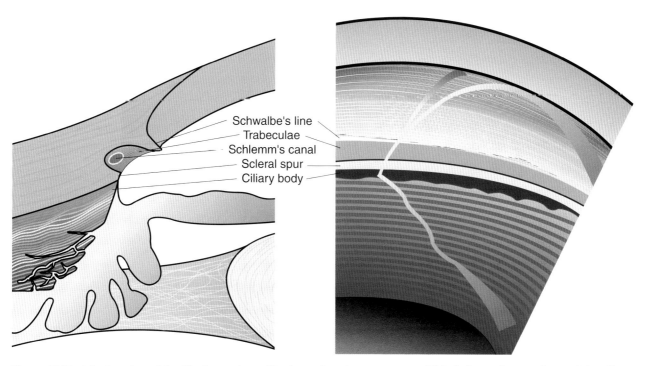

Figure 16.18   The junction of the filtering and non-filtering trabecular meshwork.   This is located posterior to Schwalbe's line, at the terminus of the two focal lines representing the anterior and posterior surfaces of the cornea. (Adapted from Gorin and Posner Slit lamp Gonioscopy, Williams and Williams.)

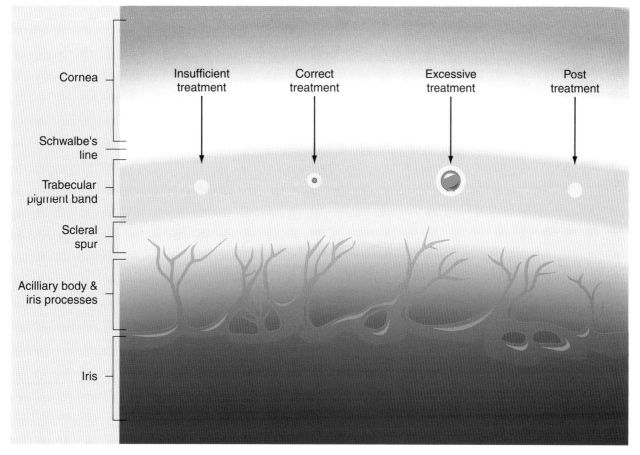

Figure 16.19   Correct level of energy delivered with argon laser trabeculoplasty.   The correct placement site is at the terminus of the arrow under the text.

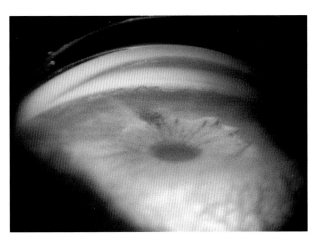

Figure 16.20 Peripheral anterior synechiae formation after argon laser trabeculoplasty.

Also, if the spot size is increased by poor focus, the irradiance decreases by the square of the difference.

Treating the eye in divided sessions or limiting laser treatment spots to 50–60 will minimize chances of a postoperative laser-induced pressure spike. The operator should be consistent in the order of treatment, treating a total of 360° in two sessions (inferior then superior, nasal then temporal, right side then left side, etc.) or 360° with fewer laser spots in one session. Historically the former treatment technique affords a better treatment effect. In eyes with small central islands of remaining visual field, the operator may wish to further subdivide the sessions to minimize the chances of a laser-induced intraocular pressure spike.

Other lasers also used in 'argon' laser trabeculoplasty differ in their laser–tissue interactions from those of argon. The frequency doubled quasi-continuous wave (high-frequency repetition) Nd:YAG (532 nm) laser's micropulses that make up each macropulse are at the thermal relaxation time of sclera. This probably decreases surface tissue denaturing and scatter, resulting in slightly deeper photon penetration. In addition, the slightly longer wavelength is slightly less well absorbed by melanin, allowing slightly deeper penetration. This will slightly decrease observed surface effects.

Postoperative care

On completion of trabeculoplasty, a final drop of apraclonidine is given to the patient. The intraocular pressure is checked at 1–2 hours post-treatment. Corticosteroids are started at q.i.d. frequency and, if a pressure spike did not occur, the patient is asked to return in 1 week to insure discontinuation of topical steroids. Non-steroidal anti-inflammatory agents are an alternative for known steroid responders. The risk of an IOP elevation of >10 mmHg after ALT with apraclonidine prophylaxis is small.

The final procedure-related visit is at 4–6 weeks postoperatively to access the effects of treatment unless the clinical situation dictates differently.

SELECTIVE LASER TRABECULOPLASTY

Developed by Mark Latina, selective laser trabeculoplasty (SLT) is another laser-based treatment of the trabecular meshwork that improves the outflow state of the eye in open-angle glaucoma. Unlike ALT, it does not produce macroscopic thermal injury in the filtering angle (Figure 16.21). This laser technique uses a Q-switched frequency doubled Nd:YAG laser (Coherent Selectra 7000 or Selectra II). The short pulse widths (3 ns) are under the thermal relaxation time for the collagen-based tissues of the filtering angle. The laser energy is spatially confined by cells containing pigment (melanin) creating fatal injury on a microscopic scale. The efficacy of this treatment is similar to that of ALT, except that the maximal effect is reached sooner and retreatment of ALT-treated eyes is possible with good effect.

Procedure

Apraclonidine (Iopidine®) or brimonidine (Alphagan®) is used pre- and postoperatively. A coated one-mirror or specialty lens is placed under topical anesthesia. Typically 270–360° are treated. The spot size is preset at 400 μm and approximately 25 non-overlapping applications are placed per 90° treated (Figure 16.22). The total energies used per application are usually in the 0.7–1.3 mJ range. Small bubble formation is a useful end point for energy levels applied.

Postoperative care

The inflammatory response to SLT is less than with argon laser trabeculoplasty. Postoperative regimens among users polled varied from q.i.d steroids for 4 days to non-steroidals on a p.r.n. (discomfort) basis over concern of blunting the macrophage response to the treatment.

LASER SUTURE LYSIS

One of the most significant advances in filtration surgery, the selective cutting of sutures after trabeculectomy, has had a profound effect on decreasing immediate postoperative hypotony and its sequelae while maintaining the benefits of full-thickness surgery. The effective window for melting of sutures without antimetabolites is 0–21 days, with effectiveness falling rapidly after 14 days. The use of antimetabolites such as 5-fluorouracil extends this greatly and sutures can be melted with good effect up to 4–6 weeks postoperatively. The use of

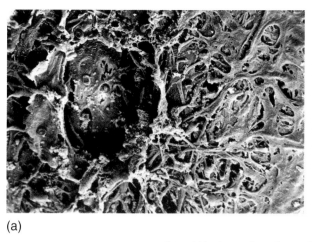

(a)

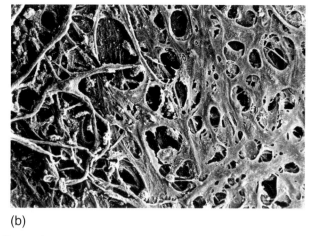

(b)

Figures 16.21   ALT versus SLT.   (a and b) The surface thermal effects of ALT versus SLT.

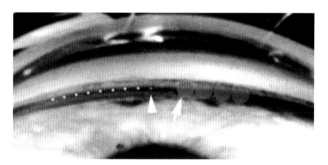

Figure 16.22   Spot size of argon laser trabeculoplasty versus selective laser trabeculoplasty.

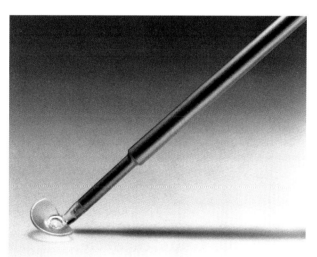

Figure 16.23   The Hoskins laser suture lysis lens.   The Hoskins laser suture lysis lens has a 120 diopter lens providing 1.2 × magnification. This decreases a 50 μm spot to about 42 μm in use. (Courtesy of Ocular Instruments.)

mitomycin C deserves special mention. This potent agent also suppresses aqueous production, and suture lysis should be undertaken with caution. In general, an increased interval to suture lysis will decrease the chances of hypotony and also decrease the effect. Suture lysis after the use of mitomycin C may even be attempted in the face of a failed filter with good results; the length of time after surgery that this may be effective is not known. There are some limits in that nylon sutures will depigment over time and will heat more slowly. Great care should be taken to avoid buttonhole formation during suture lysis after the use of mitomycin C. The technique requires the use of a continuous-wave argon or quasi-continuous wave laser (frequency doubled Nd:YAG; 532 nm), argon dye (610 nm), krypton (647.1 nm) or diode (810 nm) laser. In a postoperative eye with any blood or hemoglobin present in the subconjunctival space, the most useful lasers are those that can emit 610-nm laser light or in the red spectrum, such as krypton. This wavelength (610 nm) is poorly absorbed by hemoglobin and decreases the possibility of a conjunctival buttonhole. If hemoglobin is absent, there is some evidence that yellow (585 nm) or orange (610 nm) may limit conjunctival damage.

Patient evaluation and preparation

The number and the effect each scleral flap suture had at the time of surgery should be reviewed. Phenylephrine (2.5%) may be given to reduce congestion of the tissues before treatment. Three laser suture lysis lenses are in widest usage (Figures 16.23 to 16.25). All three lenses thin and blanch overlying tissues, allowing visualization of the sutures. All three lenses help hold the eyelid; the Hoskins and Ritch lenses have flanges for this purpose. The Hoskins and Mandelkorn laser suture lysis lenses provide magnification and smaller spot sizes which effectively increase irradiance. This should be taken into account when selecting continuous-wave power and exposure duration. Care should be taken in handling the Hoskins lens, as the neck is somewhat fragile.

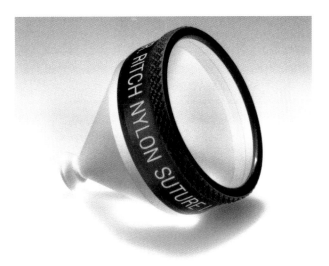

Figure 16.24   The Ritch laser suture lysis lens. The Ritch laser suture lysis lens does not provide magnification. The notch is useful for holding the eyelid but slightly cuts down the viewing field. (Courtesy of Ocular Instruments.)

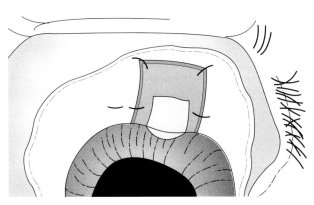

Figure 16.26   Laser suture lysis. The limbal sutures should be cut first. Premature lysis of the posterior corner sutures may cause profound hypotony.

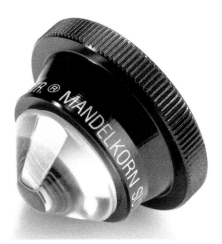

Figure 16.25   The Mandelkorn laser suture lysis lens. The Mandelkorn laser suture lysis lens provides 1.32 × magnification decreasing a 50 μm spot to 38 μm and increasing irradiance at the level of the suture 1.7 ×. (Courtesy of Ocular Instruments.)

Procedure

Topical anesthetic agents are used. The patient is asked to look down and the iridectomy is used to locate the approximate area of the scleral flap. The continuous-wave power should start low (50 μm; 0.05–0.1 s, 400 mW) with caution directly proportional to the relative potency of antimetabolite employed and amount of blood in the subconjunctival space. The laser spot should be focused on the suture to produce one long cut end which will lie flat (Figure 16.26). After successful lysis, the melted suture ends will retract; occasionally the suture

blanches but does not retract. This indicates that sufficient tension in the suture to cause retraction does not exist, and that no extra filtration can be gained by pursuing this suture. The one suture per session rule should be observed, especially when mitomycin C has been used. Additional sutures may be cut after careful evaluation a few hours after the initial attempt. In emergency situations aqueous may be released from the paracentesis created at surgery to temporize. Complications are mainly limited to small conjunctival buttonholes from the laser and hypotony with or without buttonhole formation. These may be treated with patching and with or without aqueous suppressants as the clinical situation dictates. If antimetabolites have been used, the use of a McCalister contact lens (Figure 16.27) without patching may be used to help close the conjunctival defect. This lens provides tamponade and may be tolerated for 1–2 weeks if needed. The use of aqueous suppressants is also an option with this lens. Bleb-related endophthalmitis is a continuous concern in any patient with a thin filtering bleb. The status of the scleral flap sutures should always be ascertained. If there appears to be an impending suture extrusion, this should be stopped by segmenting the suture or rounding the end.

AB EXTERNO CYCLODESTRUCTIVE PROCEDURES

Introduction

It has been over 60 years since Weve and Voght introduced diathermy and penetrating diathermy, respectively, as cyclodestructive techniques. Since then, electrolysis, beta-irradiation, cryotherapy, xenon arc, ultrasound, surgical excision and various visible and infrared lasers have been tried in an

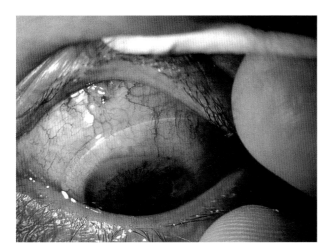

Figure 16.27 The McCalister contact lens. The McCalister contact lens provides tamponade after a full-thickness erbium:YAG laser sclerostomy. Both the laser sclerostomy and suture closing the conjunctival entry wound are visible.

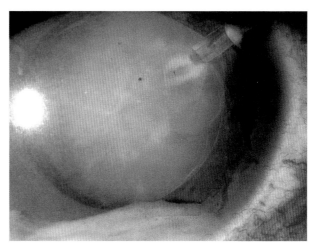

Figure 16.28 Tremendous inflammatory responses are possible after cyclophotocoagulation. (Courtesy of James Martone, MD.)

attempt to improve on this type of glaucoma surgery. In current practice, laser-based cyclodestructive procedures are useful in the treatment of glaucomas with poor surgical prognosis in which trabeculectomy with antimetabolites or aqueous drainage devices have failed. In addition, these procedures may also be used to decrease pain and to lower pressure in cases with limited visual potential. The most frequently used techniques are laser-based contact and non-contact cyclophotocoagulation using Nd:YAG or diode-based laser systems. The use of these techniques causes considerable pain, inflammation and visual loss; they should therefore be treatments of last recourse (Figure 16.28). Initial reports of sympathetic ophthalmia were in eyes with previous ocular surgery, creating controversy. Subsequently, there have been reports of sympathetic ophthalmia occurring in eyes after cyclophotocoagulation, not previously operated upon. Laser–tissue interactions vary somewhat depending on the wavelength and the peak power delivered. High-power, pulsed lasers (20 μs), such as the Microrupter series, cause more tissue disruption. Continuous-wave lasers require a longer exposure time to deliver sufficient energy to cause cyclophotocoagulation; the effects are more coagulative in nature. Distinctive pops that are heard are steam bubbles disrupting uveal tissue. The reported rates of phthisis are in excess of the occurrence of choroidal hemorrhage or loss of fixation in eyes with advanced glaucoma undergoing trabeculectomy. This argument in favor of cyclophotocoagulation should perhaps be revisited by surgeons. Although laser-based treatments produce less pain than cyclocryotherapy, they should be performed under retrobulbar anesthesia and the patients given a 3–4-day supply of moderate strength analgesic such as Vicodin.

Patient preparation

All cyclodestructive procedures are performed under retrobulbar anesthesia using a mixture of a short-acting (2–4% lidocaine) and long-acting (0.75% bupivicaine) local anesthetic. In the event that general anesthesia is used, the operator should remember to administer a retrobulbar block for postoperative comfort. Apraclonidine may also be given preoperatively if not currently used by the patient to blanch conjunctiva and minimize the chances of an IOP spike.

Contact transscleral cyclophotocoagulation

A representative diode-based unit is the Oculight SLx (Iris Medical, Mountain View, CA, Figure 16.29). These contact delivery systems use exposures much longer than the pulsed high peak power Nd:YAG systems; the tissue effects therefore tend to be somewhat less explosive and more coagulative. The use of a contact fiberoptic probe also creates a focal relative desiccation of sclera, increasing scleral transmission of laser light. The use of operator and assistant eye protection is mandatory and great care should be used when pointing the muzzle end of the fiberoptic. The patient is placed in the supine position and given retrobulbar anesthesia. An eyelid speculum is placed and the non-operative eye patched shut. Transillumination should be used to localize the ciliary body for placement of the fiberoptic. The Nd:YAG technique differs slightly from the diode technique. Generally, 8–10 applications per 90° of 4–6 J (watt × second) are placed for 360°, sparing the 3:00 and 9:00 positions. In non-Caucasian patients with increased melanin (chromophore) continuous-wave power is decreased. In addition, decreased power settings may

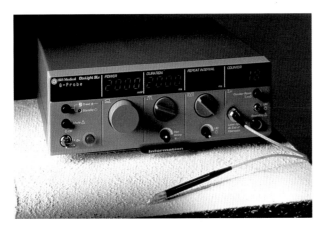

Figure 16.29 The Oculight SLX (Iris Medical, Mountain View, CA) diode photocoagulator.

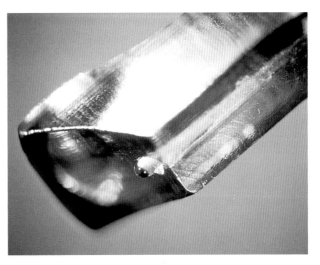

Figure 16.31 The G-probe for use with the Oculight SLX (Iris Medical, Mountain View, CA) diode photocoagulator. The probe is adapted to the contour of the limbus providing the correct orientation of the fiberoptic delivery system.

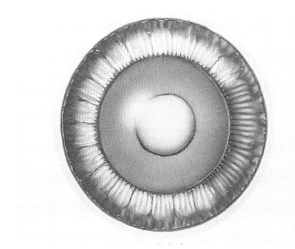

Figure 16.30 An alternative to 360° placement with sparing in the 3:00 and 9:00 positions suggested for diode laser cyclophotocoagulation.

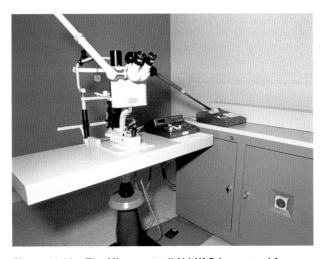

Figure 16.32 The Microrupter II Nd:YAG laser used for non-contact cyclophotocoagulation.

be needed when treating in the area of IOL haptics which are pigmented. When using a diode laser such as the Oculight SLx, suggested settings are 2.5 s at 2–2500 mW. The region spared is 45° above and below the temporal horizontal midline (Figure 16.30). Energy is delivered to the eye through the G-probe (Figure 16.31), which is a handpiece containing the fiberoptic for laser delivery. It is contoured to fit the limbus, providing the correct spacing to deliver the laser energy to the ciliary body.

Non-contact transscleral cyclophotocoagulation

Currently, the non-contact technique uses the Microrupter series lasers (Figure 16.32; Lasag, Thun, Switzerland). The Microrupter II is used in the free-running mode which delivers multiple joule, 20-µs pulses. To separate the focal points of the He:Ne aiming laser (ocular surface) and the

Nd:YAG laser (ciliary body), the focusing offset is set to 9 (Figure 16.33). A lid speculum or the Shields contact lens (Figure 16.34) may be used to facilitate treatment. Most commonly, 8–10 spots per quadrant are placed at a distance of 1–1.5 mm posterior to the limbus. The 3:00 and 9:00 are spared to avoid injury to the long posterior ciliary arteries. The operator may wish to consider transillumination of the globe for a more accurate location of the ciliary body in very long or short eyes. The energies used in most studies are in the 4–8 J range; 4–6 J are usually suggested at present. The use of the Shields lens (Figure 16.34) facilitates transfer of laser energy (eliminating conjunctival burns; Figure 16.35) and therefore the lower end of this energy range should be used to avoid overtreatment. The Shields lens also acts as a lid speculum and visual axis occluder,

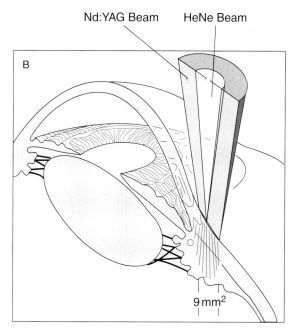

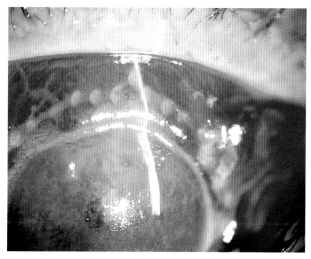

Figure 16.35 Conjunctival burns. Conjunctival burns produced by the non-contact method of cyclophotocoagulation without the use of the Shields contact lens.

Figure 16.33 Microrupter series lasers. To separate the focal points of the He:Ne aiming laser (ocular surface) and the Nd:YAG laser (ciliary body), the focusing offset is set to 9 on the Microrupter series lasers.

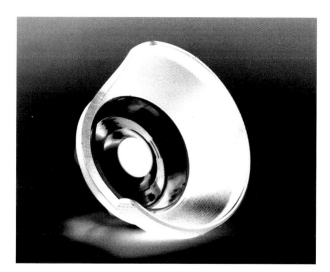

Figure 16.34 The Shields contact lens for transscleral cyclophotocoagulation. This lens compresses overlying tissues facilitating transfer of laser energy. A central opaque area shields the eye and etch marks at 1-mm interval increments allow accurate placement of laser energy. (Courtesy of Anne Coleman, MD.)

and has marks at 1-mm increments for reproducible placement of laser spots.

Postoperative care

The eye is patched shut until the postoperative day-1 examination. At this time prednisolone acetate 1% is started at 4–8 times per day based on induced inflammation. Atropine 1% is used twice

daily for cycloplegia. The ocular hypotensive medications are adjusted, based on clinical response, and the patient asked to return in 1 week and 1 month postoperatively. Eyes may be re-treated with decreased numbers of spots if the pressure is not adequately controlled at 4–6 weeks postoperatively.

ENDOSCOPIC CYCLOPHOTOCOAGULATION

The delivery of laser energy during endoscopic cyclophotocoagulation (ECP) is markedly different from transscleral delivery techniques. This technique requires an incision and viscoelastic or irrigation which allows entry of the device probe containing the endoscope and laser fiberoptic. The technique is commonly paired with cataract surgery after lens implantation but may be performed with other intraocular procedures. After completion of lens implantation, viscoelastic is used to create a space between iris and lens capsule to allow access to the ciliary processes. The ciliary processes are visualized endoscopically and the laser energy is applied (810 nm) at 500–900 mW for 0.5–2 s (Figure 16.36). This produces a whitening and shrinkage of the ciliary process (Figure 16.37). Alternatively, a painting technique to create a surface ablation of 180–200° after cataract surgery has also been described. Postoperatively, corticosteroids are included in the medical regimen and titrated to the level of observed inflammation.

AQUEOUS MISDIRECTION

In cases of aqueous misdirection, the aqueous collects posterior to the anterior hyaloid face, pushing the lens (natural or pseudophakos) and iris forward,

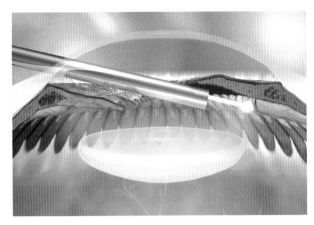

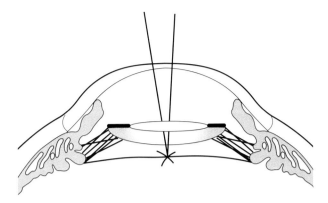

Figure 16.36 Endoscopic laser cyclophotocoagulation. Drawing showing the application of the laser energy in endoscopic laser cyclophotocoagulation (ECP) after completion of a clear cornea cataract procedure.

Figure 16.38 Aqueous misdirection. Aqueous misdirection may be stopped by disruption of the anterior hyaloid face. In pseudophakic patients with this problem, a capsulotomy should also be created.

AQUEOUS DRAINAGE IMPLANT TUBE OCCLUSIONS

Occlusions and malpositions are common complications of aqueous drainage implants. The majority of these will require operative intervention. In some cases they may be treated by laser therapy. In situations where the drainage tube has been occluded by blood, fibrin or vitreous pushed forward by choroidal effusions, treatment should wait until the transient hypotony has resolved. If the clinical situation can wait for this, then the strands of vitreous may be cut where they enter the drainage tube with a Q-switched Nd:YAG laser using 1–2-mJ pulses and an iridectomy lens (Figure 16.39). If this leaves a plug of vitreous in the drainage tube it may be dislodged by focusing and releasing a 3–5 mJ pulse focused in the sealed portion of the tube just behind the plug. This will dislodge the vitreous or fibrin into the anterior chamber or allow it to travel into the filtering capsule of the implant. If this fails, then operative intervention is warranted. Iris may also occlude the drainage tube. Evidence for iris bombé (Figure 16.12) should be sought and an iridectomy performed if needed. Iris may also be retracted by focal application of low continuous-wave power long-exposure argon laser energy.

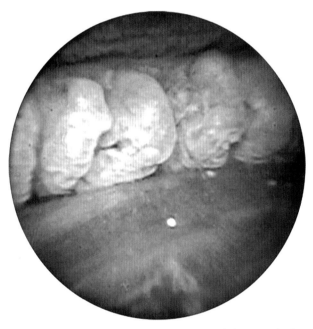

Figure 16.37 Endoscopic view of endoscopic laser cyclophotocoagulation (ECP)-treated ciliary processes.

closing the angle (Figure 16.38). Surgical disruption of the hyaloid face may allow the trapped aqueous to resume its normal pathway and relieve the anteriorly directed forces. The anterior hyaloid face may be disrupted using a Q-switched Nd:YAG laser delivering 2–4 mJ per pulse and 1–3 pulses per burst through a capsulotomy lens. This energy may be delivered through the pupil or a large iridectomy in both phakic and pseudophakic patients. In addition, if the posterior capsule is intact, a capsulotomy should also be performed.

Argon laser shrinkage of swollen ciliary processes through a large iridectomy has also been reported. The treatment should use a long low continuous wave power burn. The effects of successful treatment are dramatic with rapid restoration of normal anterior chamber depth.

REVISION OF THE FAILING FILTER

The use of the laser to lyse flap sutures as intraocular pressure rises following filtering surgery has previously been discussed. In cases where a pigmented membrane may be visualized, an argon laser may be used to revise the filtering site. In most cases, the internal ostium will be patent, pigmented tissues will be absent, and a Q-switched Nd:YAG laser will be required.

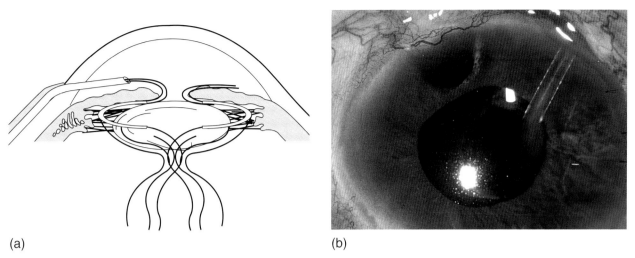

(a)   (b)

Figure 16.39   Drainage tubes occluded secondary to volume shifts.   If drainage tubes have occluded secondary to volume shifts from choroidal effusions, waiting until the hypotony resolves will place the vitreous on traction allowing it to be cut with a Nd:YAG laser. A second application will dislodge it into the anterior chamber or allow it to escape up the drainage tube into the filtering capsule.

Procedure

After topical anesthesia, an Abraham or Wise lens is placed on the eye. If mitomycin C was used, the scleral flap should be inspected for remaining sutures to cut, even if many months have passed since surgery. The main risk of revision is creating a conjunctival buttonhole. Therefore, energy is increased until optical breakdown is observed and the focus used is slightly deep to the episcleral surface. At the conclusion of the procedure a modified Seidel test with a fluorescein strip is performed. Buttonholes created may be most comfortably treated with a McCalister contact lens, with or without aqueous suppressants. The use of a Simmons shell with a disposable contact lens, symblepharon ring (medium size), or patching have also been described. Although good success has been reported when a filter has worked on an extended basis, it is the experience of the author and others that this type of revision has a low success. However, the cost and morbidity of these procedures are also low and selected patients may benefit. 'Needling' of the scleral flap would be an alternative approach to the use of lasers in this situation.

TREATMENT OF HYPOTONOUS CYCLODIALYSIS CLEFTS

Cyclodialysis clefts can be caused by blunt ocular trauma and surgical procedures involving the manipulation of iris. They seldom close spontaneously and a trial of cycloplegia with cessation of steroids will have even less success after the cleft has been present for 6 or more weeks. These clefts may be closed by the use of an argon laser.

Patient evaluation

The patient is given pilocarpine to maximally open the cyclodialysis cleft. Compression gonioscopy may also be helpful in diagnosis. If the anterior chamber has shallowed and the filtering angle is not visible, the patient is given retrobulbar anesthesia and the chamber deepened by intracameral sodium hyaluronate (plain Healon), an agent that will irrigate easily from the eye. The number, extent, and location of the clefts can now be established.

Procedure

If retrobulbar therapy was not necessary, anesthesia should be obtained with topical proparacaine. Topical anesthesia may be adequate, but this depends on the individual's discomfort threshold and the continuous-wave power required. Treatment is by the placement of overlapping laser spots on the sclera surface first. The spot size should be 100 μm and the exposure time 0.1 s. A continuous-wave power is selected that will generate a small gas bubble on the scleral surface (Figure 16.40). This will require a high power (> 1.5 W) and may cause discomfort requiring retrobulbar anesthesia. Secondly, the uveal side of the cleft is treated, starting in the depths of the cleft, as this tissue will contract, narrowing the cleft. The power delivered should be varied according to iris color with lighter-color irides receiving up to 1 W and brown receiving slightly less (800–900 mW range, initially). A marked surface effect should be seen on the uveal side of the cleft. Multiple treatments may be necessary.

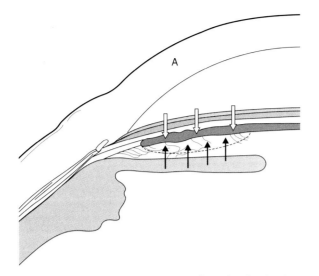

Figure 16.40   Cyclodialysis cleft.   The scleral side (larger arrows) is treated first with high-power argon laser burns. The uveal side (smaller arrows) follows at power and exposure settings that create a marked surface effect. (Adapted from Gonioscopy. Troncoso: Davis and Co., 1947.)

Postoperative care

If viscoelastic was used, it should be removed under sterile conditions by irrigation using gentle downward pressure on the posterior lip of the paracentesis. The patient is given atropine 1% three times daily and an antibiotic four times daily (if a paracentesis was made) for 3 days. The patient should also be instructed on the symptoms of an acute pressure rise and provided with an after-hours contact mechanism.

Further reading

Abraham RK. Protocol for single-session argon laser iridectomy for angle-closure glaucoma. Int Ophthalmol Clin 1981; 21: 145–66

Abraham RK, Miller GL. Outpatient argon iridectomy for angle-closure glaucoma: a 3-1/2 year study. Adv Ophthalmol 1977; 34: 186–91

Allingham RR, de Kater AW, Bellows AR, et al. Probe placement and power levels in contact transscleral neodymium:YAG cyclophotocoagulaton. Arch Ophthalmol 1990; 108: 738–42

Alward WL, Hodapp EA, Parel JM, et al. Argon laser endophotocoagulation closure of cyclodialysis clefts. Am J Ophthalmol 1988; 106: 748–9

Arden GB, Berninger T, Hogg CR, et al. A survey of color discrimination in German ophthalmologists. Changes associated with the use of lasers and operating microscopes. Ophthalmology 1991; 98: 567–75

Beckman H, Sugar HS. Neodymium laser cyclocoagulation. Arch Ophthalmol 1973; 90: 27–8

Beckman H, Sugar HS. Laser iridectomy therapy of glaucoma. Arch Ophthalmol 1973; 90: 453–5

Beckman H, Rota A, Barraco R, et al. Limbectomies, keratectomies, and keratostomies performed with a rapid pulsed carbon dioxide laser. Am J Ophthalmol 1971; 71: 1277–83

Berninger TA, Canning CR, Gunduz K, et al. Using argon laser blue light reduces ophthalmologists' color contrast sensitivity. Argon blue and surgeons vision. Arch Ophthalmol 1989; 107: 1453–8

Blok MD, Greve EL, Dunnebier EA, et al. Scleral flap sutures and the development of shallow or flat anterior chamber after trabeculectomy. Ophthalmic Surg 1993; 24: 309–13

Boettner EA, Wolter JR. Transmission of the ocular media. Ophthalmic Res 1962; 1: 776

Brancato R, Leoni G, Trabucchi G, et al. Probe placement and energy levels in continuous wave neodymium-YAG contact transscleral cyclophotocoagulation. Arch Ophthalmol 1990; 108: 679–83

Brancato R, Carassa R, Trabucchi G. Diode laser compared with argon laser for trabeculoplasty. Am J Ophthalmol 1991; 112: 50–5

Brown RH, Lynch MG, Tearse JE, et al. Neodymium:YAG vitreous surgery for phakic and pseudophakic malignant glaucoma. Arch Ophthalmol 1986; 104: 1464–6

Brown RH, Stewart RH, Lynch MG, et al. ALO 2145 reduces the IOP elevation after anterior segment laser surgery. Ophthalmology 1988; 95: 378–84

Brown SVL, Higginbotham E, Tessler H. Sympathetic ophthalmia following Nd:YAG cyclotherapy [letter]. Ophthalmic Surg 1965; 21: 736

Budenz DL, Brown SVL, Thomes JV, et al. Laser therapy for internally failing glaucoma filtration surgery. Ophthalmic Laser Ther 1986; 1: 169

Chen J, Cohn RA, Lin SC, et al. Endoscopic photocoagulation of the ciliary body for treatment of refractory glaucomas. Am J Ophthalmol 1997; 124: 787–96

Chopra H, et al. Early postoperative titration of bleb function: argon laser lysis and removable sutures in trabeculectomy. J Glaucoma 1992; 1: 54

Cohen EJ, Schwartz LW, Luskind RD, et al. Neodymium: YAG laser transscleral cyclophotocoagulation for glaucoma after penetrating keratoplasty. Ophthalmic Surg 1989; 20: 713–16

Cohen JS, Shaffer RN, Hetherington J Jr, et al. Revision of filtration surgery. Arch Ophthalmol 1977; 95: 1612–15

Cohn HC, Whalen WR, Aron-Rosa D. YAG laser treatment in a series of failed trabeculectomy. Am J Ophthalmol 1989; 108: 395

Dailey RA, Samples JR, Van Buskirk EM. Reopening filtration fistulas with neodymium:YAG laser. Am J Ophthalmol 1986; 102: 491–5

De Alwis TV. The long-term follow-up of patients treated with YAG laser to reopen closed or closing fistulae following glaucoma surgery. Eye 1993; 7: 444

Del Priore LV, Robin AL, Pollack IP. Long-term follow-up of neodymium:YAG laser angle surgery for open-angle glaucoma. Ophthalmology 1988; 95: 277–81

Del Priore LV, Robin AL, Pollack IP. Neodymium:YAG and argon laser iridotomy. Long-term follow-up in a prospective, randomized clinical trial. Ophthalmology 1988; 95: 1207–11

Drake MV. Neodymium:YAG laser iridotomy. Surv Ophthalmol 1987; 32: 171–7

Edward DP, Brown SV, Higginbotham E, et al. Sympathetic ophthalmia following neodymium:YAG cyclotherapy. Ophthalmic Surg 1989; 20: 544–6

Epstein DL, Steinert RF, Puliafito CA. Neodymium:YAG laser therapy to the anterior hyaloid in aphakic malignant glaucoma. Am J Ophthalmol 1984; 98: 137–43

Fankhauser F, van der Zypen E, Kwasniewska S, et al. Transscleral cyclophotocoagulation using a neodymium:YAG laser. Ophthalmic Surg 1986; 17: 94–100

Federman JL, Ando F, Schubert HD, et al. Contact laser for transscleral photocoagulation. Ophthalmic Surg 1987; 18: 183–4

Mittra RA, Allingham RR, Shields MB. Follow-up of argon laser trabeculoplasty: is a day-one postoperative IOP check necessary? Ophthalmic Surg Lasers 1995; 26: 410–13

Gaasterland DE, Hennings DR, Boutacoff TA, et al. Ab interno and ab externo filtering operations by laser contact surgery. Ophthalmic Surg 1987; 18: 254–7

Halkias A, Magauran DM, Joyce M. Ciliary block (malignant) glaucoma after cataract extraction with lens implanted treated with YAG laser capsulotomy and anterior hyaloidectomy. Br J Ophthalmol 1992; 76: 569–70

Hampton C, Shields MB, Miller KN, et al. Evaluation of a protocol for transscleral neodymium:YAG cyclophotocoagulation in one hundred patients. Ophthalmology 1990; 97: 910–17

Harbin TS Jr. Treatment of cyclodialysis clefts with argon laser photocoagulation. Ophthalmology 1982; 89: 1082

Haut J, Gaven I, Moulin F, et al. Study of the first hundred phakic eyes treated by peripheral iridotomy using the Nd:YAG laser. Int Ophthalmol 1986; 9: 227–35

Hawkins TA, Stewart WC. One year results of semiconductor transscleral cyclophotocoagulation in glaucoma patients. Arch Ophthalmol 1993; 111: 488–91

Herbort CP, Mermoud A, Schnyder C, et al. Anti-inflammatory effect of diclofenac drops after argon laser trabeculoplasty. Arch Ophthalmol 1993; 111: 481–3

Herschler J. Laser shrinkage of the ciliary processes: a treatment for malignant (ciliary block) glaucoma. Ophthalmology 1980; 87: 1155–9

Hill RA, Minckler DS, Lee M, et al. Apraclonidine prophylaxis for postcycloplegic IOP spikes. Ophthalmology 1991; 98: 1083–6

Hillenkamp F. Interaction between laser radiation and biological systems. In Hillenkamp F, Pratesi R, Sacchi CA, eds. Lasers in Biology and Medicine. New York: Plenum, 1980

Ho T, Fan R. Sequential argon-YAG laser iridotomies in dark irides. Br J Ophthalmol 1992; 76: 329–31

Hoskins HD, Migliazzo CV. Laser iridectomy – a technique for blue irides. Ophthalmic Surg 1984; 15: 448–90

Hoskins HD Jr, Migliazzo C. Management of failing filtering blebs with the argon laser. Ophthalmic Surg 1984; 15: 731

Hotchkiss ML, Robin AL, Pollack IP, et al. Nonsteroidal anti-inflammatory agents after argon laser trabeculoplasty: a trial with flurbiprofen and indomethacin. Ophthalmology 1984; 91: 969–76

James WA Jr, de Roetth A Jr, Forbes M, et al. Argon laser photomydriasis. Am J Ophthalmol 1976; 81: 62–70

Joondeph HC. Management of postoperative and post-traumatic cyclodialysis clefts with argon laser photocoagulation. Ophthalmic Surg 1980; 11: 186

Juzych MS, Chopra V, Banitt MR, et al. Comparison of long-term outcomes of selective laser trabeculoplasty versus argon laser trabeculoplasty in open-angle glaucoma. Ophthalmology 2004; 111: 1853–9

Kalenak JW, Parkinson JM, Kass MA, et al. Transscleral neodymium:YAG laser cyclocoagulation for uncontrolled glaucoma. Ophthalmic Surg 1990; 21: 346–51

Khuri CH. Argon laser iridectomies. Am J Ophthalmol 1973; 76: 490–3

Kimbrough RL, Trempe CS, Brockhurst RJ, et al. Angle-closure in nanophthalmos. Am J Ophthalmol 1979; 88: 572–9

Kitazawa Y, Taniguchi T, Sugiyama K. Use of apraclonidine to reduce acute IOP rise following Q-switched Nd:YAG laser iridotomy. Ophthalmic Surg 1989; 20: 49

Klapper RM. Q-switched Neodymium:YAG laser iridotomy. Ophthalmology 1984; 91: 1017

Klapper RM, Wandel T, Donnenfeld E, et al. Transscleral neodymium:YAG thermal cyclophotocoagulation in refractory glaucoma. A preliminary report. Ophthalmology 1988; 95: 719–22

Klein HZ, Shields MB, Ernest JT. Two-stage argon laser trabeculoplasty in open angle glaucoma. Am J Ophthalmol 1985; 99: 392–5

Krasnov MM. Q-switched laser iridectomy and Q-switched laser goniopuncture. Adv Ophthalmol 1977; 34: 192–6

Krasnov MM, Naumidi LP. Contact transscleral laser cyclocoagulation in glaucoma. Ann Ophthalmol 1990; 22: 354–8

Kurata F, Krupin T, Kolker AE. Reopening filtration fistulas with transconjunctival argon laser photocoagulation. Am J Ophthalmol 1984; 98: 340

Latina MA, Rankin GA. Internal and transconjunctival neodymium:YAG revision of late-failing filters. Ophthalmology 1991; 98: 215

Latina MA, Sibayan SA, Shin DH, et al. Q-switched 532-nm Nd:YAG laser trabeculoplasty (selective laser trabeculoplasty): a multicenter, pilot, clinical study. Ophthalmology 1998; 105: 2082–8; discussion 2089–90

Lerman S. Radiant Energy and the Eye. New York: Macmillan, 1980

Lesperance FA Jr. Ophthalmic Lasers: Photocoagulation, Photo-radiation, and Surgery, 3rd edn. St Louis, MO: Mosby, 1989

Lewis R, Perkins TW, Gangnon R, et al. The rarity of clinically significant rise in intraocular pressure after laser peripheral iridotomy with apraclonidine. Ophthalmology 1998; 105: 2256–9

Lieberman MF. Suture lysis by laser and goniolens. Am J Ophthalmol 1983; 95: 257

Lim AS, Tan A, Chew P, et al. Laser iridoplasty in the treatment of severe acute angle closure glaucoma. Int Ophthalmol 1993; 17: 33–6

Lima FE, Magacho L, Carvalho DM, et al. A prospective, comparative study between endoscopic cyclophotocoagulation and the Ahmed drainage implant in refractory glaucoma. J Glaucoma 2004; 13: 233–7

Little BC, Hitchings RA. Pseudophakic malignant glaucoma: Nd:YAG capsulotomy as a primary treatment. Eye 1993; 7: 102

McMillan TA, Stewart WC, Nutaitis MJ, et al. The effect of varying wavelength on subconjunctival scleral laser suture lysis in rabbits. Acta Ophthalmol (Copenh) 1992; 70: 758–61

Melamed S, Ashkenazi I, Glovinski J, et al. Tight scleral flap trabeculectomy with postoperative laser suture lysis. Am J Ophthalmol 1990; 109: 303–9

Melamed S, Ashkenazi I, Blumenthal M. Nd:YAG laser hyaloidotomy for malignant glaucoma following one-piece 7mm intraocular lens implantation. Br J Ophthalmol 1991; 75: 501

Minckler DS. Does Nd:YAG cyclotherapy cause sympathetic ophthalmia? [editorial] Ophthalmic Surg 1989; 20: 543

Morinelli EN, Sidoti PA, Heuer DK, et al. Laser suture lysis after mitomycin C trabeculectomy. Ophthalmology 1996; 103: 306–14

Nelson JS, Berns MW. Basic laser physics and tissue interactions. Contemporary Dermatology 1988; 2: 2

Noureddin BN, Wilson-Holt N, Lavin M, et al. Advanced uncontrolled glaucoma. Nd:YAG cyclophotocoagulation or tube surgery. Ophthalmology 1992; 99: 430–6

Oh Y, Katz LJ. Indications and technique for reopening closed filtering blebs using the Nd:YAG laser: a review and case series. Ophthalmic Surg 1993; 24: 617

Oram O, Gross RL, Severin TD, et al. Opening an occluded Molteno tube with the picosecond neodymium–yttrium–lithium fluoride laser. Arch Ophthalmol 1994; 112: 1023

Ormerod LD, Baerveldt G, Sunalp MA, et al. Management of the hypotonous cyclodialysis cleft. Ophthalmology 1991; 98: 1384–93

Pappa KS, Derick RJ, Weber PA, et al. Late argon suture lysis after mitomycin-C trabeculectomy. Ophthalmology 1993; 100: 1268–71

Pastor SA, Singh K, Lee DA, et al. Cyclophotocoagulation: a report by the American Academy of Ophthalmology. Ophthalmology 2001; 108: 2130–8

Partamiam LG. Treatment of a cyclodialysis cleft with argon laser photocoagulation in a patient with a shallow anterior chamber. Am J Ophthalmol 1985; 99: 5

Pavlin CJ, Ritch R, Foster FS. Ultrasound biomicroscopy in plateau iris syndrome. Am J Ophthalmol 1992; 113: 390

Perkins ES, Brown NA. Iridotomy with a ruby laser. Br J Ophthalmol 1973; 57: 487

Pollack IP, Patz A. Argon laser iridotomy: an experimental and clinical study. Ophthalmic Surg 1976; 7: 22

Potash SD, Tello C, Liebmann J, et al. Ultrasound biomicroscopy in pigment dispersion syndrome. Ophthalmology 1994; 101: 332–9

Praeger DL. The reopening of closed filtering blebs using the neodymium:YAG laser. Ophthalmology 1984; 91: 373

Quigley HA. Long-term follow-up of laser iridotomy. Ophthalmology 1981; 88: 218

Rankin GA, Latina MA. Transconjunctival Nd:YAG laser revision of failing trabeculectomy. Ophthalmic Surg 1990; 21: 365

Ritch R. Argon laser treatment for medically unresponsive attacks of angle-closure glaucoma. Am J Ophthalmol 1982; 94: 197

Ritch R. Techniques of Argon Laser Iridectomy and Iridoplasty. Palo Alto, CA: Coherent Medical Press, 1983

Ritch R. A new lens for argon laser trabeculoplasty. Ophthalmic Surg 1985; 16: 331

Ritch R. Argon laser peripheral iridoplasty: an overview. J Glaucoma 1992; 1: 206

Ritch R. Plateau iris is caused by abnormally positioned ciliary processes. J Glaucoma 1992; 1: 23

Ritch R, Palmberg P. Argon laser iridectomy in densely pigmented irides. Am J Ophthalmol 1982; 94: 800

Ritch R, Solomon IS. Glaucoma surgery. In: Esperance FA, ed. Ophthalmic Lasers, 3rd edn. St Louis, MO: Mosby, 1989

Ritch R, Potash SD, Liebmann JM. A new lens for argon laser suture lysis. Ophthalmic Surg 1994; 25: 126

Robin AL, Pollack IP. Argon laser peripheral iridotomies in the treatment of primary angle closure glaucoma: long-term follow-up. Arch Ophthalmol 1982; 100: 919

Robin AL, Pollack IP. A comparison of neodymium:YAG and argon laser iridotomies. Ophthalmology 1984; 91: 1011

Robin AL, Pollack IP, DeFaller JM. Effects of topical ALO 2145 (p-aminoclonidine hydrochloride) on intraocular pressure rise following argon laser iridotomy. Arch Ophthalmol 1987; 105: 1208

Robin AL, Pollack IP, de Fallor JM. Effect of ALO 2145 on intraocular pressure following argon laser trabeculoplasty. Arch Ophthalmol 1987; 105: 656

Savage JA, Simmons RJ. Staged glaucoma filtration surgery with planned early conversion from scleral flap to full-thickness operation using argon laser. Ophthalmic Laser Ther 1986; 1: 201

Schrems W, Belcher CDI, Tomlinson CP. Neodymium:YAG laser iridectomy: a report of 200 cases. Ophthalmic Laser Ther 1987; 2: 33

Schuman JS, Puliafito CA. Laser cyclophotocoagulation. Int Ophthalmol Clin 1990; 30: 111

Schuman JS, Puliafito CA, Allingham RR, et al. Contact transscleral continuous wave neodymium:YAG laser cyclophotocoagulation. Ophthalmology 1990; 97: 571–80

Schuman JS, Jacobson JJ, Puliafito CA, et al. Experimental use of semiconductor diode laser in contact transscleral cyclophotocoagulation in rabbits. Arch Ophthalmol 1990; 108: 1152–7

Schuman JS, Noecker RJ, Puliafito CA, et al. Energy levels and probe placement in contact transscleral semiconductor diode laser cyclophotocoagulation in human cadaver eyes. Arch Ophthalmol 1991; 109: 1534–8

Schuman JS, Bellows AR, Shingleton BJ, et al. Contact transscleral Nd:YAG laser cyclophotocoagulation: midterm results. Ophthalmology 1992; 99: 1089–94

Schuman JS, Stinson WG, Hutchinson BT, et al. Holmium laser sclerectomy. Success and complications. Ophthalmology 1993; 100: 1060–5

Schwartz AL, Love DC, Schwartz MA. Longterm follow-up of argon laser trabeculoplasty for uncontrolled open angle glaucoma. Arch Ophthalmol 1985; 103: 1482

Schwartz AL, Weiss H. Bleb leak with hypotony after laser suture lysis and trabeculectomy with mitomycin-C. Arch Ophthalmol 1992; 110: 1049

Shahinian LJ, Egbert PR, Williams AS. Histologic study of healing after ab interno laser sclerostomy. Am J Ophthalmol 1992; 114: 216

Shields MB, Wilkerson MH, Echelman DA. A comparison of two energy levels for noncontact transscleral neodymium-YAG cyclophotocoagulation. Arch Ophthalmol 1993; 111: 484

Shingleton BJ, Richter CU, Dharma SK, et al. Long-term efficacy of argon laser trabeculoplasty, a ten-year follow-up study. Ophthalmology 1993; 100: 1324–9

Simmons RJ. Discussion of Herschler J. Laser shrinkage of ciliary processes: a treatment for malignant glaucoma. Ophthalmology 1980; 87: 1158

Simmons RB, Blasini M, Shields MB, et al. Comparison of transscleral neodymium:YAG cyclophotocoagulation with and without a contact lens in human autopsy eyes. Am J Ophthalmol 1990; 109: 174–9

Simmons RB, Shields MB, Blasini M, et al. Transscleral Nd:YAG laser cyclophotocoagulation with a contact lens. Am J Ophthalmol 1991; 112: 671–7

Sliney DH, Mainster MA. Potential laser hazards to the clinician during photocoagulation. Am J Ophthalmol 1987; 103: 758

Smith J. Argon laser trabeculoplasty: comparison of bichromatic and monochromatic wavelengths. Ophthalmology 1984; 91: 355

Spaeth GL, Baez K. Argon laser trabeculoplasty controls one third of cases of progressive, uncontrolled, open angle glaucoma for 5 years. Arch Ophthalmol 1992; 110: 491

Spurny RC, Lederer CM Jr. Krypton laser trabeculoplasty. Arch Ophthalmol 1984; 102: 1626

Starita RJ, Klapper RM. Neodymium:YAG photodisruption of the anterior hyaloid face in aphakic flat chamber: a diagnostic and therapeutic tool. Int Ophthalmol Clin 1985; 25: 119

Stetz D, Smith HJ, Ritch R. A simplified technique for laser iridectomy in blue irides. Am J Ophthalmol 1983; 96: 249

Tello C, Chi T, Shepps G, et al, Ultrasound biomicroscopy in pseudophakic malignant glaucoma. Ophthalmology 1993; 100: 1330–4

The Glaucoma Laser Trial Research Group. The Glaucoma Laser Trial (GLT). 2. Results of argon laser trabeculoplasty versus topical medicines. Ophthalmology 1990; 97: 1403

Thomas JV. Pupilloplasty and photomydriasis. In: Belcher CD, Thomas JV, Simmons RJ, eds. Photocoagulation in Glaucoma and Anterior Segment Disease. Baltimore, MD: Williams & Wilkins, 1984

Ticho U, Ivry M. Reopening of occluded filtering blebs by argon laser photocoagulation. Am J Ophthalmol 1977; 84: 413

Tomey KF, Traverso CE, Shammas IV. Neodymium:YAG laser iridotomy in the treatment and prevention of angle closure glaucoma: a review of 373 eyes. Arch Ophthalmol 1987; 105: 476

Tomlinson CP, Brigham M, Belcher CD III. Suture manipulation with the argon laser. Ophthalmic Laser Ther 1987; 2: 151

Trope GE, Ma S. Mid-term effects of neodymium:YAG transscleral cyclocoagulation in glaucoma. Ophthalmology 1990; 97: 73

Van Buskirk EM. Reopening filtration fistulas with the argon laser. Am J Ophthalmol 1982; 94: 1

Van Rens GH. Transconjunctival reopening of an occluded filtration fistula with the Q-switched neodymium:YAG laser. Doc Ophthalmol 1988; 70: 205

Vogel A, Dlugos C, Nuffer R, et al. Optical properties of human sclera and their consequences for transscleral laser applications. Lasers Surg Med 1991; 11: 331–40

Walsh JT, Flotte TJ, Deutsch TF. Er:YAG laser ablation of tissue: effect of pulse duration and tissue type on thermal damage. Lasers Surg Med 1989; 9: 314

Weber PA, Henry MA, Kapetansky FM, et al. Argon laser treatment of the ciliary processes in aphakic glaucoma with flat anterior chamber. Am J Ophthalmol 1984; 97: 82–5

Wetzel W, Haring G, Brinkmann R, et al. Laser sclerostomy ab externo using the erbium:YAG laser. First results of a clinical study. Ger J Ophthalmol 1994; 3: 112–15

Wilensky JT, Welch D, Mirolovich M. Transscleral cyclocoagulation using a neodymium:YAG laser. Ophthalmic Surg 1985; 16: 95

Wilson RP, Javitt JC. Ab interno laser sclerostomy in aphakic patients with glaucoma and chronic inflammation. Am J Ophthalmol 1990; 110: 178

Wise JB. Ten-year results of laser trabeculoplasty. Eye 1987; 1: 45

Wise JB, Munnerlyn CR, Erickson PJ. A high-efficiency laser iridotomy-sphincterotomy lens. Am J Ophthalmol 1986; 101: 546

Yassur Y, David R, Rosenblatt I, et al. Iridotomy with red krypton laser. Br J Ophthalmol 1986; 70: 295–7

17 Filtering surgery

Jeffrey D Henderer, Richard P Wilson

INTRODUCTION

For roughly 100 years, attempts have been made to lower intraocular pressure by surgically establishing continual filtration of aqueous from the anterior chamber to the subconjunctival space. A wide variety of techniques were used until the early 1970s when 'trabeculectomy' as described by Cairns in 1968 became the preferred technique for glaucoma filtering surgery. The continued popularity of trabeculectomy has been due to a lower postoperative complication rate compared to previous procedures. Its safety is due to the partial-thickness scleral flap overlying the filtration site, thereby providing some resistance to flow and decreasing the incidence of early postoperative complications due to the over-filtration that had often accompanied 'full thickness' procedures. Because of the decreased complication rate, trabeculectomy has become the filtering procedure of choice, and over the past 20 years much of the work done in glaucoma surgery has been directed towards modifications of the basic procedure, attempting to further lower the complication rate and increase the success rate. In this chapter, a basic trabeculectomy technique is presented with attention to the details of its performance. Modifications of the technique are also presented, including various suture techniques and the use of antimetabolites.

GENERAL PRINCIPLES

Filtering surgery is usually indicated when the patient's glaucoma is observed to worsen at the present level of intraocular pressure, usually after establishing maximum tolerated medical therapy, and possibly following laser trabeculoplasty. Surgery may also be indicated when the target intraocular pressure has not been achieved by other means and the disease is expected to worsen. In some

cases, such as low-tension glaucoma, it may be difficult to achieve the low intraocular pressure necessary to stabilize the disease with medicine or laser, thereby leading to earlier surgery.

The goal of guarded filtering surgery is to create a partial thickness scleral flap at the limbus overlying a hole punched through the remaining eye wall, effectively connecting the anterior chamber to the outside world. The scleral flap is sutured back into place, with tension on the sutures adjusted to allow a calculated flow out of the hole. The aqueous then collects under the conjunctiva, elevating it and forming a 'bleb.' The success of the surgery depends on a constant leak of aqueous through the scleral opening, and the integrity of the conjunctival bleb, so there is no leak of aqueous onto the ocular surface. For this reason, during filtering surgery, the conjunctiva should be handled as little as possible and as meticulously as possible. The conjunctiva overlying the area of the filtration site should never be touched. Non-toothed forceps, such as utility forceps or Pierce–Hoskins forceps, should be used when handling conjunctiva.

Bleeding conjunctival and scleral vessels must be painstakingly cauterized. Even slight oozing, which would be of little significance in other types of ocular surgery, can significantly decrease the chance of successful glaucoma filtering surgery, by promoting scarring of the scleral flap or limiting the size and functional capacity of the filtration bleb. A 23-gauge needle tip cautery may be used for precise cauterization of small vessels, and may also be used within the anterior chamber to stop bleeding of iris or ciliary body vessels.

The surgeon must make certain prior to entering into the anterior chamber that the scleral flap is dissected anteriorly enough so that the sclerostomy site will enter the anterior chamber and will not be over the ciliary body. Careful observation is required in patients with altered limbal anatomy from previous surgery. When a limbus-based conjunctival flap is being developed in such a patient, careful and patient dissection is often required to extend the dissection anteriorly enough for appropriate placement of the filtration site.

After initial suturing of the scleral flap, the surgeon should re-form the anterior chamber to a normal depth and pressure and then always evaluate the amount of filtration obtained prior to closing the conjunctiva. As described in the following text, further manipulation can be done to adjust filtration to a specific level of outflow, rather than simply placing a predetermined number of sutures in the scleral flap for every case. This intraoperative adjustment is crucial for obtaining a consistently successful result.

TECHNIQUES

Preparation

After sterile prepping and draping, the lid speculum should be inserted with care so that the speculum does not cause pressure on the globe. A traction suture should be placed in such a way as to maximally infraduct the globe, exposing conjunctiva as far superiorly and posteriorly as possible, especially if a limbus-based conjunctival flap is being used. This is crucial for making the conjunctival incision as far posterior as possible, preferably 10 mm posterior to the limbus, so that the area of the postoperative filtering bleb will not be limited by scar tissue from the conjunctival incision. Either a corneal traction suture or a superior rectus bridle suture may be used. The corneal traction suture has the advantage of avoiding the rare instance of scleral perforation which may occur with the larger needle and less well visualized needle pass of the superior rectus

bridle suture, and also avoids bleeding at the superior rectus and postoperative ptosis that may occur rarely with the superior rectus bridle suture. However, the corneal traction suture has the disadvantage that dissection through the Tenon's capsule is more laborious. Also, the other disadvantage of the corneal traction suture is the possibility, especially in myopes with pliable sclera, that when the eye is forcibly infraducted near the end of the surgery for closure of the limbus-based conjunctival flap, the traction at the superior limbus will distort the anatomy enough at the filtration site that the wound cleft will gape with outflow of aqueous and inability to maintain a formed chamber during conjunctival wound closure. In general, we prefer a superior rectus bridle suture for limbus-based conjunctival flaps and a corneal traction suture, if needed, for fornix-based flaps.

Placement of a corneal traction suture is best done with a 6-0 or 7-0 Vicryl suture on an S-29 needle through superior peripheral clear cornea (Figure 17.1b). Care should be taken not to enter the anterior chamber. If the filtration site is to be off-set either superonasally or superotemporally, then the traction suture should be centered in the quadrant to be used. The globe needs minimal stabilization during passage of this suture, with a cellulose sponge being sufficient to hold the globe steady for needle passage. With either suture technique, the surgeon should remember at all times to resist the tendency to grasp conjunctiva on the superior bulbar portion of the globe anywhere near the planned filtration site.

A superior rectus bridle suture is best done with a 4-0 silk suture on a taper-point needle. The superior rectus muscle can be grasped with a toothed forceps by either infraducting the globe with a muscle hook pressing into the inferior fornix

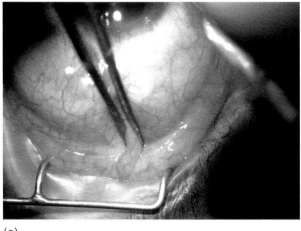

(a)

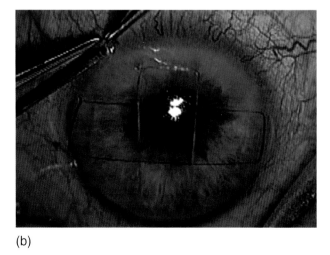

(b)

Figure 17.1 Blunt dissection and traction suture. (a) A muscle hook is used to turn the eye as far as possible before the superior rectus is grasped. This allows the suture line with its foreign body reaction to be as far as possible from the site of filtration. (b) A 7-0 Vicryl corneal traction suture has been placed in front of the eventual scleral flap location and the eye rotated inferiorly. The black horizontal mattress suture is an anterior chamber-maintaining suture (see Figure 17.20).

and grasping the muscle posteriorly under direct visualization (Figure 17.1a), or by sliding the closed forceps into the superior fornix and then opening the forceps, rotating it perpendicularly to the globe, and with firm downward pressure grasping the superior rectus. The globe can then be infraducted and the bridle suture placed underneath the muscle. Since toothed forceps are necessary for grasping the superior rectus, a conjunctival buttonhole may occur, but it will be far posteriorly in the area of the conjunctival incision.

Conjunctival flap dissection

There is no consensus among surgeons as to whether a limbus-based or fornix-based conjunctival flap is associated with a better surgical result. The surgeon who only occasionally performs filtering surgery may feel more comfortable with a fornix-based approach, because the surgical field is easier to see, and perhaps have more assurance that the scleral flap dissection and anterior chamber entry is positioned appropriately anteriorly. A significant disadvantage of the fornix-based approach is the higher chance of a wound leak when closing the conjunctiva at the end of the case. Prior to the widespread use of antimetabolites, a small leak was usually of no consequence, except for perhaps resulting in a less extensive bleb. However, with the use of antimetabolites, such a leak may have much more grave consequences. The leak may take much longer to seal or not seal at all, putting the patient at risk of blebitis, flat anterior chamber, and hypotony with or without choroidal detachment. A further disadvantage of the fornix-based approach is that a wound leak may be induced if laser suture lysis or digital ocular compression is needed in the early postoperative period. Using the conjunctival suturing technique developed by Dr James Wise has been a great help in reducing the likelihood of

limbal leaks. Nonetheless, the use of the limbus-based flap with its intact limbal conjunctival barrier reduces the concerns encountered with a limbal incision, often making it the approach of choice, at least when antimetabolites are to be used.

When using a limbus-based conjunctival flap, the conjunctiva is incised with Westcott scissors at least 10 mm posterior to the superior limbus. The incision is extended in either direction for a total of about 10–15 mm of length, taking care that the entire length of the incision remains at least 10 mm posterior to the limbus. If a corneal traction suture is used, then the Tenon's capsule is grasped with a non-toothed forceps, such as the Pierce–Hoskins, by both the assistant and the surgeon in order to tent it upward, taking care not to include the superior rectus muscle. The Tenon's capsule is then incised with the Westcott scissors down to bare sclera anterior to the superior rectus insertion and the Tenon's incision is extended for at least the entire length of the conjunctival incision and perhaps 1–2 mm further on either side to allow comfortable stretching of the tissue forward. The conjunctival–Tenon's flap complex can then be reflected downward over the cornea with the assistance of both sharp and blunt dissection with Westcott scissors through the episcleral attachments about a millimeter posterior to the conjunctival limbal insertion. This dissection should always be done under direct visualization with the flap stretched anteriorly, thereby making an inadvertent buttonhole incision much less likely. Once the episcleral attachments have been incised, the remainder of the forward dissection can be done bluntly with a cellulose sponge, in order to decrease the likelihood of buttonhole formation (Figure 17.2a). However, it is important to make certain that the Tenon's fibers are dissected as far forward into the corneoscleral sulcus as possible. In some patients, such as young patients or African-American patients, the Tenon's

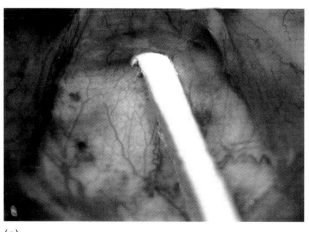

(a)

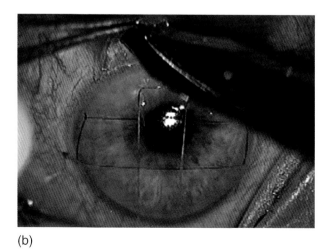

(b)

Figure 17.2　Blunt dissection.　(a) A sponge is used to bluntly dissect down to the limbus, minimizing the chance of a buttonhole. (b) Blunt Wescott scissors and non-toothed forceps are used to undermine a fornix-based conjunctival and Tenon's flap. The hemorrhage outlines the extent of the dissection.

may be too thick for the dissection to be completed with the cellulose sponge and therefore the final remaining fibers must be dissected with a 67 blade tip oriented perpendicularly to the scleral surface and 'scraped' circumferentially along the base of the Tenon's attachments. The remaining tissue can then be pushed forward into the sulcus as desired. Patient and complete anterior dissection of the conjunctival flap is crucial to allow sufficient exposure to perform the proper scleral flap dissection.

If a superior rectus bridle suture is used, the only difference from the technique just described is with the conjunctival and Tenon's incision. With the bridle suture, the surgeon should grasp conjunctiva only with the non-toothed forceps just anterior to the bridle suture and pull the conjunctiva toward the patient's feet to put the tissue on stretch and then incise it with the blunt Westcott scissors. The Tenon's is grasped in a like manner but without the need for an assistant to also grasp this tissue since it is, in effect, already held by the bridle suture. As this Tenon's incision is done over the superior rectus, care should be taken not to cut into muscle. The incision is then extended as previously described.

If a fornix-based conjunctival flap approach is elected, a limbal conjunctival incision of about 6–8 mm is initiated by tenting the conjunctiva near the limbus with non-toothed forceps and the incision is begun with the Westcott scissors (Figure 17.2b). This is carefully extended along the limbus for the full length of the peritomy. The Tenon's is incised in a like manner. Blunt dissection with the blunt Westcott scissors should be done posteriorly underneath the Tenon's, along the length of the limbal incision, to allow for good posterior exposure, to encourage larger posterior bleb development, and to allow posterior placement of antimetabolites, if necessary (Figure 17.2b). We have had good success using a fornix-based trabeculectomy technique

popularized by Peng Khaw, MD. We now recommend dissecting enough of a conjunctival flap to permit much of the superior quadrant to serve a bleb. It may also be helpful to dissect posteriorly enough to puncture the posterior Tenon's insertion near the superior rectus insertion. This large dissection, combined with a broad application of antimetabolite and posteriorly directed flow from the scleral flap promotes a low, diffuse bleb that is much less likely to break down over time and pose an infection risk.

Scleral flap dissection

The size and shape of the scleral flap is of some significance. Most surgeons prefer either a square, rectangular or triangular flap with the anterior base of the flap being 2–4 mm with the length likewise ranging from 2 to 4 mm. Depending on the placement of the underlying scleral punch, rectangular and triangular flaps can promote sideways flow or posterior flow. Khaw's theory holds that sideways flow more commonly leads to eventual bleb breakdown at the limbus and so, with his technique, the goal is to create posteriorly directed flow through the flap to form a low, diffuse bleb. To achieve this, a large rectangular flap with a central punch is needed. Prior to dissection of the flap, the surgeon should confirm its appropriate placement anteriorly at the limbus and then, if desired, outline the desired dimensions with the needle-point cautery (Figure 17.3a). A 67 blade should then be used to outline the scleral flap with a scleral incision of one-half to two-thirds scleral thickness (Figure 17.3b). The posterior-most aspect of the scleral flap is then grasped with non-toothed forceps and the flap is dissected forward with the blade held almost flat against the sclera (Figure 17.4). During this dissection, the scleral flap should be pulled continually anteriorly with the forceps so that the dissection is

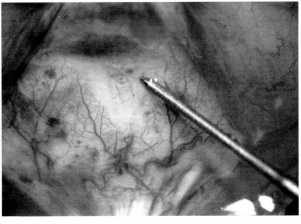

(a)

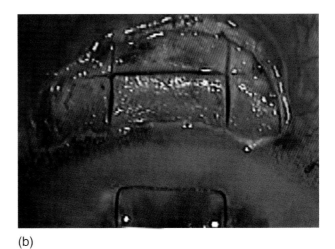

(b)

Figure 17.3 Scleral flap. (a) Cautery is used to outline the scleral flap. (b) A 67 blade is used to outline a partial-thickness scleral flap.

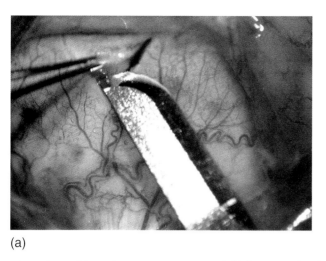
(a)

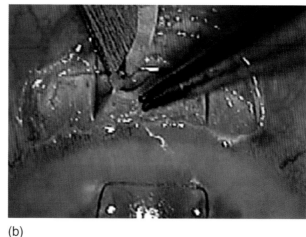
(b)

Figure 17.4 Dissecting the scleral flap. (a) The posterior tip of the scleral flap is grasped firmly and lifted toward the ceiling and anteriorly. The best surgical plane will be found at the base of the fibers where the sclera pulls apart. (b) The scleral flap is dissected with the 67 blade using traction from a forceps to facilitate visualization.

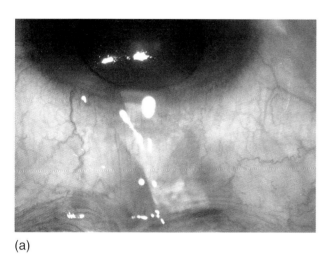
(a)

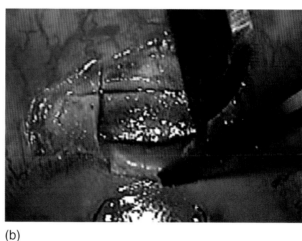
(b)

Figure 17.5 Dissecting the scleral flap. (a) The dissection is carried forward until the knife blade can be seen in clear cornea anterior to the limbus. (b) The scleral flap is dissected well into clear cornea with the 67 blade.

done with the tip of the blade under direct visualization. As the dissection continues anteriorly, the thickness of the flap can continually be assessed and modified as necessary. With a triangular flap, if a particularly low postoperative pressure is believed necessary, the anterior portion of the flap can be made thinner. If it is especially important to avoid over-filtration in a particular patient, the surgeon can make certain that the scleral flap remains quite thick. In general, we much prefer a thick flap to a thin one. The dissection should be continued anteriorly until the cornea is seen in the bed of the flap, and/or until the knife blade can be visualized in clear cornea (Figure 17.5). A third approach has been advocated by Paul Palmberg, who has developed a 'safety-valve' scleral flap dissection that attempts to prevent flow for an intraocular pressure of < 5 mmHg.

Paracentesis track

After completion of the scleral flap dissection, a clear cornea paracentesis track is made (Figure 17.6a). One way is to fixate the globe by firmly grasping the sclera with a 0.12 millimeter forceps, taking care not to touch the conjunctiva. A 27- or 30-gauge, 5/8-inch sharp needle on a 1 or 3 ml syringe is then passed through clear cornea, attempting to make a self-sealing track about 2 mm long. The track should be begun just on the clear corneal side of the limbus and is produced without ever pointing the needle downward. The needle must always be oriented parallel to the plane of the iris with the bevel up. The correct technique involves rotating the globe superiorly with the fixating hand as much as pushing the needle forward. The entry into the anterior chamber should be over iris, not lens, but the surgeon must make certain that the full bevel of the

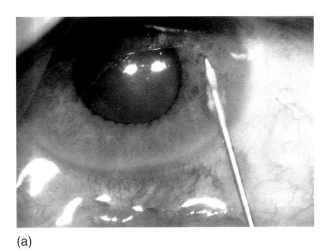

(a)

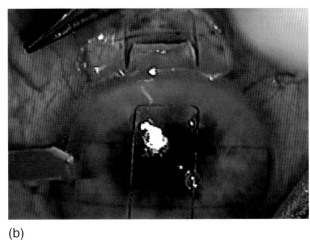

(b)

Figure 17.6 Making a paracentesis track. (a) A paracentesis track is made with a 27 gauge needle before the eye is entered for the trabeculectomy block. Subsequent filling of the anterior chamber with balanced salt solution is done through a 30-gauge needle. (b) A paracentesis is made with a sharp-pointed blade as for cataract surgery.

needle tip is within the anterior chamber before withdrawing it. A second technique is to create a paracentesis with a sharp-pointed blade essentially in the same fashion as for cataract surgery (Figure 17.6b). In general, the location of the track is left to the preference of the surgeon. Some prefer to always make the track on the side of the dominant hand with the track being placed superiorly and oriented toward the inferior limbus. Others prefer to always place the track with a more horizontal orientation temporally, requiring use of either hand, depending on which eye is undergoing the surgery. We recommend placing this incision in temporal clear cornea to facilitate postoperative access to the eye if the anterior chamber must be re-formed in the early postoperative period.

Corneoscleral block excision

The size of the opening into the anterior chamber is not of tremendous importance. However, the proximity of the opening to the edge of the scleral flap is of crucial importance. No matter what flap construction is used, the opening should be as anterior into the cornea as the flap will permit. This avoids the underlying ciliary body. When using a triangular flap in a patient who may need a particularly low pressure with a high-flow filter, the surgeon may wish to excise the corneoscleral block up to the very edge of the scleral flap. Certainly this will then require tight suturing of the scleral flap over that area and will increase the risk of overfiltration, but may be necessary in selected patients. For a more conservative filter, the block excision may be positioned centrally underneath the flap with perhaps a millimeter of tissue remaining between the internal opening and the edge of the scleral flap. Also, the surgeon can preferentially orient the direction of the filtration by off-setting the block excision

much closer to one side of the scleral flap than the other. Often for a right-hand-dominant surgeon, this may mean off-setting the internal block excision to the left edge of the scleral flap, relative to the surgeon's view, so that placement of scleral flap sutures will be with a more easily controlled forehand pass of the suture. When using a rectangular flap, we recommend the opening be made in the center of the base of the flap. One punch is often sufficient, but if more flow is desired, additional punches can be made directly posteriorly to the initial one. This forms a 'channel' directed at the posterior lip of the scleral flap and promotes the desired posterior flow. We rarely extend the opening more than halfway back to the floor of the flap.

There are several different techniques of excising the corneoscleral block of tissue. One technique involves excision of the block with a sharp-pointed blade and Vannas scissors and another uses a sharp-pointed blade and a punch, such as the Kelly Descemet punch or the Luntz–Dodick punch. If a limbus-based conjunctival flap has been used, the assistant will need to stretch it anteriorly over the cornea to maintain a clear view for the surgeon. The surgeon then grasps the posterior aspect of the scleral flap with the non-dominant hand, reflects it anteriorly, and, with the dominant hand, makes as vertical an incision as possible (perpendicular to the iris) with the sharp-pointed blade into the anterior chamber through clear cornea at, and parallel to, the base of the scleral flap (Figure 17.7b). This incision should be 1–3 mm long, depending upon how big an internal block of tissue the surgeon wishes to excise. Care must be taken to make certain that this incision is full thickness into the anterior chamber. If a punch is to be used, it should be positioned through the incision so that a full-thickness block of corneoscleral tissue will be excised. The punch should be made so that the tissue is excised

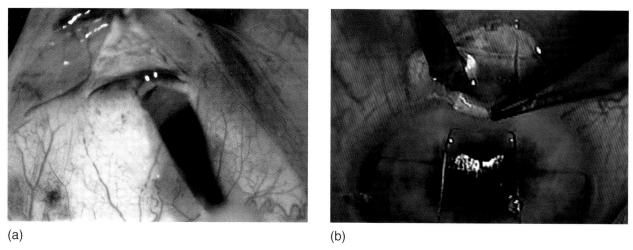

(a) (b)

Figure 17.7 Trabeculectomy block. (a) A superblade is used to make the anterior–posterior incisions for the trabeculectomy block. (b) A sharp-pointed blade is used to make an incision in the floor of the flap into the anterior chamber. It is helpful to make this incision as perpendicular to the cornea as possible to facilitate the subsequent scleral punch.

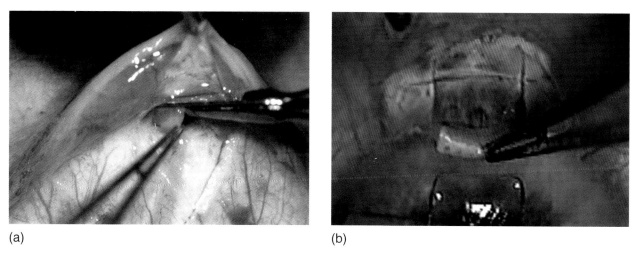

(a) (b)

Figure 17.8 The corneoscleral excision. (a) The trabeculectomy block is completed with Vannas scissors. (b) The Kelly Descemet punch is used to remove a block of tissue. To promote posteriorly directed flow, it is helpful to make the punch in the center of the flap and to punch posteriorly until about half-way to the posterior lip of the scleral flap.

from the posterior lip of the anteriorly placed incision. The punch should be positioned wherever the surgeon desires. As mentioned previously the punch can be close to the edge of the scleral flap (off-setting the excision towards the dominant hand as desired by the surgeon) or centrally. Several punches may be required to obtain the desired size of opening (Figure 17.8b). Care should be taken that a thin lip of Descemet membrane does not remain over what would otherwise appear to be a full-thickness opening. If the initial sharp-pointed blade incision into the anterior chamber was appropriately positioned through clear cornea, the opening produced by the punch will be through clear cornea and perhaps trabecular meshwork, but remain anterior to scleral spur. This anterior block excision greatly reduces the risk of bleeding or blockage of the filtration opening by ciliary body or iris, as may occur with a more posterior entry site.

The other common technique of corneoscleral block excision is done by two parallel, radial, full-thickness incisions with the sharp-pointed blade (Figure 17.7a). These two incisions determine the width of the block to be excised and should be positioned as described above, according to the surgeon's desire to direct outflow toward one side of the flap or the other, and according to the amount of aqueous egress desired. Vannas scissors are then positioned parallel to the limbus with one tip of the Vannas scissors through one of the radial incisions into the anterior chamber. Care should be taken to make certain that the tip is completely in the anterior chamber so that a full-thickness cut will be made. The scissors are then slid as far posteriorly as possible and oriented perpendicular to the plane of tissue and a full-thickness cut is made. If the radial incisions were begun in clear cornea and extended posteriorly just into the transition zone of blue limbal tissue, then the posterior Vannas incision will remain anterior to the scleral spur. The assistant must maintain anterior traction on the scleral flap while the surgeon then grasps the posterior edge of the corneoscleral block and places it on posterior stretch. A firm stretch is required. This will deform the peripheral cornea, but it is necessary to make certain that the anterior extent of the block incision will be appropriately far enough anterior. The Vannas scissors are then slid as far anteriorly as possible, maintaining the orientation of the blades parallel to the limbus. Also, the lower blade should be more anterior than the upper blade, so that the remaining corneal edge will be beveled posteriorly, leaving no posterior corneal ledge for iris to adhere to, should the chamber shallow postoperatively (Figure 17.8a).

Iridectomy

A peripheral iridectomy is generally required in all phakic cases, even if there is a previous iridectomy at another site. The only instance in which an iridectomy is not required is if the filtration site is positioned directly over a previous peripheral iridectomy or sector iridectomy and there is no iris tissue visible through the internal opening. Otherwise, a peripheral iridectomy must be done after excision of the corneoscleral tissue. The iris will often balloon into the filtration site or must be grasped with a 0.12 forceps and brought into the corneoscleral opening. Vannas scissors should be used for the iridectomy with the blades oriented flush against the sclera and parallel to the limbus (Figure 17.9). Care should be taken to have the assistant keep conjunctiva and Tenon's away from the blades in the case of a limbus-based conjunctival flap. The surgeon should make certain to excise enough iris tissue so that the edge of the iridectomy is free from the corneoscleral opening. It is better to err on the side of a larger iridectomy than necessary, or otherwise the iridectomy may be only of partial thickness, especially in African-American patients who have thick irides. Infrequently, there may be transient bleeding from iris vessels. In the vast majority of cases, this lasts less than a minute. The surgeon can simply continue irrigation with balanced salt solution through the filtration site to prevent residual blood remaining in the anterior chamber, or can use the 23-guage cautery tip to stop the bleeding.

Scleral flap closure

Prior to closure of the scleral flap, the filtration site should be irrigated with balanced salt solution, and the surgeon should verify that there is no residual bleeding and that there is a clear filtration opening not blocked by Descemet's membrane, iris, ciliary body, or vitreous (Figure 17.10). The scleral flap is then reposited in its bed and closed with interrupted 10-0 nylon sutures. As this is the principal step that will serve to regulate the amount of aqueous outflow, flap suturing should be a carefully thought-out process. The intent is to understand exactly how much each suture contributes to restricting outflow, for when it comes time to perform suture lysis, the surgeon must know which suture to cut and what the likely effect will be. It does no good if the initial flap sutures are 'tight' and subsequent ones are 'loose', to cut one of the 'loose' ones postoperatively. There will probably be no increase in outflow. Preferably, the suture tension should be loosest for the initial sutures (ideally set to a tension that allows sufficient flow to reach eventual desired postoperative intraocular pressure) and tighter for subsequent ones. The process can then be reversed when it comes time for suture lysis, permitting a controlled lowering of intraocular pressure. If the flap is square or rectangular, a suture should be placed in each posterior cornea of the flap. A triangular flap may be closed with one nylon suture at the apex. These sutures do not have to be particularly tight, but do function

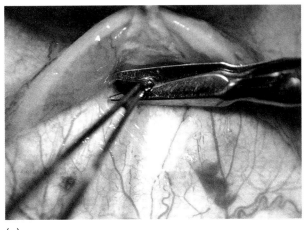

(a)

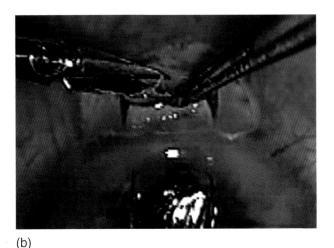

(b)

Figure 17.9   Iridectomy.   (a,b) An iridectomy is made with Vannas scissors.

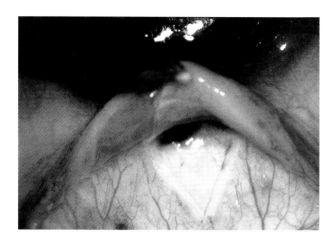

Figure 17.10 Inspecting the filtration site. Before scleral flap closure, the filtration site should be inspected for residual bleeding or blockage of the filtration opening.

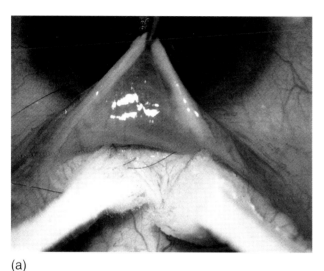

(a)

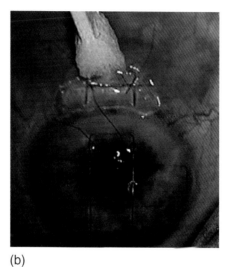

(b)

Figure 17.11 Testing for aqueous flow. (a) Testing for aqueous flow through the trabeculectomy is done with Weckcell spears after each suture has been placed so as to set the intraocular pressure at several levels. When antifibrosis agents are used, there should be almost no leakage at intraocular pressures less than 10, and only a slow ooze at levels from 10 to 15. (b) The aqueous flow is assessed with a Weckcell spear. The intent is to have flow only along the posterior lip of the scleral flap.

to both maintain the flap in its bed and, especially for rectangular flaps with posteriorly directed flow, will provide enough tension to permit the titration of the desired postoperative intraocular pressure. If extensive cautery was required to cauterize scleral perforating vessels, the scleral bed edges may have retracted; the flap in this case should not be pulled tight enough to result in complete apposition of the flap to its original bed edge, or postoperative astigmatism might occur. The sutures should be only of partial thickness through the scleral flap. Otherwise, a stretch or 'claw' hole may result, especially if the flap is thin, and it may be very difficult to gain control over flow of aqueous through this defect (hence our preference for thick flaps).

Once the flap is sutured into its bed, the anterior chamber is re-formed through the previously placed clear cornea paracentesis track. The goal of this step is to overinflate the eye and then evaluate the flow through the flap, and wait to see what the intraocular pressure will be at equilibrium when

flow has essentially stopped. The surgeon should evaluate the extent of aqueous egress around the edges of the scleral flap.

The area is dried with a cellulose sponge and checked for spontaneous aqueous flow (Figure 17.11b). This is the time when the surgeon can 'set' the suture tension to titrate the desired postoperative intraocular pressure. To facilitate this, we highly recommend the use of adjustable knots for these sutures. If there is copious egress of aqueous, it may be necessary to tighten the sutures, or place additional sutures, to more firmly appose the edge of the flap to the edge of the bed. The surgeon should remember to make these suture passes of partial thickness through the flap, as described above. The sutures should be trimmed at the knot so that, in the case of a low or flat bleb postoperatively, the loose ends will not protrude into the conjunctiva and cause a conjunctival buttonhole leak. It is not necessary to bury the knots into the sclera, but we prefer it, to avoid loose ends.

Once the eventual desired postoperative intra-ocular pressure has been set with the initial sutures, externalized, releasable scleral-flap sutures may be placed as described later in this chapter. This will temporarily cause less flow in the immediate post-operative period, will help protect against hypotony and, upon postoperative removal, will permit a fur-ther reduction in intracular pressure when desired. The three steps of suture placement, anterior cham-ber re-formation, and evaluation of aqueous out-flow and level of intraocular pressure (assessed by palpation or amount of pressure needed to deform the corneal light reflex with a 30-gauge cannula) are patiently and continually repeated after each new suture is placed until the anterior chamber remains deep after re-formation with the desired intra-ocular pressure and with a continual but slow and controlled egress of aqueous from the edge of the flap (Figure 17.11a).

In some cases, such as patients with a shallow anterior chamber and chronic angle closure (who are at risk for flat chamber), or young adults with significant myopia and thin sclera who are at risk for hypotony maculopathy (especially if mitomycin is used) the surgeon may wish to have minimal or no egress of aqueous visible and use suture lysis to regulate the intraocular pressure in the postopera-tive period. However, the surgeon should make certain that outflow can be induced by applying light pressure with the cellulose sponge on the scleral-bed side of the edge of the flap. In cases in which the egress of aqueous is less than the surgeon believes necessary, short bursts of cautery with the needle-point cautery can be applied into the cleft at the edge of the flap in order to make the edges gape and allow aqueous outflow (Figure 17.12). Special care should be taken to initially apply this cautery in a very short burst, since excessive retraction of tissue may occur, making it difficult to suture the edges close enough to prevent over-filtration.

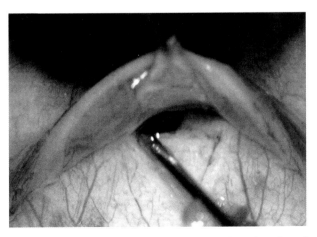

Figure 17.12 If the block is not close enough to the edge of the flap, cautery can be used to shrink the sclera to lessen overlap.

Rather than using cautery to increase outflow, the surgeon may wish to simply remove the sutures already placed, replacing them with looser sutures. The number of sutures required to obtain the desired level of outflow may be highly variable from patient to patient, depending on many factors including the amount of flow desired (which will depend upon the type of glaucoma and the charac-teristics of the patient), the thickness of the scleral flap, and the proximity of the corneoscleral opening to the edge of the flap. In some cases, the posterior corner or apex sutures may be all that is required, while in other cases 6–8 sutures may be necessary for control of the amount of aqueous egress. For a rectangular flap using a central punch, we rarely use more than one suture at each flap corner and one releasable suture in the center of the posterior lip of the flap. The tension on the two corner sutures is set to permit the desired long-term intraocular pressure and the tension on the releasable suture is set to regulate the initial postoperative intraocular pressure. The intraoperative evaluation and mani-pulation of the amount of aqueous egress is crucial for obtaining consistently good results, minimizing early postoperative complications, and avoiding unwanted surprises which may occur if the sur-geon simply places a predetermined, standard number of sutures without evaluating or adjusting the flow rate intraoperatively (Figure 17.13). The judgment of the correct amount of aqueous egress requires experience. This aspect of the surgery is a large part of the 'art' of glaucoma filtering surgery, and the glaucoma surgeon should strive to develop a 'feel' for the correct amount of outflow for each particular case.

Conjunctival flap closure

If a fornix-based conjunctival flap has been created, the limbal incision site should be de-epithelialized by scraping with a 67 blade or by cautery. Conjun-ctiva should then be stretched anteriorly with the goal of suturing both Tenon's and the conjunctiva back into position at the limbus. For short limbal incisions the closure can be as simple as suturing either end of the peritomy with an anterior anchor-ing suture of 10-0 nylon through peripheral clear cornea. A small running or purse-string-type suture will probably be required to close any gaping of conjunctiva beyond the anchoring suture. The other end of the conjunctival flap is then very tightly stretched and also sutured anteriorly with an anchoring suture. As at the other end of the wound, a small running closure may be required to prevent leakage distal to the anchoring suture, especially if a posterior relaxing incision had initially been made at that end of the conjunctival incision. Longer conjunctival peritomies often will not be watertight unless the entire peritomy is sutured in

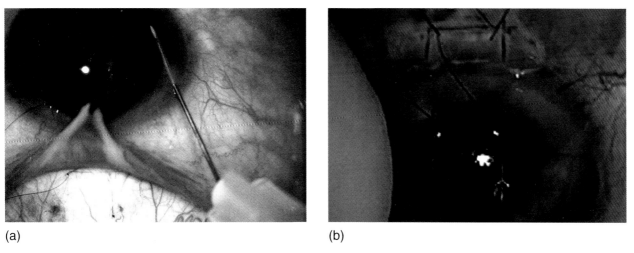

(a)   (b)

Figure 17.13 Re-forming the anterior chamber. (a) After placement of scleral flap sutures, the anterior chamber is re-formed via the paracentesis track, and the amount of filtration is observed and modified as judged necessary. (b) The tension on the two corner sutures should be adjusted using sliding knots to permit enough flow, so that at equilibrium the eventual desired postoperative IOP is achieved. This photograph shows the two adjustable sutures in place. The IOP is being estimated by palpation after re-forming the anterior chamber and waiting for equilibrium.

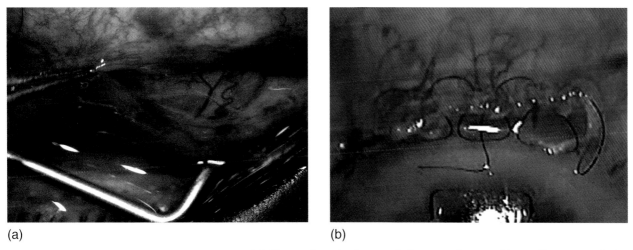

(a)   (b)

Figure 17.14 Closing the conjunctival wound. (a) The conjunctival wound closure is hastened by pulling up with the needle until the taut suture elevates the suture line at the point where the wound has been closed. A Pierce–Hoskins forceps is used to grasp both sides of the wound just anterior to the point where the taut suture is holding up the wound. (b) The Wise closure technique uses partly overlapping mattress sutures to secure as much of the limbus as possible. The effect is to create a series of 'triangles'. The central corneal pass is made deep to the releasable suture seen here passing under the conjunctival edge perpendicular to the limbus.

place at the limbus. This can be done with multiple interrupted mattress sutures, or the running, overlapping mattress suture technique of James Wise (Figure 17.14b and Figure 17.15b). We strongly suggest using 8-0 nylon on a BV needle as this provides a good balance of suture strength and a small, yet stiff, needle to tightly close the incision without causing buttonholes at the limbus. We have found vascular needles are too weak to suture in the cornea and a TG-140 needle is too large, so that a buttonhole forms with each conjunctival pass. The anterior chamber should be re-formed and slight pressure applied to the edge of the scleral flap if necessary to produce a filtration bleb, so that the conjunctival closure can be checked

for leakage. Fluorescein may need to be applied to detect any small leak.

As is the case for closure of the fornix-based flap, there is no uniform agreement among surgeons as to the best suturing technique for the limbus-based conjunctival closure. If the conjunctival incision was appropriately high in the superior fornix, a single layer, unlocked running closure with 10-0 nylon on a cutting needle and using small, closely spaced bites incorporating Tenon's and conjunctiva is quite adequate. However, we also utilize a two-layer closure, closing Tenon's and conjunctiva in separate layers. Tenon's may be closed with a running locked suture which can then be externalized through conjunctiva at the end of the

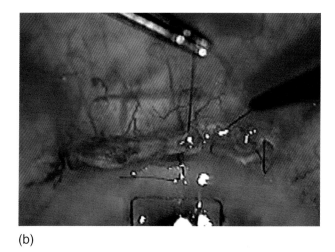

(a)   (b)

Figure 17.15 Closing the conjunctival wound. (a) The suture tension is then relaxed and the needle passed under and just ahead of the Pierce–Hoskins forceps. The forceps are not released until the needle holder grabs the needle on the other side of the suture line and is ready to make the next pass. These two steps are repeated rapidly until the wound is closed. (b) The slack is taken up to cinch the mattress sutures tight to the cornea.

Tenon's closure and run in the opposite direction as a standard unlocked running closure for the conjunctival closure (Figures 17.14a, 17.15a). Many different types of suture have been advocated for this closure including 9-0 Vicryl, 10-0 Vicryl, 9-0 PDS, and 10-0 nylon. Vascular needles have been very popular as well, and we have found 8-0 Vicryl on a BV needle to work well for limbus-based flaps. Our favorite technique is to use monofilament 9-0 Vicryl on a cutting needle, as it permits the suture to be 'cinched' down at the end of the double layer closure, adding an extra level of protection against leaks. Regardless of the suture used, a tightly closed, two-layer closure should prevent wound leak and lessen inflammation at the wound site.

A final comparison of the resultant bleb from the two surgery techniques is seen in Figure 17.16. Neither eye received intraoperative anitmetabolite, but both received a total of 10 mg of postoperative subconjunctival 5-fluorouracil. The bleb in Figure 17.16a has developed one bleb leak with blebitis. It seems unlikely that the bleb in Figure 17.16b will be as prone to this complication.

MODIFICATIONS

Releasable sutures

In cases in which the surgeon desires only minimal initial filtration, externalized releasable sutures should be considered. In these instances, and perhaps when antimetabolites are used, the surgeon may plan on tightly closing the scleral flap initially with a more aggressive outflow produced later from removal of the releasable suture when it is determined that a more copious drainage is necessary and safe. This lessens the likelihood of early postoperative complications of overfiltration and flat chamber. Many surgeons also believe that removal of the externalized releasable suture is easier and safer than employing the analogous technique of postoperative laser suture lysis. The two techniques described below may be used with either limbus-based or fornix-based conjunctival flaps.

For the first technique, the initial pass of the 10-0 nylon suture begins on the clear cornea side of the limbus no more than about 1 mm onto clear cornea (Figure 17.17a). The needle is passed about half-thickness through cornea and sclera, exiting the sclera near the edge of the scleral flap (Figure 17.18a). The next pass is through the scleral flap into the edge of the scleral bed using the technique as described previously for routine scleral-flap closure (Figure 17.19a). The final pass of the suture is done back-handed simply reversing the initial pass of the suture, following a path roughly parallel to the initial suture pass, but far enough apart so that when the suture is eventually cut, there is enough suture exposed to be easily grasped (Figure 17.20a). The two ends of the suture are now exposed on peripheral clear cornea and are tied tightly with the ends trimmed at the knot (Figure 17.21a). One, or possibly two, of this type of suture may be placed on either side of the flap. The suture may be released in the postoperative period when deemed appropriate by the surgeon. This is done at the slit lamp under topical anesthesia by simply cutting through the exposed suture with a sharp-pointed blade or Vannas scissors and removing it with a slow, steady pull. This suture works quite well, but can cause significant postoperative astigmatism, can be irritating and can be difficult to remove, as there is a 90° angle between the scleral flap pass and the corneal exit site. When attempting to remove the suture, it should be pulled

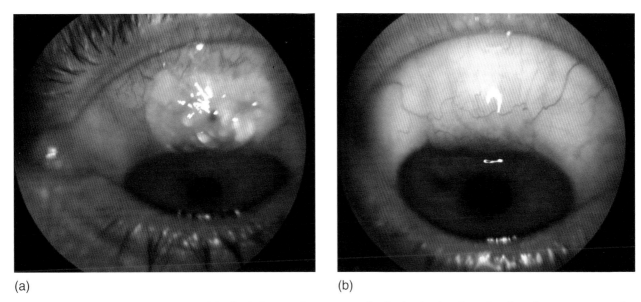

(a) (b)

Figure 17.16 Comparison of blebs. (a) The left eye of a patient who had a limbus-based trabeculectomy, triangular scleral flap and 10 mg of postoperative 5-fluorouracil delivered in two subconjunctival injections. No intraoperative antimetabolite was used. Note the large avascular bleb. The IOP is 12 on one medicine and there has been one bleb leak with blebitis. (b) The right eye of the same patient after receiving a fornix-based trabeculectomy and a rectangular scleral flap designed for posteriorly directed flow. 10 mg of postoperative 5-fluorouracil was delivered in two subconjunctival injections and no intraoperative antimetabolite was used. Note the low, diffuse, mildly vascular bleb. After removing the releasable suture, the IOP was 10 on no medication.

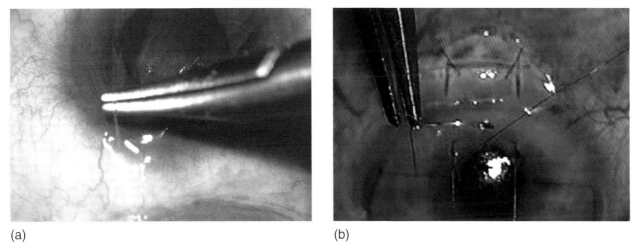

(a) (b)

Figure 17.17 The releasable suture. (a) This kind of releasable suture starts in the cornea approximately 2 mm away from the trabeculectomy flap and 1 mm in front of the limbus. (b) The alternative releasable suture starts in the cornea parallel to the limbus and exits in front of the middle of the flap.

down toward the floor, not out toward the slit lamp, to reduce the likelihood of breakage.

The second technique is astigmatically neutral, is not irritating and is easy to remove during the first 1–3 weeks postoperatively before fibrosis through the subconjunctival loop locks it in place. For a fornix-based rectangular flap, the initial pass is made in clear cornea entering about a millimeter anterior to the limbus about the location of the edge of the scleral flap. The suture is directed parallel to the limbus and exits the cornea in about the middle of the flap (Figure 17.17b). A second pass is made entering the cornea adjacent to the previous exit site and directed to exit in the base of the scleral flap (Figure 17.18b). This should be a shallow pass. The next pass approximates the posterior lip of the flap to its bed (Figure 17.19b). A four-wrap throw is then made grasping the suture as it lies on the scleral flap (Figure 17.20b). The end of the suture is not pulled through, so that a loop forms (Figure 17.21b). Once the tension on the throw is adjusted, the needle tag end is cut short. The four wraps prevent the 'knot' from unraveling and yet allow the suture to be removed by grasping the 'elbow' in the suture as it lies on the cornea. The tag end is cut flush to the corneal surface.

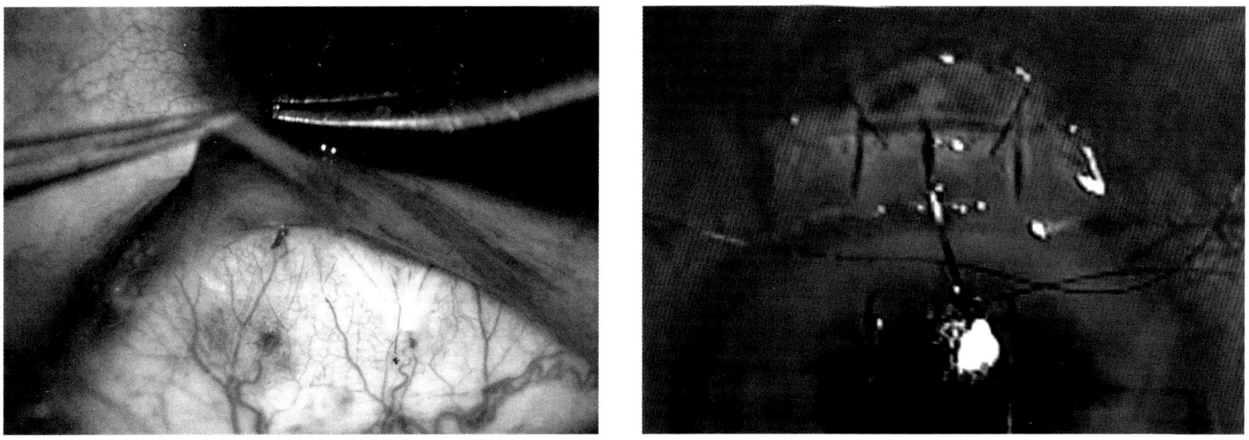

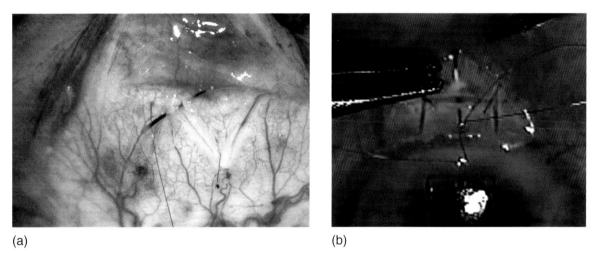

(a) (b)

Figure 17.18 The releasable suture. (a) The suture needle emerges on the other side of the limbus. (b) The next bite enters the cornea adjacent to the exit site of the first bite, but is a shallow pass headed toward the base of the scleral flap. Care is taken not to perforate the flap creating a fistula. The net effect is to leave a small 'elbow' of suture lying on the surface of the cornea that can be grasped later to remove the suture.

(a) (b)

Figure 17.19 The releasable suture. (a) A routine bite is taken in the trabeculectomy flap over where the block is closest to the edge of the flap. (b) A routine bite is then taken to approximate the posterior edge of the scleral flap with the posterior lip.

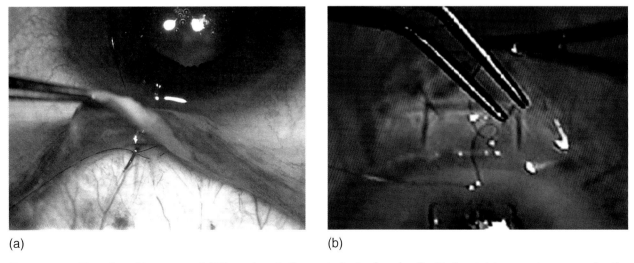

(a) (b)

Figure 17.20 The releasable suture. (a) The suture is then exteriorized under the limbus taking care to pass under the suture from the first pass, or not to touch it at all. This is important so as not to restrict pulling the suture from the track closest to the trabeculectomy when it is released. (b) A four-wrap throw is then made and the loop of suture on top of the scleral flap is grasped.

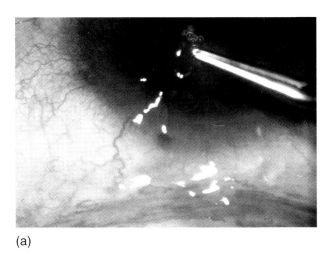 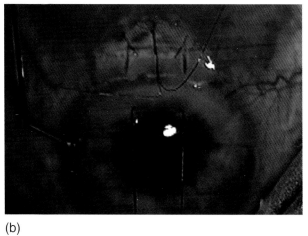

(a)   (b)

Figure 17.21 Completion of the releasable suture. (a) The releasable suture is now tied with four throws on the first knot. (b) The loop is not pulled through, but is left as a loop. The final knot is seen here. Tension on the four-wrap throw can be adjusted to permit flow consistent with the desired initial postoperative IOP. The needle and corneal tag ends are then cut short and flush to the cornea with the Vannas scissors.

Anterior chamber-maintaining suture

In patients with a posterior chamber intraocular lens, the surgeon may wish to consider intraoperative placement of an anterior chamber maintenance suture in order to eliminate concern over a postoperative flat chamber. This suture should be placed at the beginning of the procedure, before the eye is entered, when the eye is still firm and the anterior chamber is deep. A 9-0 nylon suture, double-armed with a straight needle, is passed from limbus to limbus to form a barrier to forward movement of the lens. The initial entry of the needle should be directed perpendicularly to the curve of the peripheral cornea just inside the conjunctiva. The entry point should be at the 8:30 o'clock position for a right-handed surgeon and the 3:30 o'clock position for a left-handed surgeon so that the intraocular pass of the needle will be in a forehand fashion. The needle is then passed across the anterior chamber just above the iris and lens and is externalized just on the corneal side of the limbus. The other arm of the suture is passed with a similar course parallel to the initial pass with the entry site 2–3 mm superior to the initial suture pass (Figure 17.22). The two free ends are then tied tightly with four or five throws to prevent slippage of the knot. The suture must be cinched tight enough to slightly deform the peripheral cornea at the entry and exit sites of the suture. The suture is trimmed flush with the knot. The patient is kept on topical antibiotics postoperatively as long as this suture is in place. The suture may be removed at any time that the surgeon believes the risk of postoperative flat chamber has passed.

Antimetabolites

Certain patients have been shown to have a poor success rate with the basic trabeculectomy technique described above. The predominant risk factors for failure include neovascular glaucoma, aphakia, and previous intraocular surgery with residual scar tissue remaining. Many other factors are also known to predispose patients to failure of filtration surgery. Over the past decade the antimetabolites 5-fluorouracil (5-FU) and mitomycin have been used to improve the success rate of filtering surgery in these patients. 5-FU is administered via both postopcrative subconjunctival injections, and topical application at the time of surgery. Mitomycin requires intraoperative application. There is no consensus among glaucoma surgeons as to the ideal method of intraoperative mitomycin application. Differences of opinion exist as to the ideal vehicle for mitomycin application, the concentration of mitomycin to be used, and the ideal application time. Peng Khaw has shown little additional release of drug from a cellulose sponge beyond three minutes of application. Regardless of the differing opinions over specific aspects of mitomycin usage, certain important principles will always apply. Whenever mitomycin is to be used, it must be applied prior to entry into the anterior chamber. If the surgeon prefers to place the mitomycin after dissection of the scleral flap, particular care must be taken not to enter the anterior chamber when extending the flap dissection anteriorly. Also, care must be taken to make certain that mitomycin does not come into contact with the edges of the conjunctival wound, especially if a fornix-based conjunctival flap has been dissected. When employing mitomycin with a fornix-based conjunctival approach, the surgeon must make certain that the limbal peritomy is broad enough and the dissection posterior enough to allow placement of the mitomycin sponge without contact to the wound edges. When using mitomycin, the surgeon should carefully titrate the amount of filtration so as to have control over the amount of

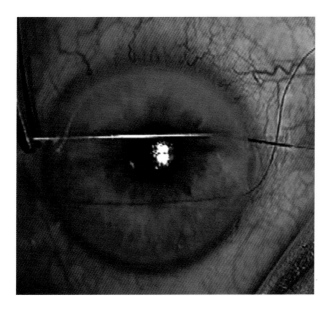

Figure 17.22 Anterior chamber-maintaining suture. The anterior chamber-maintaining suture is double-armed 9-0 nylon on a straight Keith needle. The needle often needs to be bent near the suture insertion to facilitate grasping of the suture with the needle holder and passing it while avoiding the nose. The two arms are passed parallel to each other, exiting temporally (much easier because of the nose). In this photograph, the inferior pass has been made from photograph right to left. The superior pass is almost complete. The bent end of the needle is seen on the right, partly in the anterior chamber, and the needle holder is now being used to pull the needle across the anterior chamber. Counter traction can be applied by grasping the suture on the nasal side with a tying forceps to prevent a sudden springing of the needle base posteriorly against the IOL when it enters the anterior chamber. A view of the finished suture can be seen in Figure 17.1.

aqueous filtration obtained at the end of the case. This can be accomplished by modifications in dissection of the scleral flap, placement of the corneoscleral filtration site, and closure of the scleral flap, as discussed in detail previously. As Paul Palmberg has commented, it is particularly important to realize that antimetabolites do not cause immediate postoperative hypotony. Nor do they enable flow. They have no effect whatsoever on the scleral flap, but only allow whatever conditions are created at the time of surgery to be 'fixed'. If the flap is poorly constructed so that it does not leak, no amount of antimetabolite will permit flow. If the flap is too loose, antimetabolites will inhibit any healing that might have eventually slowed down the aqueous flow, and hypotony will be assured.

Mitomycin may be applied with a cellulose sponge that has been thinned to approximately half of its original thickness and approximately half of its original length. The sponge is saturated with mitomycin, placed over the site of the intended filtration site, and the conjunctiva and Tenon's is draped carefully over the sponge (Figures 17.23, 17.24a). Our preferred technique, however, is to use three or more 1–2-mm plegets of cellulose sponge placed over a broad area of the superior sclera. We do not place the antimetabolite anywhere near the location of the as-yet-to-be-formed scleral flap, but instead generally place one sponge on either side of the superior rectus and one sponge at about the muscle insertion. The cut conjunctival edge is held off the scleral surface to minimize its contact with the antimetabolite (Figure 17.24b). This broad application of antimetabolite attempts to prevent areas of focal bleb ischemia that are at high risk for subsequent breakdown and leak. We recommend either

the use of the James Wise conjunctival closure technique with a fornix-based conjunctival flap, or the use of a limbus-based conjunctival flap when employing mitomycin, using a concentration of mitomycin of 0.4 mg/ml with an application time of 1–4 minutes. The length of application is individualized for each patient, depending on the characteristics of the patient, the type of glaucoma, and the health of the ocular tissues at the surgery site. The sponge is then removed from the field and the area of application is vigorously irrigated with approximately 10–15 ml of balanced salt solutions (BSS). With this technique, the mitomycin is applied prior to dissection of the scleral flap. This eliminates any chance of entering the anterior chamber prior to the mitomycin application and lessens the likelihood of a prolonged hypotony which may occur if mitomycin placement underneath the scleral flap results in complete ischemia with no healing at all in the bed of the flap, or mitomycin penetrates the thinned scleral bed and ablates part of the ciliary body.

SUMMARY

In many patients, glaucoma filtration surgery can halt or at least retard what would otherwise be relentlessly progressive vision loss from glaucoma. Filtration surgery requires diligent attention to details of performance. The planned approach and intraoperative execution of the procedure must be individualized for each given patient in order to maximize the likelihood of the desired result of glaucoma filtration surgery, preserved vision and preserved quality of life.

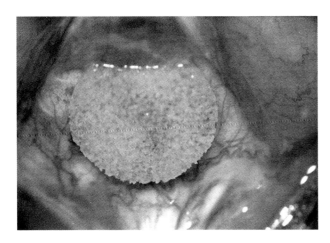

Figure 17.23 Application of mitomycin. The sponge supplied as a light shield also makes an excellent vehicle for the mitomycin soak, when it is trimmed to fit into the limbus. Alternatively, several small square pieces of sponge can be used to 'pack' the site of the future bleb.

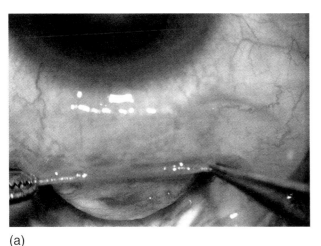

(a)

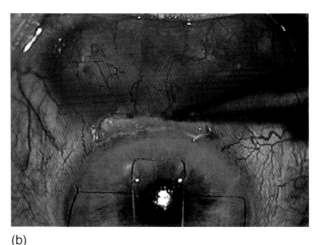

(b)

Figure 17.24 Mitomycin. (a) The conjunctival–Tenon's flap is pulled posteriorly over the mitomycin-soaked sponge with the edge of the conjunctival wound reflected forward to eliminate any chance of contact with the sponge. (b) The fornix-based conjunctival–Tenon's flap is pulled anteriorly over the three pieces of antimetabolite-soaked sponge. The sponges are placed well posteriorly to the site of the intended scleral flap at the limbus. The size and/or number of sponges is adjusted to apply the antimetabolite over a broad area, to promote the formation of a broad, low, diffuse bleb.

Further reading

Allen RC, Bellows AR, Hutchinson TST, Murphy SD. Filtration surgery in the treatment of neovascular glaucoma. Ophthalmology 1982; 89: 1181

Bellows AR, Johnston MA. Surgical management of chronic glaucoma in aphakia. Ophthalmology 1983; 90: 807

Cairns JE. Trabeculectomy – preliminary report of a new method. Am J Ophthalmol 1968; 66: 673

Chen CW, Huang HT, Barr JS, Lee CC. Trabeculectomy with simultaneous topical application of mitomycin-C in refractory glaucoma. J Ocular Pharmacol 1990; 6: 175

Heuer DK, Parrish RK, Gressel MG, et al. 6-Fluorouracil and glaucoma filtering surgery II. A pilot study. Ophthalmology 1984; 91: 384–94

Heuer DK, Gressel MG, Parrish RK. Trabeculectomy in aphakic eyes. Ophthalmology 1984; 91: 1045

Heuer DK, Parrish RK, Gressel MG, et al. 5-Fluorouracil and glaucoma filtering surgery III. Intermediate follow-up of a pilot study. Ophthalmology 1986; 93: 1537

Inaba Z. Long-term results of trabeculectomy on the Japanese: an analysis by life-table method. Jpn J Ophthalmol 1982; 26: 336–73

Katz LJ, Spaeth GL. Filtration surgery. In: Ritch R, Shield MB, Krupin T, eds. The Glaucomas. St Louis, MO: Mosby, 1989: 653

Khaw PT. Advances in glaucoma surgery: evolution of antimetabolite adjunctive therapy. J Glaucoma 2001; 10(5 Suppl 1): S81–4

Kimbrough RL, Stewart RM, Decker WL, Praeger TL. Trabeculectomy: square or triangular scleral flap. Ophthalmic Surg 1982; 13: 753

Kronfeld P. The rise of the filter operations. Surv Ophthalmol 1972; 17: 68

Liss RP, Scholes GN, Crandall AS. Glaucoma filtration surgery: new horizontal mattress closure of conjunctival incision. Ophthalmic Surg 1991; 22: 298

Luntz M, Freedman J. Fornix-based conjunctival flap in glaucoma filtration surgery. Ophthalmic Surg 1980; 11: 516

Palmer SS. Mitomycin as adjunct chemotherapy with trabeculectomy. Ophthalmology 1991; 98: 317

Quigley HA. Slipknots for trabeculectomy flap closure. Ophthalmic Surg 1985; 16: 56

Reichert R, Stewart W, Shields MB. Limbus-based vs fornix based conjunctival flaps in trabeculectomy. Ophthalmic Surg 1987; 18: 672

Schwartz AL, Anderson DR. Trabecular surgery. Arch Ophthalmol 1974; 92: 134

Shuster JN, Krupin T, Kolker AE, et al. Limbus-based vs fornix-based conjunctival flaps in trabeculectomy. Arch Ophthalmol 1984; 102: 361

Singh G. Effect of size of trabeculectomy on intraocular pressure. Glaucoma 1983; 5: 192

Starita RJ, Fellman RL, Spaeth GL, Poryzees EM. Effect of varying size of scleral flap and corneal block on trabeculectomy. Ophthalmic Surg 1984; 15: 454

Traverso CE, Tomey KF, Antonios S. Limbal- vs. fornix-based conjunctival trabeculectomy flaps. Am J Ophthalmol 1987; 104: 28

Wilson RP, Moster MR. The chamber-retaining suture revisited. Ophthalmic Surg 1990; 21: 625

Wise JB. Mitomycin-compatible suture technique for fornix-based conjunctival flaps in glaucoma filtration surgery. Arch Ophthalmol 1993; 111: 992–7

18 Non-penetrating surgery

Baseer U Khan, Iqbal Ike Ahmed

INTRODUCTION

Although initially proposed in the 1950s by Epstein and Krasnov, non-penetrating glaucoma surgery (NPGS) emerged in the 1990s as a surgical alternative to the standard trabeculectomy. The promise of NPGS, according to its proponents, is an increased safety profile with equal efficacy of IOP lowering as compared to the standard trabeculectomy. In the absence of a full-thickness sclerostomy, filtration occurring in NPGS takes place across semi-permeable ocular structures, which provide a constant resistance to aqueous outflow. This circumvents large IOP fluctuations during the early post-operative period that can occur with trabeculectomy, which can lead to serious complications. Furthermore, in the absence of penetration in the anterior chamber, sudden decompression and the associated complications as well as intraocular inflammation, hyphema and infection are significantly reduced. Blebs that result from non-penetrating approaches are typically diffuse and low-lying as opposed to cystic and avascular blebs that are prone to leak and become infected as has been reported with trabeculectomy.

Currently, there are two procedures that are described as being NPGS: deep sclerectomy (DS) and viscocanalostomy (VC). The common principles as well as the difference between each procedure are presented in Figure 18.1.

MECHANISM OF ACTION

While the mechanism of IOP lowering is clear in standard trabeculectomy, there is debate as to how IOP is reduced by NGPS: first, where the filtration takes place; and second, where aqueous drainage occurs.

With respect to filtration, Grant demonstrated that 75% of the outflow resistance exists at the juxtacanalicular trabecular meshwork (JCT), which is also where the altered resistance exists in primary open-angle glaucoma. Some surgeons consider that stripping of the inner wall of Schlemm's canal (SC), which is also thought to remove the JCT in that region, is the principal mechanism of filtration in NPGS. This is clinically correlated with the increased percolation of aqueous noted after peeling of the inner wall of SC intraoperatively. Others have argued that microperforations are created in the trabeculo-Descemet's window (TDW) during the surgical dissection of the deeper sclerocorneal flap and the peeling of the inner wall of SC. The physiological repair of these microperforations may result in elevated IOP postoperatively requiring laser goniopuncture of the TDW. A final theory is that aqueous filters through the TDW analogous to fluid movement across a semipermeable membrane. Experimental studies in rabbits have demonstrated limited ability for the TDW to function in this manner. However, the effect is probably more significant in humans in whom Descemet's membrane is anatomically different and thinner.

Aqueous drainage is proposed to occur in a variety of mechanisms in NPGS. In DS, the superficial scleral flap is sewn loosely to the adjacent sclera to allow aqueous to seep from the scleral lake to the subconjunctival space, resulting in the formation of a bleb. In addition, ultrasound biomicroscopy studies have demonstrated hypoechoic areas in the supraciliary area deep to the aqueous lake as well as in the adjacent sclera, suggesting that aqueous drainage also occurs via uveoscleral and transscleral pathways (Figure 18.18). The additional drainage that occurs through these secondary pathways, as well as a lower flow rate, is probably why DS produces blebs that are lower compared to those of standard trabeculectomy despite achieving comparable IOP lowering.

In contrast to DS, the superficial scleral flap is securely sutured to the surrounding sclera

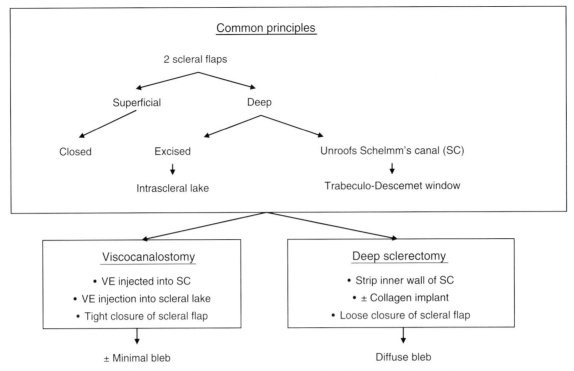

Figure 18.1   Common principles and difference between procedures for non-penetrating glaucoma surgery.

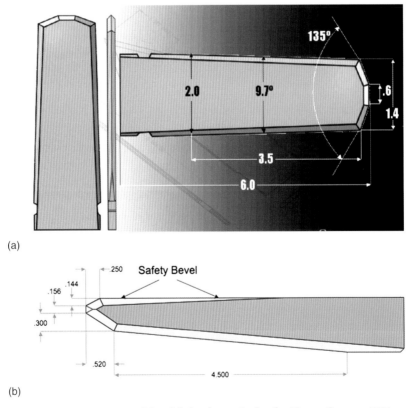

(a)

(b)

Figure 18.2   Diamond blades designed for NPGS.   (a) A schematic for the 'SuperCrescent' Diamond Blade used to create lamellar planar dissections. The key design features of this blade include the square leading facet, which distributes force over a greater area than traditional diamond blades, which are a multiplicity of facets. This allows superior control of flap dissection while still providing tactile feedback to the surgeon. (b) The 'Safety Trifacet' Diamond Blade used to create radial incisions and paracentesis. It features a 'safety bevel' that is non-cutting and can be safely apposed to tissue. The ultrathin design of both blades, at 100 μm (versus the conventional 200 μm) displaces less tissue and makes these blades less likely to stretch and distort tissue causing tissue tags and irregular surfaces. Both blades also feature a 30° cutting angle which delivers 57% more power than the industry standard 45° cutting edge.

producing a watertight closure in VC. In addition to the uveoscleral and transscleral routes, drainage is thought to occur through a mechanically altered SC. The injection of a high-viscosity viscoelastic material into the cut ends of SC results in the dilatation of the canal and possibly the creation of multiple micro-ruptures of inner and outer endothelial walls, the combined result of which is in an increased capacitance of SC and an associated lowering of IOP.

PATIENT SELECTION

Generally, NPGS is indicated in any patient with open-angle glaucoma who is considered for a standard trabeculectomy. Specific indications to perform NPGS are derived from clinical scenarios in which there is a high risk of an adverse event occurring, associated with performing a standard trabeculectomy as outlined below and in Table 18.1.

Owing to associated complications, standard trabeculectomy is generally indicated only when a patient has failed the maximum-tolerated medical therapy. Unfortunately, usage of multiple topical agents is associated with low-grade conjunctival inflammation and scarring, which reduces the long-term efficacy of the surgery. The superior safety profile of NPGS over standard trabeculectomy makes surgical

intervention a reasonable option before exhausting all medical options. Particular consideration should be given in conditions that have large diurnal IOP variations, such as pigment dispersion syndrome and pseudoexfoliation syndrome, where surgical intervention may be superior to medical management in controlling IOP fluctuations. Furthermore, NPGS, particularly VC, is less dependent on the relative health of the conjunctiva.

NPGS, which avoids sudden decompression of the eye, would be indicated in patients in whom there would be a high risk of choroidal effusion or hemorrhage if undergoing a standard trabeculectomy, especially if the patient were monocular. NPGS is also indicated in patients at risk of postoperative hypotony.

The absence of penetration into the anterior chamber reduces the amount of post-operative inflammation, thus reducing the risk of post-operative cataract formation – particularly beneficial for young patients. Finally, the bleb morphology of NPGS, absent (VC) or low lying (SC), allows for continued contact lens wear post-operatively and theoretically reduces the long-term risk of blebitis and contact lens-related bleb problems, which is a greater concern in younger patients.

NPGS is generally contraindicated in eyes in which the trabecular meshwork has been obstructed

Table 18.1   Patient selection

Indications	Contraindications
All open-angle glaucomas (especially if)	Trabecular meshwork obstructed
Early surgical intervention required	Extensive synecial angle closure
Monocular patient	Neovascular glaucoma
Large diurnal fluctuations	Occludable angles*
pigment dispersion glaucoma	Altered anatomy
pseudo-exfoliation glaucoma	Thin sclera
High risk of choroidal effusions or hemorrhages	Significant limbal scarring
axial myopia	previous scleral tunnel
hypertension	previous extracapsular cataract extraction
previously vitrectomized eye	
atherosclerosis	
history of choroidal effusion or hemorrhage	
increased episcleral venous pressure	
High risk of postoperative hypotony	
young patients	
high myopes	
males	
Uveitic glaucoma without extensive PAS	
Young patients	

*NGPS can be combined with cataract surgery or peripheral iridotomy.

or damaged or when there are structural abnormalities and anomalies in the limbal and paralimbal regions. Of note, argon laser trabeculoplasty and selective laser trabeculoplasty are not contraindications to NPGS.

TECHNIQUE

Instruments and devices

Aside from the regular instrumentation required to perform trabeculectomies, there are a few additional instruments that are beneficial when performing NPGS. Diamond blades are particularly suited to performing NPGS, given the high degree of accuracy that is required when creating the scleral flaps. Two diamond blades have been specifically designed for NPGS (Figure 18.2).

Peeling of the inner wall of SC is facilitated by forceps specifically designed for that purpose, the most common being the Mermoud forceps (Figure 18.3). Maintenance of the scleral lake, which has been shown to greatly improve the efficacy of DS, is accomplished with a space-maintaining device. The AquaFlow™ Collagen Drainage Device (Staar Surgical, Monrovia, CA) is the most commonly used implant (Table 18.2). Other devices include the SKGEL® implant (Corneal, Paris, France), which is an absorbable reticulated collagen implant, and the T-Flux™ implant (Ioltech, France), which is biocompatible but non-absorbable.

In VC, cannulation of the cut ends of SC requires the use of a 150 μm diameter polished cannula (Greishaber, Switzerland) (Figure 18.4). Subsequent to cannulation, a viscoelastic agent is injected. Studies have shown Healon 5 (Advanced Medical Optics, Santa Ana, CA) to be most effective in achieving the desired results.

Procedure

NPGS can be performed under topical (authors' preference), peribulbar or retrobulbar anesthesia. The common elements of both procedures are illustrated in Figures 18.5–18.13. The steps specific for DS are presented in Figures 18.3, 18.14, 18.15, and those for VC in Figures 18.4, 18.16, 18.17. Of note, many surgeons combine techniques used in VC (i.e. injection of viscoelastic into Schlemm's canal) with DS.

If performing phacoemulsification concurrently, the phacoemulsification should be performed first. In order to perform NPGS immediately following phacoemulsification, it is imperative that the anterior chamber be adequately pressurized to facilitate proper scleral dissection. Viscoelastic should be left in the anterior chamber after the insertion of the IOL, and removed following the excision of the deep flap with an irrigation syringe (i.e. 27-gauge cannula) instead of the mechanical irrigation and aspiration which could raise the IOP and result in rupture of the TDW.

Intraoperative complications

Complications related to the superficial flap can be managed similarly to flap complications encountered during trabeculectomy. The most significant intraoperative complication that may occur during NPGS is inadvertent perforation of the TDW, which can be classified as either a microperforation or a macroperforation. Microperforations are often occult and result in a small and localized leak

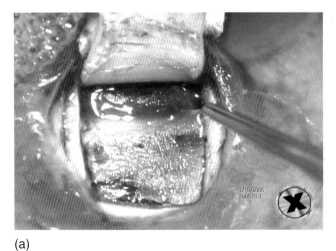

(a)

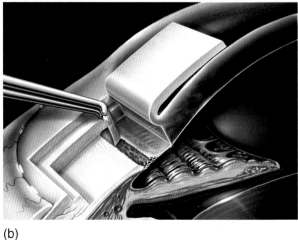

(b)

Figure 18.3 DS – Peeling of the inner wall of Schlemm's canal. (a) After the removal of the deeper scleral flap, the inner wall of SC is peeled with specially designed forceps. (b) It will often come in one strip spanning the width of the dissection, appearing as a transparent tubular structure once peeled. Upon successful completion of this step, the surgeon will notice an immediate increase in the percolation of fluid through the TDM.

Table 18.2 Implants for DS: types and usage	
Implant	**Number of clinical trials**
Staar AquaFlow collagen drainage device (absorbable collagen implant)	20
SKGEL implant (absorbable reticulated collagen implant)	3
T-Flux implant (biocompatible, non-absorbable)	3

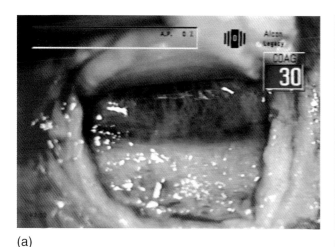
(a)

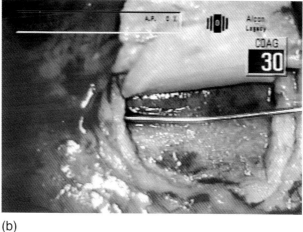
(b)

Figure 18.4   VC – Intubation of Schlemm's canal.   A paracentesis is performed to create a mild degree of hypotony in order that blood is refluxed from SC, thereby allowing for the localization of the cut ends (a). SC is then intubated with a Grieshaber cannula (b) and high-viscosity viscoelastic material is injected into each cut end five to six times – widening SC and thus improving flow through SC.

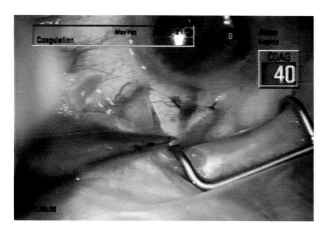

Figure 18.5   Creation of fornix-based conjunctival flap. After the application of anesthetic, a fornix-based flap is created in the superior temporal or nasal quadrant.

of aqueous with no loss of anterior chamber depth or iris prolapse, and as such are effectively inconsequential and may even contribute to enhanced IOL lowering. Macroperforations are grossly evident violations of the TDW and result in anterior chamber instability. This often necessitates conversion to standard trabeculectomy, although some surgeons have managed to tamponade the perforation with a collagen implant (Aquaflow™ device).

POSTOPERATIVE MANAGEMENT

Immediate

The post-operative management of NPGS is similar to that following a standard trabeculectomy. Patients are placed on topical antibiotics and steroids. Subconjunctival antimetabolite injections are used in a parallel manner with respect to indication, technique, timing and dosing. The major distinction in the post-operative care in NPGS from standard trabeculectomy is the contraindication of ocular massage by either the surgeon or the patient – this may rupture the TDW. Some surgeons also administer pilocarpine post-operatively to prevent iris apposition to the TDW.

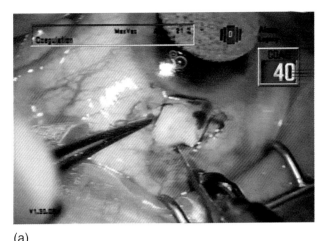

(a)

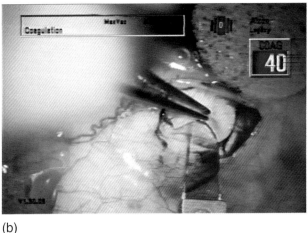

(b)

Figure 18.6 Creation of the superficial flap. (a) After undermining surrounding conjunctiva and achieving hemostasis with minimal to no cautery, the outline of the superficial scleral flap is scored. In DS, the flap is 5 mm × 5 mm square, whereas in VC it is a parabolic flap that enhances the watertight closure. It is imperative in both VC and DS that the superficial flap be carried 1–2 mm into clear cornea. (b) The thickness of the superficial flap should be 33–50% of scleral thickness.

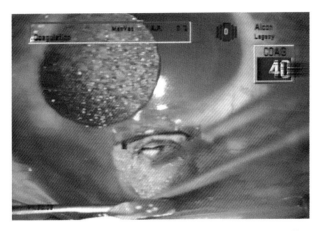

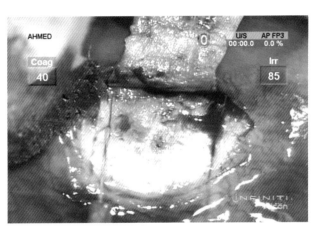

Figure 18.7 Application of mitomycin C. Traditionally, the use of mitomycin C (MMC) and other antimetabolites was avoided in NPGS. However, more surgeons are using antibmetabolite therapy as an adjunctive therapy with NPGS. Most surgeons will apply MMC at the completion of the superficial flap. Note that the MMC-soaked sponge is being held under the superficial flap while the edge of the conjunctival flap is being elevated to preclude wound leaks.

Figure 18.8 Outline of the deep flap. The next step is the creation of the deeper flap at 90% scleral thickness, which represents the most technically challenging step of NPGS, and should be performed under high magnification. The dimensions of the deeper flap are slightly smaller than those of the superficial flap. In DS it is a 4 mm × 4 mm square flap, whereas it is a smaller parabola in VC. Here the outline of the deeper flap has been scored with the 'Safety Trifact' diamond blade.

Long term

In DS, the collagen implant typically dissolves by 9 months, after which time the scleral lake will maintain itself (Figure 18.18), providing the important conduit of aqueous flow. Late increases in IOP are related to increased resistance at the TDW (healing of microperforations), intrascleral lake fibrosis, or episcleral fibrosis (Table 18.3). If IOP increases above target postoperatively, laser goniopuncture (Figures 18.19, 18.20) should be attempted first, and is required in 10–63% of cases (Table 18.4). Although this effectively converts NPGS to a penetrating procedure, performed in the

safety of the postoperative period after bleb formation, it dramatically reduces the concern for hypotony-related problems. Intrascleral or episcleral fibrosis should be considered and managed as in trabeculectomy, with antimetabolite and needling.

Rarely, an acute rise in IOP after NPGS can occur due to iris adherence or incarceration at the TDW in the early postoperative period or following goniopuncture – particularly if the openings are too large or placed too posteriorly. Iris incarceration can be managed with Nd:YAG synechiolysis and/or argon laser peripheral iridoplasty. Failing laser treatment, the iris can be swept away with

Table 18.3 Postoperative IOP elevation – causes and management

	TDW fibrosis	Iris incarceration	Bleb encapsulation	Bleb fibrosis
IOP	↑	↑↑↑	↑	↑
Postoperative time	Late	Early	Early	Mid–late
TDW configuration	Concave	PAS	Convex	Concave or convex
Bleb	Low, small	Low, small	Large, tense	Flat, thickened
Management	Nd:YAG Goniopuncture	Synechiolysis and/ or iridoplasty	Medication ± needling	Needling

TDW, trabeculo-Descemet's window.

Table 18.4 Literature review of goniopuncture

	Author			
	El Sayed	Mermoud	Shaarawy	Ahmed
Surgery	DS	DSCI	VC	DSCI
Incidence (%)	10.3	41	37	63
Mean time* (months)	9.6	9.9	9.4	6.7
IOP change (mmHg)	↓7.4	22.0 → 12.5	20.0 → 12.6	19.6 → 13.5

DS, deep sclerectomy; DSCI, deep sclerectomy with collagen implant; VC, viscocanalostomy.
*Time from surgery to time of goniopuncture.

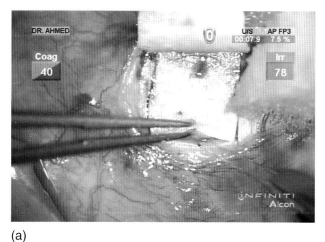

(a)

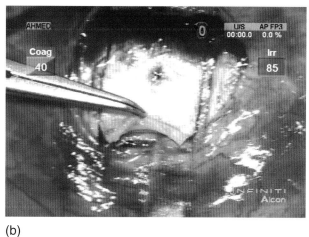

(b)

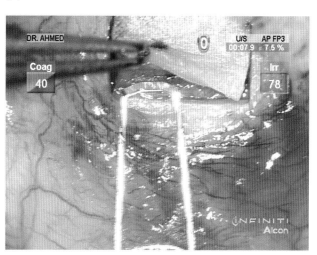

(c)

Figure 18.9 Starting the deeper flap dissection. (a) Beginning posteriorly, the sclera is incised. Some surgeons advocate cutting down to the suprachoroidal space, hence creating a full-thickness scleral incision, in order to help determine the 90% thickness depth, which leaves approximately a 75–100-μm bed. (b) and (c) At the correct depth, the surgeon will notice the irregular arrangement of scleral fibers with the deep purple hue of the choroid clearly visible. Note in (b) that the suprachoroidal space was intentionally entered posteriorly to help determine the appropriate depth of the dissection.

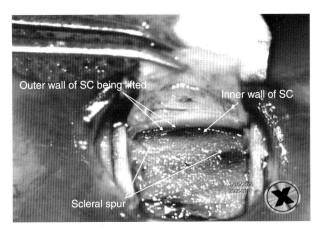

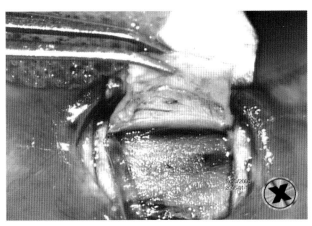

Figure 18.10 Continuing the deep flap dissection. At the correct depth, advancing the flap anteriorly, the scleral fibers in the dissection bed change from a random arrangement, to an organized arrangement circumferential to the limbus; this represents the glistening white scleral spur which is just posterior to SC. Continuing the dissection forward at this level will unroof SC beyond which is a natural plane between Descemet's membrane and the overlying stroma requiring little, or no force to advance.

Figure 18.11 Finishing the deep flap dissection. The dissection must continue at least 1 mm into clear cornea to create an adequate TDM. Vertical relaxing incisions are required at the lateral edges of the flap to carry the flap into the cornea. Great care must be taken not to rupture DM which is susceptible to trauma at this step – this is facilitated using a 'Safety Trifacet' diamond blade. The TDW may be bulging forward if the IOP is very elevated, increasing the risk of inadvertent rupture; therefore, it would be prudent to perform a paracentesis in this circumstance.

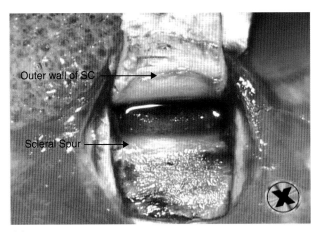

(a)

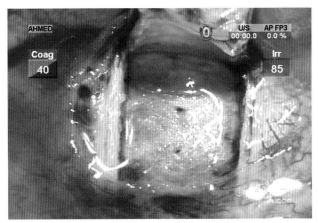

(b)

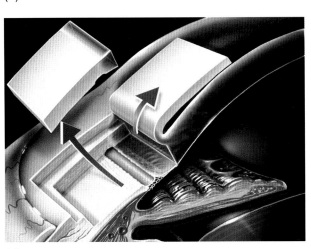

(c)

Figure 18.12 Complete deep flap dissection. Upon completion of the deep dissection, the surgeon will notice the percolation of fluid on the surface of the TDM window. Note the outer wall of SC on the undersurface of the deep flap (a). This figure also illustrates the change in scleral fiber arrangement at the scleral spur as well as the desired anterior extent of the deep dissection. Note the smooth undersurface of the deep flap beyond the SC (b) indicative of the natural cleavage plane between DM and the overlying stroma. (c) Schematic view of this dissection.

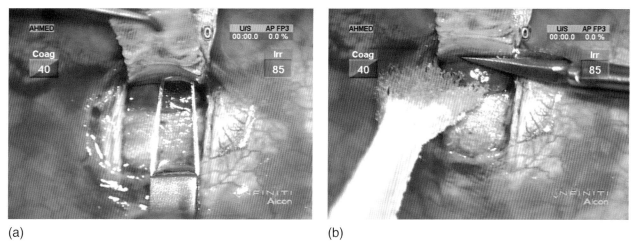

(a)   (b)

Figure 18.13 Removing the deeper flap. The deep flap must be excised to create space for the scleral lake. Removal of the flap is facilitated by the scoring of the undersurface of the flap (a) prior to using fine Vanna scissors (b).

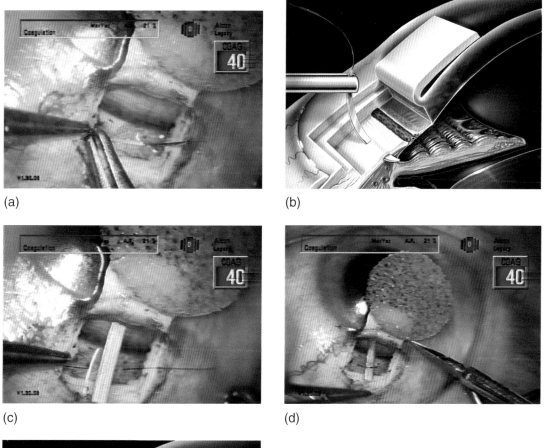

(a)   (b)

(c)   (d)

(e)

Figure 18.14 DS – Placement of collagen implant. (a,b) To fixate the collagen implant which will maintain the scleral lake, a 10-0 nylon suture is preplaced in the scleral bed. This suture is passed full thickness through the remaining sclera but remains in the suprachoroidal space. Collagen implants have also been shown to reduce inflammation adjacent to the scleral flap and bleb by activating collagenase. The collagen implant is placed in a centripetal orientation (c) and then tied into place (d). Some surgeons will also leave the implant longer than the flap such that the posterior extent of the implant protrudes beyond the posterior edge of the flap, thereby further promoting the drainage of aqueous into the subconjunctival space (e).

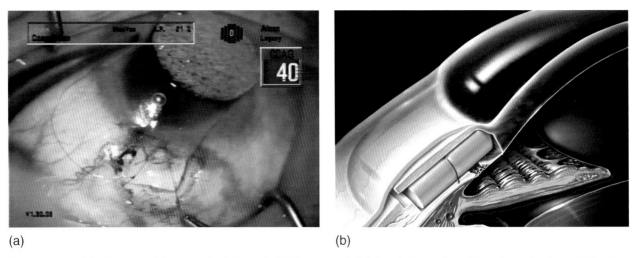

(a)   (b)

Figure 18.15   DS – Closure of the superficial flap.   (a,b) The superficial flap is then closed loosely using two 10-0 nylon sutures to promote bleb formation. Note the gap between the flap and adjacent sclera indicating the relative tension of the sutures (a).

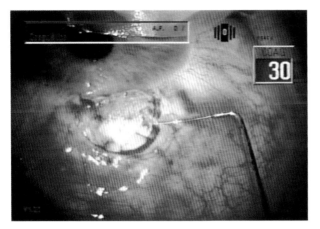

Figure 18.16   VC – Closure of the superficial flap.   The superficial flap is then reflected back into place and sewn tightly. Finally, high-viscosity viscoelastic is injected underneath the flap to maintain the scleral lake. High-viscosity viscoelastics have been shown to prevent fibrinogen migration, thus minimizing scar formation, which could obliterate the scleral lake over time.

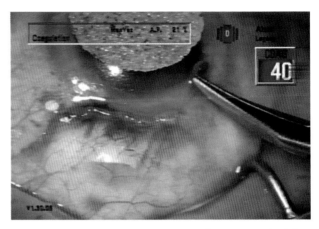

Figure 18.17   Conjunctival closure.   The conjunctival flap is closed in the usual fashion for both procedures. The authors prefer a 10-0 Vicryl suture on a vascular needle, passed in horizontal mattress fashion across the extent of the incision.

a 27-gauge needle inserted into the anterior chamber at the limbus.

Review of literature

Early NPGS studies, primarily evaluating VC or DS without an implant, suggested lesser efficacy in lowering IOP as compared to MMC trabeculectomy. However, refinements to technique such as space-maintaining devices, antimetabolite use, and post-operative modulation with Nd:YAG goniopuncture, have resulted in comparable if not superior IOP lowering while maintaining an excellent safety profile, particularly in DS with collagen implant. The IOP-lowering efficacy of VC is probably not as great as in DS with an implant. In the review of current

literature, it is worth noting that some studies have considered postoperative laser goniopuncture a failure, citing that this effectively converts NPGS into a penetrating procedure. Proponents of NPGS have countered that the need for post-operative modulation of flow with goniopuncture is no different from the need to perform argon suture lysis which, although effectively converting a guarded procedure to full thickness, is not associated with the same risks as full-thickness procedures. Currently, long-term data on NPGS are evolving which suggest that altered bleb morphology achieved with NPGS (shallow and diffuse in DS, and non-existent in VC) reduces the risk for late leakage, blebitis and endophthalmitis. A review of major studies evaluating NPGS is presented in Tables 18.5 and 18.6.

Table 18.5 Outcomes of Non Penetrating Glaucoma Surgery and Trabeculectomy

Authors	Year	Design	Surgery	Adjunctive Antimetabolite	GP (% required)	n (eyes)	Follow up	Mean preop IOP	Mean postop IOP	Mean # preop medications	Mean # postop medications	% complete success (qualified)	Definition of success
Gimbel et al	1999	NR	VC + Phaco	No	No	55	6	≈20	≈15	NR	NR	NR	NR
Mermoud et al	1999	Prospective, non randomized	DSC / Trab	POp 5FU / POp 5FU	Yes (23) NA	44 / 44	14 ± 6 / 16 ± 8	27 ± 4 / 25 ± 7	14 ± 4 / 12 ± 4	2.2 ± 0.8 / NR	0.36 ± 0.7 / 0.75 ± 1.1	69 (95) / 57 (95)	< 21
Stegmann et al	1999	Prospective	VC		No	214	35	47 ± 13	17 ± 8	0	≈0.17	82.7 (89)	≤ 22
Drüsedau et al	2000	NR	VC	No	No	59	12	28 ± 7	19 ± 8	2.4 ± 0.8	0.7 ± 0.7	36 (79)	< 21
El Sayyad et al	2000	Prospective, randomized	Trab / DS	POp 5FU / POp 5FU	NA / Yes (10)	39 / 39	12 / 12	28 ± 5 / 28 ± 6	14 ± 5 / 16 ± 4	2.6 ± 0.6 / 2.4 ± 0.7	0.3 ± 0.5 / 0.3 ± 0.4	85 (95) / 79 (92)	≤ 21
Jonescu-Cuypers et al	2001	Prospective, randomized	VC / Trab	No	No / NA	10 / 10	6 / 6	31 ± 7 / 28 ± 6	18 ± 5 / 15 ± 3	NR	NR	0 (NR) / 50 (NR)	< 20
Hamel et al	2001	Prospective, non randomized	DSCI	POp 5FU	Yes (71)	21	44 ± 17	26 ± 6	11 ± 6	2.3 ± 0.9	0.9 ± 0.9	38 (81)	< 21
Sunaric-Mégevand et al	2001	Prospective	VC	No	Yes (9)	67	23 ± 9	24 ± 7	14 ± 3	NR	1.2	52 (36)	< 20
Amrebsin et al	2002	Prospective, non randomized	Trab / DSCI	POp 5FU / POp 5FU	NA / Yes (45)	25 / 25	24 / 24	29 ± 9 / 23 ± 6	13 ± 5 / 14 ± 5	1.8 ± 1.1 / 2.5 ± 0.8	1.2 ± 1.1 / 1.0 ± 1.0	45 (90) / 40 (90)	< 21
Kozobolis et al	2002	Prospective, randomized	DS / DS	POp 5FU IOp MMC+POp 5FU / No	No / No	40 / 40	36 / 36	26 ± 4 / 28 ± 5	19 ± 3 / 16 ± 2	3.2 ± 0.8 / 3.0 ± 0.6	1.0 ± 1.0 / 0.6 ± 0.7	43 (73) / 50 (90)	< 21
Lüke et al	2002	Prospective, randomized	Trab / VC	No / No	NA / No	30 / 30	12 / 12	27 ± 7 / 27 ± 7	15 ± 4 / 17 ± 5	2.5 ± 1.1 / 2.9 ± 0.9	0.6 ± 1.0 / 1.1 ± 1.2	57 (87) / 30 (57)	< 22
O'Brart et al	2002	Prospective, randomized	VC / Trab	POp 5FU IOp MMC or 5FU + POp FU	No / NA	25 / 25	12 / 12	24.2 / 24	20 / 13	NR	NR	64 (NR) / 100 (NR)	< 21
Tanito et al	2002	Prospective, retrospective	VC+Phaco / Trab+Phaco	No / No	No / NA	57 / 57	6 / 6	21 ± 3 / 21 ± 3	16 ± 3 / 16 ± 4	1.7 ± 0.1 / 1.6 ± 0.1	0.2 ± 0.1 / 0.4 ± 0.1	95 / 98	< 21
Wishart et al	2002	Prospective	VC / VC+Phaco	No	No	10 / 1	36	25 ± 6	16 ± 4	2.4 ± 0.8	0.1	93 (100)	< 21
Ates et al	2003	Prospective	DSTF	No	Yes (12)	25	16 ± 4	26 ± 4	17 ± 4	2.2 ± 0.8	0.9 ± 0.9	39 (83)	< 21

Table 18.5 (Continued)

Authors	Year	Design	Surgery	Adjunctive Antimetabolite	GP (% required)	n (eyes)	Follow up	Mean preop IOP	Mean postop IOP	Mean # preop medications	Mean # postop medications	% complete success (qualified)	Definition of success
Carassa et al	2003	Prospective, randomized	Trab	POp 5FU	NA	25	24	23	14	3.1 ± 0.8	NR	80 (NR)	< 22
			VC	No	No	24	24	25	16	3.1 ± 0.7		76 (NR)	
Kobayashi et al	2003	Prospective, randomized	Trab	IOp MMC	NA	25	12	25 ± 3	13 ± 4	3.1 ± 0.3	0.4 ± 0.9	88 (96)	< 20
			VC	No	Yes (56)	25	2	25 ± 2	17 ± 2	3.2 ± 0.2	0.7 ± 0.9	60 (92)	
Lüke et al	2003	Prospective, randomized	VC	No	No	20	12	27 ± 6	17 ± 6	3.0 ± 1.1	0.7 ± 0.1	40 (85)	< 22
			VCSK	No	No	20	12	26 ± 3	17 ± 3	2.8 ± 1.1	0.6 ± 1.0	40 (85)	
Shaarawy et al	2003	Prospective, non randomized	VC	POp 5FU	Yes (37)	57	34 ± 11	25 ± 4	13 ± 4	NR	NR	60 (90)	≤ 21
Wishart et al	2003	Prospective, non randomized	DS	No	No	52	36 ± 12	28 ± 5	17 v 6	2.3 ± 0.7	0.2	≈68 (NR)	≤ 21
			DS+Phaco	No	No	35	35 ± 12	24 ± 7	15 ± 3	2.0 ± 0.9	0.1	≈96 (NR)	
			VC	No	No	27	36 ± 18	26 ± 9	17 ± 3	1.4 ± 0.9	0.1	≈90 (NR)	
			VC+Phaco	No	No	78	32 ± 12	24 ± 5	17 ± 3	2.2 ± 0.8	0.1	≈94 (NR)	
Cillino et al	2004	Prospective, randomized	Trab	No	NA	33	24	32.1 ± 2.7	14 ± 1	2.3 ± 0.1	0.7 ± 0.2	56 (89)	≤ 21
			DS	No	No	17	24	30.2 ± 2.9	18 ± 1	2.7 ± 0.2	0.6 ± 0.2	53 (77)	
Neudorfer et al	2004	Prospective, randomized	DSCI	No	No	13	24	27 ± 3	18 ± 3	2.9 ± 0.6	1.8 ± 0.9	2.0 NR	NR
			DSCI	IOp MMC		13	24	32 ± 6	16 ± 6	3.7 ± 0.6	1.5	NR	
Park et al	2004	Prospective	VC+Phaco	No	No	10 3	18 ± 6	20 ± 3	16 ± 2	14 ± 0.9	0.0 ± 0.5	61 (85)	< 21
Ravinet et al	2004	Prospective, randomized	DS	POp MMC	Yes (36) Yes	11	24	24 ± 8	12 ± 4	2.2 ± 1.0	0.2 ± 0.4	91 (100)	≤ 21
			DSTF	POp MMC	(64)	11	24	28 ± 14	13 ± 3	2.5 ± 0.9	0.4 ± 0.7	100 (100)	
Shaarawy et al	2004	Prospective	DSCI	POp 5FU	Yes (51)	10 5	64	27 ± 8	12 ± 3	2.3 ± 0.7	0.5 ± 0.7	57 (91)	< 21
Yalvac et al	2004	Prospective, randomized	VC	No	No	25	36	36 ± 8	16 ± 7	3.1 ± 0.4	1.5 ± 0.3	35 (79)	< 21
			Trab		NA	25	36	38 ± 9	18 ± 5	3.0 ± 0.5	0.5 ± 0.1	55 (73)	
Yarangümeli et al	2004	Prospective, randomized	Trab	No	NA	22	18 ± 6	39 ± 12	10 ± 4	3.6 ± 0.5	0.8 ± 1.2	64 (95)	≤ 18
			VC		Yes (5)	22	17 ± 6	39 ± 13	13 ± 4	3.6 ± 0.6	1.3 ± 1.2	59 (91)	
Anand et al	2005	Restropsective	DSSK	POp 5FU IOp MMC+POp 5FU	Yes (81) Yes	19	12	25	16	2.0	NR	67 (NR)	< 18
			DSSK		(45)	52	12	26	13	2.3		86 (NR)	
Cillino et al	2005	Prospective, randomized	Trab	IOp MMC	NA	21	12	28 ± 6	16 ± 4	NR	NR	71 (100)	≤ 21
			DS	IOp MMC	Yes (22)	19	12	30 ± 6	15 ± 4			79 (100)	

Table 18.5 (Continued)

Authors	Year	Design	Surgery	Adjunctive Antimetabolite	GP (% required)	n (eyes)	Follow up	Mean preop IOP	Mean postop IOP	Mean # preop medications	Mean # postop medications	% complete success (qualified)	Definition of success
Devloo et al	2005	Retrospective	DS DSASI	No No	Yes (30) Yes (50)	69 24	16 ± 9 15 ± 6	24 ± 6 26 ± 7	16 ± 6 16 ± 6	1.8 ± 0.6 1.8 ± 0.9	0.8 ± 0.8 0.5 ± 0.7	41 (82) 54 (75)	< 21
Funnell et al	2005	Retrospective	Trab+Phaco DS+Phaco	IOp MMC+POp 5FU IOp MMC+POp 5FU	NA Yes (52)	38 59	19 ± 8 16 ± 9	≈20 ≈21	≈12 ≈11	NRs	NR	≈77 (NF) ≈78 (NR)	< 19
Khairy et al	2006	Prospective, non randomized	DS	POp 5FU	Yes (5)	43	28 ± 8	25 ± 6	19 ± 5	2.1 ± 0.9	0.7 ± 1.1	NR	NR
Lachkar et al	2004	Retrospective	DS	POp 5FU	Yes (47)	25 8	72	25 ± 6	16 ± 4	2.0 ± 0.6	0.9 ± 0.9	66 (80)	< 21
Shaarawy and Mermoud	2005	Prospective, randomized	DS DSCI	POp 5FU POp 5FU	Yes (46) Yes (46)	13 13	48 48	24 ± 7 25 ± 6	16 ± 3 10 ± 4	2.2 2.2	1.1 0.4	38 (69) 69 (100)	< 21
Wevill et al	2005	Prospective	DSCI[1]	POp MMC	Yes (22)	23	36 ± 20	26 ± 9	17 ± 2	NR	NR	77 (100)	≤ 21

DS: deep sclerectomy, DSCI: deep sclerectomy with collagen implant, VC: viscocanalostomy, Trab: trabeculectomy, Phaco: phacoemulsification, DSASI: deep sclerectomy with autologous scleral implant, DSSK: Deep sclerectomy with SKGEL implant, DSTF: Deep scleretomy with T-Flux implant, IOp: Intraoperative, POp: Postoperative, IOp: Intraoperative, 5FU: 5-fluorouracil, GP: goniopuncture, NR: not reported, NA: not applicable.

[1] A 1-0 chromic suture was used as a collagen implant.

Table 18.6 Complications Associated with Non-Penetrating Glaucoma Surgery and Trabeculectomy

Authors	Year	Design	Surgery	n (eyes)	Hyphema %	Hypotony %	Flat/Shallow AC %	Choroidal detachment %	Bleb fibrosis %	Bleb encapsulation %	Induced cataract %	Late cataract progression %
Gimbel et al	1999	NR	VC + Phaco	55	NR	0	NR	0	NR	NR	NA	NA
Mermoud et al	1999	Prospective, non randomized	DSCI / Trab	44 / 44	2 / 34	0 / 18	0 / 18	5 / 20	23 / 18	11 / 11	0 / 14	9 / 11
Stegmann et al	1999	Prospective	VC	21 / 4	2	0	0	0	0	0	0*	0*
Drüsedau et al	2000	NR	VC	59	2	0	0	0	0	0	0	2
El Sayyad et al	2000	Propsective, randomized	Trab / DS	39 / 39	8 / 3	3 / 0	8 / 0	NR	NR	NR	NR	3 / 0
Jonescu-Cuypers et al	2001	Prospective, randomized	VC / Trab	10 / 10	0 / 0	0 / 0	0 / 0	0 / 0	0 / 0	0 / 0	0 / 0	0 / 0
Hamel et al	2001	Prospective, non randomized	DSCI	21	19	38	NR	NR	NR	24	0	14
Sunaric-Mégevand et al	2001	Prospective	VC	67	7	0	0	0	NR	NR	<1	NR
Amrebsin et al	2002	Prospective, non randomized	Trab / DSCI	25 / 25	30 / 15	10 / 10	20 / 0	30 / 0	NR	NR	10 / 0	15 / 10
Kozobolis et al	2002	Prospective, randomized	DS / DS	40 / 40	11 / 15	0 / 0	NR	13 / 15	20 / 13	NR	NR	NR
Lüke et al	2002	Prospective, randomized	Trab / VC	30 / 30	27 / 10	37 / 20	23 / 0	20 / 0	NR	NR	NR	0 / 7
O'Brart et al	2002	Prospective, randomized	VC / Trab	25 / 25	9 / 28	NR	9 / 32	NR	NR	13 / 16	NR	0 / 20
Tanito et al	2002	Prospective, retrospective	VC+Phaco / Trab+Phaco	57 / 57	14 / 21	0 / 0	0 / 0	0 / 0	NR	NR	NA	NA
Wishart et al	2002	Prospective	VC / VC+Phaco	101	5	0	0	7	NR	NR	0 / NA	0 / NA
Ates et al	2003	Prospective	DSTF	25	0	0	0	0	NR	NR	0	0
Carassa et al	2003	Prospective, randomized	Trab / VC	25 / 24	4 / 13	20 / 0	NR	4 / 0	NR	NR	NR	NR
Kobayashi et al	2003	Prospective, randomized	VC / Trab	25 / 25	24 / 0	20 / 0	16 / 0	N	8 / 0	NR	NR	8 / 0
Lüke et al	2003	Prospective, randomized	VC / VCSK	20 / 20	15 / 10	NR	15 / 10	0 / 5	NA	NA	0 / 0	0 / 0

Table 18.6 (Continued)

Authors	Year	Design	Surgery	n (eyes)	Hyphema %	Hypotony %	Flat/Shallow AC %	Choroidal detachment %	Bleb fibrosis %	Bleb encapsulation %	Induced cataract %	Late cataract progression %
Shaarawy et al	2003	Prospective, non randomized	VC	57	35	4	0	16	NR	4	0	9
Wishart et al	2003	Prospective, non randomized	DS DS+Phaco VC VC+Phaco	52 35 27 78	1 1 19 5	NR	0 0 4 0	6 3 4 5	NR	NR	NR NA NR NA	NR NA NR NA
Cillino et al	2004	Prospective, randomized	Trab DS	18 17	28 18	28 0	39 6	22 0	NR	NR	NR	NR
Shaarawy et al	2004	Prospective	DSCI	105	9	1	0	7	12	20	0	23
Neudorfer et al	2004	Prospective, randomized	DSCI DSCI	13 13	8 15	0 0	NR	8 8	NR	NR	NR	8 15
Park et al	2004	Prospective	VC+Phaco	103	53	0	NR	0	NR	NR	NA	NA
Ravinet et al	2004	Prospective, randomized	DS DSTF	11 11	27 18	NR	0 0	9 0	NR	54 54	0	9 18
Shaarawy and Mermoud	2005	Prospective, randomized	DS DSCI	13 13	0 8	0 0	0 0	0 0	NR	NR	NR	38 31
Yalvac et al	2004	Prospective, randomized	VC Trab	25 25	4 8	1 7	NR	NR	NR	4 12	NR	8 35
Yarangümeli et al	2004	Prospective, randomized	Trab VC	22 22	5 5	23 23	9 5	NR	NR	NR	NR	32 9
Anand et al	2005	Restropsective	DSSK DSSK	19 52	14 2	NR NR	0 5	NR NR	NR NR	15 0	NR NR	1 0
Cillino et al	2005	Prospective, randomized	Trab DS	21 19	43 21	38 0	43 5	29 5	NR	NR	NR	NR
Devloo et al	2005	Retrospective	DS DSASI	69 24	0 0	1 1	0 0	0 0	NR	3 4	0 0	1 0
Funnell et al	2005	Retrospective	Trab+Phaco DS+Phaco	38 59	5 6	0 3	8 0	0 3	NR	NR	NA	NA
Khairy et al	2005	Prospective, non randomized	DS	43	1	0	1	0	NR	5	0	0
Lachkar et al	2005	Retrospective	DS	258	1	NR	1	0	NR	NR	NR	2
Wevill et al	2005	Prospective	DSCI[1]	23	13	0	0	0	0	0	0	4

DS: deep sclerectomy, DSCI: deep sclerectomy with collagen implant, VC: viscocanalostomy, Trab: trabeculectomy, Phaco: phacoemulsification, DSASI: deep sclerectomy with SKGEL implant, DSTF: Deep sclerotomy with T-Flux implant, PCp: Postoperative, IOp: Intraoperative, 5FU: 5-fluorouracil, GP: goniopuncture, NR: not reported, NA: not applicable.

[1] A 1-0 chromic suture was used as a collagen implant.

* in patients under 40 years of age.

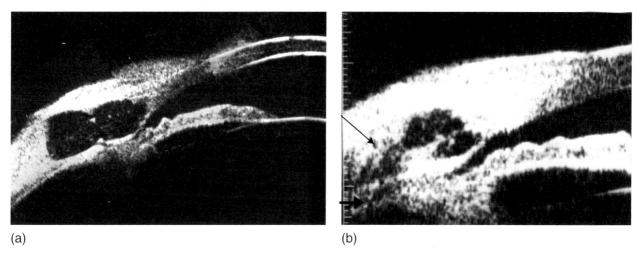

(a)   (b)

Figure 18.18   UBM analysis of scleral lake.   (a) A composite UBM view, taken at 1 week post-NPGS, along the length of the collagen implant, which appears as a hypoechoic structure. Note the indentation around the implant where the fixation suture is placed. (b) A composite UBM, taken at 9 months post-NPGS, along the same axis demonstrating almost total dissolution of the collagen implant, preservation of the scleral lake, and hypoechoic areas in the supraciliary (large arrow) and scleral region (small arrow) adjacent to the scleral lake.

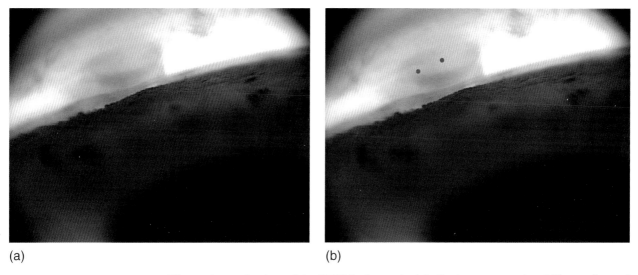

(a)   (b)

Figure 18.19   Goniopuncture.   The gonioscopic view of the TDW is shown in (a). Goniopuncture should be performed in the anterior portion of the TDM as indicated by the red circles in (b). Goniopuncture is performed using a YAG laser set to the free-running Q-switch mode, delivering 4–8 shots, at 4–8 mJ to create one or two holes in the TDW at any time after 2 weeks postoperatively. The TDW must be sufficiently thin and anteriorly dissected in order to perform goniopuncture, highlighting the need for accurate dissection of the deep flap.

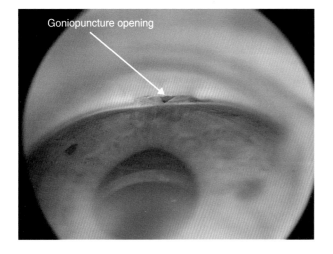

Figure 18.20 Goniopuncture. This figure demonstrates the appearance of the opening created by goniopuncture. The opening in this case was placed posterior to the ideal location where goniopuncture should be performed. Despite this, iris incarceration did not develop.

SUMMARY

NPGS has emerged as a viable and potentially superior alternative to the standard trabeculectomy in the surgical management of glaucoma. Published data have clearly demonstrated its superior safety profile as compared to trabeculectomy. Furthermore, the addition of space-maintaining devices, antimetabolite use and Nd:YAG goniopuncture to surgical technique and post-operative care management regimes have enabled NPGS to provide comparable IOP-lowering efficacy. The high degree of technical skill and surgical precision required to properly perform NPGS has resulted in a greater understanding of Schlemm's canal and outflow anatomy. This knowledge is being utilized to develop further innovations in NPGS and other novel procedures.

Further reading

Ambresin A, Shaarawy T, Mermoud A. Deep sclerectomy with collagen implant in one eye compared with trabeculectomy in the other eye of the same patient. J Glaucoma 2002; 11: 214–20

Anand N, Atherley C. Deep sclerectomy augmented with mitomycin C. Eye 2005; 19: 442–50

Ates H, Uretmen O, Andac K, Azarsiz SS. Deep sclerectomy with a nonabsorbable implant (T-Flux): preliminary results. Can J Ophthalmol 2003; 38: 482–8

Cairns JE. Trabeculectomy. Preliminary report of a new method. Am J Ophthalmol 1968; 66: 673–9

Carassa RG, Bettin P, Fiori M, Brancato R. Viscocanalostomy versus trabeculectomy in white adults affected by open-angle glaucoma: a 2-year randomized, controlled trial. Ophthalmology 2003; 110: 882–7

Chiselita D. Non-penetrating deep sclerectomy versus trabeculectomy in primary open-angle glaucoma surgery. Eye 2001; 15: 197–201

Cillino S, Pace FD, Casuccio A, et al. Deep sclerectomy versus punch trabeculectomy with or without phacoemulsification: a randomized clinical trial. J Glaucoma 2004; 13: 500–6

Cillino S, Di Pace F, Casuccio A, Lodato G. Deep sclerectomy versus punch trabeculectomy: effect of low-dosage mitomycin C. Ophthalmologica 2005; 219: 281–6

Dahan E, Drusedau MU. Non-penetrating filtration surgery for glaucoma: control by surgery only. J Cataract Refract Surg 2000; 26: 695–701

Dahan E, Shaarawy T, Mermoud A, et al. Non-penetrating glaucoma surgery. In: MY, Duker JS, eds. Ophthalmology, 2nd edn. St, Louis, MO: Mosby, 2004

Delarive T, Rossier A, Rossier S, et al. Aqueous dynamic and histological findings after deep sclerectomy with collagen implant in an animal model. Br J Ophthalmol 2003; 87: 1340–4

D'Eliseo D, Pastena B, Longanesi L, et al. Comparison of deep sclerectomy with implant and combined glaucoma surgery. Ophthalmologica 2003; 217: 208–11

Detry-Morel M. Non penetrating deep sclerectomy (NPDS) with SKGEL implant and/or 5-fluorouracile (5-FU). Bull Soc Belge Ophtalmol 2001; 280: 23–32

Devloo S, Deghislage C, Van Malderen L, et al. Non-penetrating deep sclerectomy without or with autologous scleral implant in open-angle glaucoma: medium-term results. Graefes Arch Clin Exp Ophthalmol 2005; 8: 1–7

Drüsedau MU, von Wolff K, Bull H, von Barsewisch B. Viscocanalostomy for primary open-angle glaucoma: the Grass Pantow experience. J Cataract Refract Surg 2000; 26: 1367–73

El Sayyad F, Helal M, El-Kholify H, et al. Nonpenetrating deep sclerectomy versus trabeculectomy in bilateral primary open-angle glaucoma. Ophthalmology 2000; 107: 1671–4

Epstein E. Fibrosing response to aqueous. Its relation to glaucoma. Br J Ophthalmol 1959; 43: 641–7

Funnell CL, Clowes M, Anand N. Combined cataract and glaucoma surgery with mitomycin C: phacoemulsification–trabeculectomy compared to phacoemulsification–deep sclerectomy. Br J Ophthalmol 2005; 89: 694–8

Fyodorov SN, Ioffe DI, Ronkina TI. Deep sclerectomy: technique and mechanism of a new glaucomatous procedure. Glaucoma 1984; 6: 281–3

Gianoli F, Schnyder CC, Bovey E, Mermoud A. Combined surgery for cataract and glaucoma: phacoemulsification and deep sclerectomy compared with phacoemulsification and trabeculectomy. J Cataract Refract Surg 1999; 25: 340–6

Gimbel HV, Penno EE, Ferensowicz M. Combined cataract surgery, intraocular lens implantation, and viscocanalostomy. J Cataract Refract Surg 1999; 25: 1370–5

Goldsmith JA, Ahmed IK, Crandall AS. Nonpenetrating glaucoma surgery. Ophthalmol Clin North Am 2005; 18: 443–60

Hamel M, Shaarawy T, Mermoud A. Deep sclerectomy with collagen implant in patients with glaucoma and high myopia. J Cataract Refract Surg 2001; 27: 1410–17

Iester M, Ravinet E, Mermoud A. Postoperative subconjunctival mitomycin-C injection after non-penetrating glaucoma surgery. J Ocul Pharmacol Ther 2002; 18: 307–12

Jehn AB, Bohnke M, Mojon DS. Deep sclerectomy with collagen implant: initial experience. Ophthalmologica 2002; 216: 235–8

Johnson DH, Johnson M. How does nonpenetrating glaucoma surgery work? Aqueous outflow resistance and glaucoma surgery. J Glaucoma 2001; 10: 55–67

Jonescu-Cuypers C, Jacobi P, Konen W, Krieglstein G. Primary viscocanalostomy versus trabeculectomy in white patients with open-angle glaucoma: a randomized clinical trial. Ophthalmology 2001; 108: 254–8

Karlen ME, Sanchez E, Schnyder CC, et al. Deep sclerectomy with collagen implant: medium term results. Br J Ophthalmol 1999; 83: 6–11

Kazakova D, Roters S, Schnyder CC, et al. Ultrasound biomicroscopy images: long-term results after deep sclerectomy with collagen implant. Graefes Arch Clin Exp Ophthalmol 2002; 240: 918–23

Khairy HA, Green FD, Nassar MK, Azuara-Blanco A. Control of intraocular pressure after deep sclerectomy. Eye 2006; 20: 336–40

Kobayashi H, Kobayashi K, Okinami S. A comparison of the intraocular pressure-lowering effect and safety of viscocanalostomy and trabeculectomy with mitomycin C in bilateral open-angle glaucoma. Graefes Arch Clin Exp Ophthalmol 2003; 241: 359–66

Koslov VI, Bagrov SN, Anisimova SY, et al. Non-penetrating deep sclerectomy with collagen. Ophthalmic Surg 1990; 3: 44–6

Kozlova T, Zagorski ZF, Rakowska E. A simplified technique for non-penetrating deep sclerectomy. Eur J Ophthalmol 2002; 12: 188–92

Kozobolis VP, Christodoulakis EV, Tzanakis N, et al. Primary deep sclerectomy versus primary deep sclerectomy with the use of mitomycin C in primary open-angle glaucoma. J Glaucoma 2002; 11: 287–93

Krasnov MM. Externalization of Schlemm's canal (sinusotomy) in glaucoma. Br J Ophthalmol 1968; 52: 157–61

Lachkar Y, Neverauskiene J, Jeanteur-Lunel MN, et al. Nonpenetrating deep sclerectomy: a 6-year retrospective study. Eur J Ophthalmol 2004; 14: 26–36

Libre PE. Nonpenetrating filtering surgery and goniopuncture (staged trabeculectomy) for episcleral venous pressure glaucoma. Am J Ophthalmol 2003; 136: 1172–4

Lüke C, Dietlein TS, Jacobi PC, et al. A prospective randomized trial of viscocanalostomy versus trabeculectomy in open-angle glaucoma: a 1-year follow-up study. J Glaucoma 2002; 11: 294–9

Lüke C, Dietlein TS, Jacobi PC, et al. A prospective randomised trial of viscocanalostomy with and without implantation of a reticulated hyaluronic acid implant (SKGEL) in open angle glaucoma. Br J Ophthalmol 2003; 87: 599–603

Mermoud A, Karlen ME, Schnyder CC, et al. Nd:Yag goniopuncture after deep sclerectomy with collagen implant. Ophthalmic Surg Lasers 1999; 30: 120–5

Mermoud A, Schnyder CC, Sickenberg M, et al. Comparison of deep sclerectomy with collagen implant and trabeculectomy in open-angle glaucoma. J Cataract Refract Surg 1999; 25: 323–31

Neudorfer M, Sadetzki S, Anisimova S, Geyer O. Nonpenetrating deep sclerectomy with the use of adjunctive mitomycin C. Ophthalmic Surg Lasers Imaging 2004; 35: 6–12

O'Brart DP, Rowlands E, Islam N, Noury AM. A randomised, prospective study comparing trabeculectomy augmented with antimetabolites with a viscocanalostomy technique for the management of open angle glaucoma uncontrolled by medical therapy. Br J Ophthalmol 2002; 86: 748–54

O'Brart DP, Shiew M, Edmunds B. A randomised, prospective study comparing trabeculectomy with viscocanalostomy with adjunctive antimetabolite usage for the management of open angle glaucoma uncontrolled by medical therapy. Br J Ophthalmol 2004; 88: 1012–17

Park M, Tanito M, Nishikawa M, et al. Combined viscocanalostomy and cataract surgery compared with cataract surgery in Japanese patients with glaucoma. J Glaucoma 2004; 13: 55–61

Ravinet E, Bovey E, Mermoud A. T-Flux implant versus Healon GV in deep sclerectomy. J Glaucoma 2004; 13: 46–50

Sanchez E, Schnyder CC, Sickenberg M, et al. Deep sclerectomy: results with and without collagen implant. Int Ophthalmol 1996–97; 20: 157–62

Shaarawy T, Mermoud A. Deep sclerectomy in one eye vs deep sclerectomy with collagen implant in the contralateral

eye of the same patient: long-term follow-up. Eye 2005; 19: 298–302

Shaarawy T, Karlen M, Schnyder C, et al. Five-year results of deep sclerectomy with collagen implant. J Cataract Refract Surg 2001; 27: 1770–8

Shaarawy T, Nguyen C, Schnyder C, Mermoud A. Five year results of viscocanalostomy. Br J Ophthalmol 2003; 87: 441–5

Shaarawy T, Mansouri K, Schnyder C, et al. Long-term results of deep sclerectomy with collagen implant. J Cataract Refract Surg 2004; 30: 1225–31

Shaarawy T, Nguyen C, Schnyder C, Mermoud A. Comparative study between deep sclerectomy with and without collagen implant: long term follow up. Br J Ophthalmol 2004; 88: 95–8

Stegmann R, Pienaar A, Miller D. Viscocanalostomy for open-angle glaucoma in black African patients. J Cataract Refract Surg 1999; 25: 316–22

Sugar HS. Experimental trabeculectomy in glaucoma. Am J Ophthalmol 1961; 51: 623–7

Sunaric-Megevand G, Leuenberger PM. Results of viscocanalostomy for primary open-angle glaucoma. Am J Ophthalmol 2001; 132: 221–8

Tanito M, Park M, Nishikawa M, et al. Comparison of surgical outcomes of combined viscocanalostomy and cataract surgery with combined trabeculotomy and cataract surgery. Am J Ophthalmol 2002; 134: 513–20

Uretmen O, Ates H, Guven S, Andac K. Comparison of outcomes of viscocanalostomy and phacoviscocanalostomy. Can J Ophthalmol 2003; 38: 580–6

Vuori ML. Complications of neodymium:YAG laser goniopuncture after deep sclerectomy. Acta Ophthalmol Scand 2003; 81: 573–6

Wevill MT, Meyer D, Van Aswegen E. A pilot study of deep sclerectomy with implantation of chromic suture material as a collagen implant: medium-term results. Eye 2005; 19: 549–54

Wild GJ, Kent AR, Peng Q. Dilation of Schlemm's canal in viscocanalostomy: comparison of 2 viscoelastic substances. J Cataract Refract Surg 2001; 27: 1294–7

Wishart MS, Shergill T, Porooshani H. Viscocanalostomy and phacoviscocanalostomy: long-term results. J Cataract Refract Surg 2002; 28: 745–51

Wishart PK, Wishart MS, Porooshani H. Viscocanalostomy and deep sclerectomy for the surgical treatment of glaucoma: a longterm follow-up. Acta Ophthalmol Scand 2003; 81: 343–8

Yalvac IS, Sahin M, Eksioglu U, et al. Primary viscocanalostomy versus trabeculectomy for primary open-angle glaucoma: three-year prospective randomized clinical trial. J Cataract Refract Surg 2004; 30: 2050–7

Yarangümeli A, Gureser S, Koz OG, et al. Viscocanalostomy versus trabeculectomy in patients with bilateral high-tension glaucoma. Int Ophthalmol 2004; 25: 207–13

Yarangümeli A, Koz OG, Alp MN, et al. Viscocanalostomy with mitomycin-C: a preliminary study. Eur J Ophthalmol 2005; 15: 202–8

Zimmerman TJ, Kooner KS, Ford VJ, et al. Trabeculectomy vs. non-penetrating trabeculectomy: a retrospective study of two procedures in phakic patients with glaucoma. Ophthalmic Surg 1984; 15: 734–40

19 Aqueous shunts

Anne L Coleman, JoAnn A Giaconi

INTRODUCTION

Aqueous shunts are drainage devices designed to lower intraocular pressure by draining aqueous humor from the interior of the eye to an encapsulated reservoir near the equator of the globe. In general, aqueous shunts have been used in eyes with poor surgical prognoses, as listed in Table 19.1. The devices consist of one or more plates connected to a tube; the tube not only serves as the means of egress of aqueous from the eye but also prevents the opening into the eye from closing. Although there have been several devices used to keep an opening in the eye patent, Anthony Molteno was the first to design an implant that helped with the formation of a posterior episcleral filtering bleb.

Most aqueous shunts have a similar design. There is a silicone or Silastic tube that is placed into the eye (through the limbus or pars plana) and through which aqueous humor passes into the episcleral–subconjunctival space near the globe's equator. In this area there is an episcleral plate that is designed to help form and maintain a filtering bleb. Three key design features distinguish different implants: (1) the presence of a valve or mechanism to restrict the flow of aqueous humor from the eye; (2) the surface area of the episcleral plate; and (3) the material used.

The restriction of flow of aqueous humor from the eye is important in the prevention of immediate postoperative hypotony and its attendant complications. Implants that do not have such a mechanism, the Molteno, Baerveldt, and Schocket band implants, are usually inserted in either a two-stage procedure, where encapsulation of the bleb is allowed to occur before a second surgery to actually insert the tube into the eye, or a one-stage procedure, where the flow of aqueous is restricted by a suture ligature around the tube or an internal stent. Several aqueous shunts, specifically the Krupin Valve implant, Joseph implant, White pump-shunt, Optimed Glaucoma Pressure Regulator, and Ahmed Glaucoma Valve implant, have pressure-sensitive valves or internal mechanisms to restrict the flow of aqueous from the eye, with the goal being to prevent ocular hypotony in the immediate postoperative period. Prata and co-authors reported that the Ahmed and Krupin implants function as flow-restricting devices at flow rates of 2–25 µl/min. *In vitro* tests with human plasma showed that the Ahmed and Krupin implants had greater resistance (change in pressure/change in flow) than partially ligated Baerveldt implants.

The surface area of the episcleral plate may influence the amount of intraocular pressure reduction because of its effect on filtering bleb size. In animal eyes with Molteno implants, Minckler and co-authors found that the pressure within the filtration bleb surrounding the episcleral plate was similar to the pressure in the anterior chamber. Since the main resistance to aqueous flow and pressure reduction is the capsular wall surrounding the episcleral plate, a potential advantage of a larger filtration bleb is a larger surface area for diffusion. Heuer and co-authors have reported that there is a greater reduction in intraocular pressure

Table 19.1 Clinical indications for aqueous shunts
1. Prior failed glaucoma filtering surgery
2. Aphakic/pseudo-phakic glaucoma
3. Neovascular glaucoma
4. Uveitic glaucoma
5. Congenital glaucoma after failed angle surgery
6. Prior penetrating keratoplasty
7. Angle closure glaucoma
8. Epithelial downgrowth
9. ICE syndrome

in eyes with the double-plate Molteno implant compared to the single-plate Molteno implant, and Mills and co-authors found 2-year success rates of 67% and 85% for single and double-plate Molteno implants, respectively. Although Lloyd and co-authors reported the percentage decrease in intraocular pressure to be similar for the Baerveldt 500 mm^2 and 350 mm^2 implants, eyes with the larger implant required an average of 0.6 fewer medications postoperatively. Thus, a larger surface area may be beneficial in terms of intraocular pressure reduction. Whether better intraocular pressure reduction is associated with more post-operative complications is not clear. Heuer and co-authors reported that double-plate Molteno implants are associated with more complications than single-plate implants, while Lloyd and co-authors did not find a statistically significant difference in the number of complications between 350 mm^2 and 500 mm^2 Baerveldt implants.

Even though aqueous shunts are made of relatively non-reactive substances such as polypropylene, silicone, Silastic (a soft, pliable plastic), and polymethyl methacrylate, they do stimulate the formation of a collagenous and fibrovascular capsule around the episcleral plate. Histopathologically, this capsular wall has been described as a collagenous meshwork that progressively becomes denser from inside to out. The thickness of this capsule is important in the resistance of aqueous flow from the episcleral plate to the surrounding vasculature. Excessive fibrous reaction around the bleb appears to be the major cause of long-term drainage device failure. In a rabbit model, Ayyala and colleagues have shown that polypropylene end-plates are more inflammatory than silicone ones, and that the rigidity and shape of the end-plate may promote inflammation. Currently, investigators are attempting to modify the surface of the episcleral plate to help prevent the formation of a thick capsule, but no studies have been published to date on the effects of such modifications in humans. Antifibrotic agents such as mitomycin C and 5-fluorouracil have been tried at the time of surgery to decrease fibrous reaction. Several studies have shown no advantage of these antifibrotic agents compared to controls, whereas the incidence of complications such as late hypotony, flat anterior chamber, and conjunctival melts causing tube and plate erosions were higher.

At the present time, it is not clear whether the commercially available devices (Table 19.2) exhibit similar efficacy or if one device has certain advantages over the others. Currently, there is an ongoing prospective, randomized trial in humans comparing the Baerveldt and Ahmed drainage devices in patients. Results obtained with the various devices are summarized in Table 19.3.

Complications associated with aqueous shunts can be categorized as those associated with the

Table 19.2   Commercially available aqueous shunts (year introduced)
Non-valved implants
Single-plate and double-plate Molteno implants (1979)
Baerveldt implant (1990)
Valved implants
Krupin Valve disc implant (1990)
Ahmed Glaucoma Valve implants (1993)

reduction of intraocular pressure, with the functioning and placement of the tube, with the episcleral plate and the response of surrounding tissues to it, and with intraocular surgery per se. A complete list of complications is provided in Table 19.4. Information about most of the specific complications is given with Figures 19.1–19.38. Suprachoroidal hemorrhage is a complication that can occur in any eye predisposed to develop them, regardless of the presence of a device to restrict flow. Ocular hypotony may also occur with both valved and non-valved devices where flow is restricted. Ocular hypotony may occur because of inadequate restriction of aqueous flow, leakage of aqueous around the tube, or the decreased production of aqueous humor by the ciliary body. Phthisis bulbi has been reported in 2–18% of eyes following shunt placement, with neovascular glaucoma having a greater risk. Complications associated with intraocular surgery per se also occur with glaucoma drainage devices. The incidence of retinal detachment has been reported as 0–14%, and that of vitreous hemorrhage is 0–11% (vitreous hemorrhages may be secondary to underlying disease such as proliferative diabetic retinopathy). The incidence of epiretinal membranes and/or cystoid macular edema have been reported in 0–14% of eyes, and that of endophthalmitis after Molteno, Baerveldt, Ahmed or Krupin implants is 0–3%.

The Ex-Press Mini Glaucoma Shunt (CibaVision, Duluth, GA) was FDA approved in 2002. It is a stainless-steel 'tube' with a 27-gauge shaft, 2.96 mm in length with a 0.4-mm internal diameter. It features a patented flow-restricting device within its lumen. To implant one, a small conjunctival incision is made 10 mm from the limbus after which a 25-gauge needle is used to make a limbal incision. The device loaded onto an introducer is then placed through the limbal incision. Currently, there is little peer-reviewed literature on the device. Contraindications to its use include angle-closure, neovascular, uveitic, congenital/juvenile glaucomas, as well as severe dry eye or blepharitis. Reported complications have included hypotony, conjunctival erosion over the device, and lack of IOP control due to bleb scarring.

Table 19.3 Cumulative probability of success of different types of aqueous shunt

Study	Type of shunt	Number of eyes (patients)	Diagnoses (no. of eyes)	Follow-up time (mean ± SD; months)	Cumulative probability of success/time	Definition of success
Lloyd, Sedlak et al., 1994	Molteno single-plate	96 (96)	Aphakia/IOL (50) Failed filter (12) NVG (18) <13 yrs old (16)	47.4 ± 18.2 59.8 ± 6.6 33.8 ± 24.7 65.7 ± 8.4	74.2%/2 years 58%/2 years 57%/2 years 68%/2 years	(1) IOP ≤ 21 and > 5 mmHg with or without meds (2) No further glaucoma surgery (3) No devastating complications (4) No loss of light perception
Mermoud et al., 1993	Molteno single-plate	60 (54)	NVG (60)	24.7 ± 9.4	53%/2 years	(1) IOP ≤ 21 mmHg with or without meds (2) No further glaucoma surgery (3) No development of phthisis bulbi (4) No loss of light perception
Hill et al., 1993	Molteno single-plate or double-plate in one-stage implantation	10 (10)	Uveitic glaucoma	28 ± 17	79%/2 years	(1) IOP ≤ 21 and > 5 mmHg with or without meds (2) No further glaucoma surgery (3) No development of phthisis bulbi (4) No loss of light perception
Mills et al., 1996	Molteno single-plate or double-plate	77 (71)	Aphakic/IOL (24) NVG (20) Uveitic (12) Failed filter (9) Traumatic (8) Congenital (4)	Median 44 months (range 6–107)	54%/5 years	(1) IOP ≤ 22 with or without meds (2) No further glaucoma surgery (3) No devastating complications (4) No loss of light perception
Heuer et al., 1992	Molteno single-plate	37 (37)	OAG (15) ACG (21) Uveitic (5) Congenital (4) Traumatic (4) Uncertain (1)	14.9 ± 68.9	46%/2 years	(1) IOP ≤ 21 and ≥ 6 mmHg with or without meds (2) No further glaucoma surgery (3) No devastating complications
Heuer et al., 1992	Molteno double-plate	38 (38)	OAG (18) ACG (17) Uveitic (8) Congenital (4) Traumatic (3) Uncertain (1)	16.4 ± 6.8	71%/2 years	(1) IOP ≤ 21 and ≥ 6 mmHg with or without meds (2) No further glaucoma surgery (3) No devastating complications
Lloyd, Baerveldt, Heuer et al., 1994	Baerveldt implant (200 or 350 mm²)	13 (13)	Aphakic/IOL (10)	16.2 ± 7.6	67%/18 months	(1) IOP ≤ 21 and ≥ 6 mmHg with or without meds (2) No further glaucoma surgery (3) No devastating complications (4) No loss of light perception

Continued

Table 19.3 Continued

Study	Type of shunt	Number of eyes (patients)	Diagnoses (no. of eyes)	Follow-up time (mean ± SD; months)	Cumulative probability of success/time	Definition of success
Lloyd, Baerveldt, Fellenbaum et al., 1994	Baerveldt implant (350 mm²)	37 (37)	Aphakic/IOL (33) Failed filter (4)	15.5 ± 4.8	93%/18 months	(1) IOP ≤ 21 and ≥ 6 mmHg with or without meds (2) No further glaucoma surgery (3) No devastating complications (4) No loss of light perception
Lloyd, Baerveldt, Fellenbaum et al., 1994	Baerveldt implant (500 mm²)	36 (36)	Aphakic/IOL (31) Failed filter (5)	14.1 ± 5.4	88%/18 months	(1) IOP ≤ 21 and ≥ 6 mmHg with or without meds (2) No further glaucoma surgery (3) No devastating complications (4) No loss of light perception
Siegner et al., 1995	Baerveldt implant (200, 250, 350 or 500 mm²)	103 (100)	NVG (34) Congenital (15) Uveitic (11) OAG (16) ACG (7) PKP (9) Traumatic (7) CMG (4)	13.6 ± 0.9	60.3%/2 years	(1) IOP ≤ 21 and ≥ 5 mmHg with or without meds (2) No further glaucoma surgery (3) No loss of light perception
Hodkin et al., 1995	Baerveldt implant (350 mm²)	50 (50)	Aphakic/IOL (35) Failed filter (12) NVG (7) Age <13 yrs old (3) PKP (13) Phakic (5)	13.7 ± 19.2	70%/18 months	(1) IOP ≤ 21 mmHg with or without meds (2) No further glaucoma surgery (3) No development of phthisis bulbi (4) No loss of light perception
Fellenbaum et al., 1994	Krupin eye valve with disc	25 (25)	OAG (11) ACG (7) NVG (3) CMG (2) ICE (2)	13.2, range 4–19	66%/1 year	(1) IOP < 22 and > 5 mmHg with or without meds (2) No further glaucoma surgery (3) No devastating complications
Coleman et al., 1995	Ahmed Glaucoma Valve	60 (60)	OAG (18) PKP (16) NVG (14) Congenital (6) Uveitic (5) ACG (1)	Median 9.3, range 3–22	78%/1 year	(1) IOP <22 and > 4 mmHg with or without meds (2) Less than 20% reduction in IOP from preop value if preop IOP < 22 mmHg (3) No further glaucoma surgery (4) No devastating complications

IOL, intraocular lens; NVG, neovascular glaucoma; OAG, open-angle glaucoma; ACG, angle-closure glaucoma; PKP, penetrating keratoplasty; CMG, chronic mixed glaucoma; ICE, iridocorneal endothelial syndrome.

Table 19.4 Complications

1. Complications associated with reduction of intraocular pressure
   a. Flat anterior chamber
   b. Serous choroidal effusions
   c. Suprachoroidal hemorrhage
   d. Ocular hypotony
   e. Phthisis bulbi
2. Complications associated with the functioning and placement of the tube
   a. Tube blockage
   b. Tube retraction or malposition
   c. Tube erosion
   d. Tube–lens touch
   e. Tube–corneal touch
   f. Corneal decompensation/edema
   g. Corneal graft failure
   h. Anterior uveitis
3. Complications associated with the episcleral plate
   a. Implant extrusion or erosion
   b. Bleb encapsulation
   c. Motility disturbances
4. Complications associated with intraocular surgery *per se*
   a. Retinal detachment and/or vitreous hemorrhage
   b. Endophthalmitis
   c. Malignant glaucoma or aqueous misdirection
   d. Pupillary block
   e. Epiretinal membrane and/or cystoid macular edema

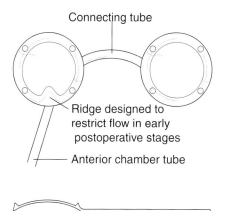

Figure 19.2 The double-plate Molteno implant. Double-plate Molteno implants consist of a single-plate Molteno implant connected with a 10 mm long silicone tube to another circular episcleral plate. The surface area of $270\,mm^2$ is twice that of the single-plate Molteno implant ($265\,mm^2$ for the pressure ridge design), and the plates are positioned on both sides of a rectus muscle. Right and left-eyed double-plate Molteno implants are available. The pressure ridge (marked) is a modification found on both single and double-plate implants. The ridge increases the resistance of aqueous flow from the eye during the first postoperative week by enabling swollen Tenon's tissue to create a temporary seal over the implant. This seal increases aqueous flow resistance from the eye in the immediate postoperative period.

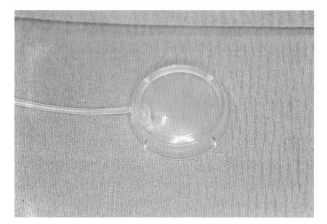

Figure 19.1 The Molteno implant. Single-plate Molteno implants (Molteno Ophthalmic Limited, New Zealand) consist of a circular, rigid polypropylene episcleral plate and a silicone tube. The tube opens onto the surface of the convex, episcleral plate, and its inner diameter is 0.34 mm. The plate's diameter is 13 mm. One side of the single-plate Molteno implant has a surface area of $135\,mm^2$ ($133\,mm^2$ for the pressure ridge design).

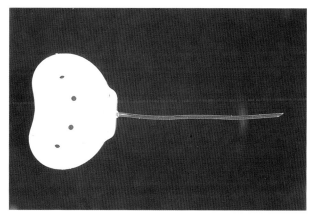

Figure 19.3 The Baerveldt implant. The Baerveldt implant (Advanced Medical Optics, Santa Ana, CA) consists of a silicone tube and episcleral plate. The episcleral plate is impregnated with barium, making it radiopaque. Fenestration holes are a part of the plate design in order to minimize bleb height and its associated problems. Bleb height is minimized by the growth of fibrovascular tissue through these holes. The plate is currently available in three sizes: 250, 350, and $425\,mm^2$. The internal diameter of the tube is 0.3 mm. When implanted, the plate is generally placed underneath two adjacent rectus muscles.

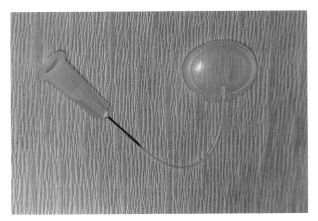

Figure 19.4 The Krupin Valve disc implant. The Krupin Valve disc implant (EagleVision, Memphis, TN) consists of a Silastic tube attached to the convex, anterior surface of a silicone disc. The disc is oval, measures 13 mm posteriorly and 18 mm horizontally, and has a surface area of 184 mm^2. The internal diameter of the tube is 0.38 mm. The valve mechanism consists of horizontal and vertical slits in the distal end of the Silastic tube. The slits are designed to open at a pressure of 11 mmHg and close at a pressure of 9 mmHg.

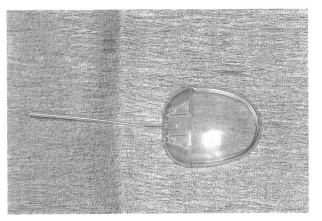

Figure 19.6 The Ahmed Glaucoma Valve. The Ahmed Glaucoma Valve implant (New World Medical, Inc., Rancho Cucamonga, CA) has a silicone tube and silicone elastomer membrane valve. The episcleral plate is available either in rigid polypropylene (shown here) or flexible silicone, and comes in single and double-plate models. The inner diameter of the tube is 0.3 mm. A single plate has a surface area of 184 mm^2. In both models, the plate is shaped similar to a horseshoe crab and measures 16 mm posteriorly and 13 mm horizontally. Pediatric-sized plates are also available with a surface area of 96 mm^2. The opening pressure of the Ahmed Glaucoma Valve implant is theoretically 8 mmHg.

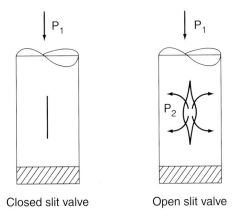

Closed slit valve   Open slit valve

Figure 19.5 Function of a slit valve. The slit valve opens when the pressure in the eye and tube (P_1) is greater than the pressure outside the eye and tube (P_2). The Krupin Valve disc implant has a theoretical opening pressure between 10 and 12 mmHg and a closing pressure between 8 and 10 mmHg.

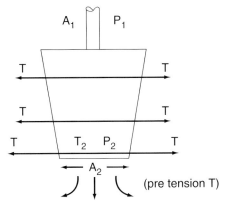

Figure 19.7 Function of the Ahmed Glaucoma Valve. The valve-like mechanism of the Ahmed Glaucoma Valve implant consists of a silicone membrane folded over on itself and placed on stretch so that there is tension across the membrane (T). The tension on the membrane is adjusted so that the opening pressure is 8–10 mmHg. The membrane is shaped so that it has a larger area at the entrance of the tube (inlet or A_1) and a smaller area where the fluid exits (outlet or A_2). Because of this venturi-shaped chamber, compared to slit valves a smaller pressure differential is needed between the inside (P_1) and outside (P_2) of the eye allows for fluid to exit the eye than in slit valves. When P_1-P_2 is greater than T, the membranes open and aqueous flows through the valve.

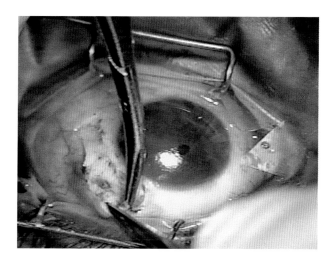

Figure 19.8 Peritomy. A limbus-based or fornix-based (as shown here) conjunctival incision is made after the placement of a traction suture through the peripheral cornea or under a rectus muscle. The length of the conjunctival incision depends on the implant to be inserted. A double-plate implant requires exposure of two quadrants while a single-plate implant requires exposure of one quadrant. The identification of the rectus muscles in a quadrant helps with the insertion of Baerveldt and Krupin Valve disc implants. The sclera in the quadrant is exposed by dissection in the sub-Tenon's space so that the implant can be placed posterior to the insertions of the rectus muscles. The episcleral vessels are cauterized as needed.

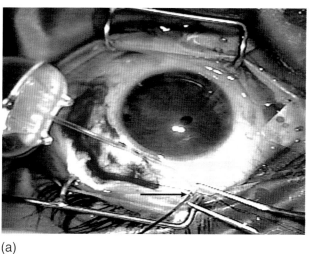

(a)

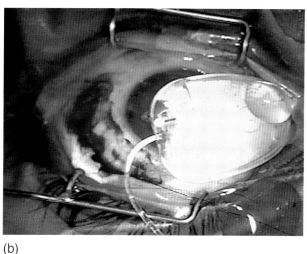

(b)

Figure 19.9 Preparation of the implant. The tube of the Ahmed Glaucoma Valve implant shown here is irrigated with a 27-gauge cannula. (a) The arrow points to the cannula in the end of the tube. (b) Irrigation of fluid through the cannula. The implant may be soaked in an antibiotic solution prior to implantation. The tube should then be irrigated with balanced saline solution prior to suturing the plate to episclera. The irrigation of the tube is important with the Molteno, Baerveldt, and Krupin implants in order to check the patency of the tube. Irrigation of the tube in the Ahmed Glaucoma Valve implant not only checks patency but also helps to break the capillary attraction of the silicone membranes so that the valve-like mechanism can function.

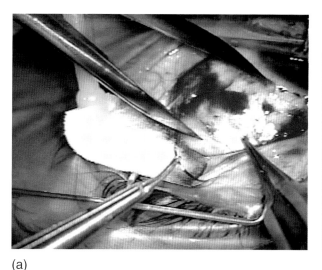

(a)

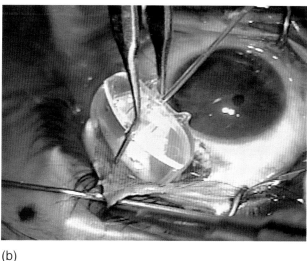

(b)

Figure 19.10 Insertion of the plate. The episcleral plate should be secured 8–10 mm posterior to the limbus with non-absorbable sutures (5-0 to 9-0 Supramid, nylon, polypropylene or mersilene). The holes present on the anterior edge of Molteno,

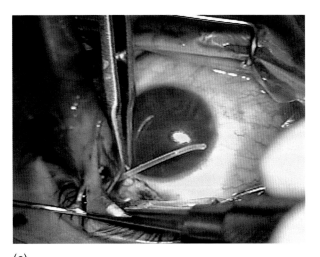

(c)

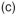

Figure 19.10 Continued Baerveldt and Ahmed implants are used to help fixate the implant. If a double-plate Molteno is used, one plate should be on either side of a rectus muscle. The connecting silicone tube may be placed over or under the rectus muscle. Shown here: (a) A caliper is used to measure 10 mm from the limbus. The suture used to secure the plate may be pre-placed at the 10-mm mark; in this case one needle of a double-armed 9-0 nylon suture is placed through half-thickness sclera in the mid-portion of the quadrant. (b) The insertion is started, using a smooth forceps to grasp the device. (c) The plate easily slips into the prepared sub-Tenon's pocket.

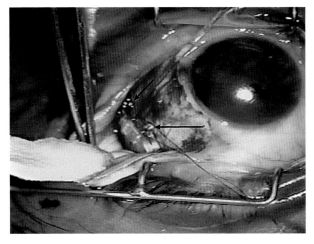

Figure 19.11 Fixating the implant to the sclera. The fixation holes (arrows) of the Ahmed Glaucoma Valve implant are used to fixate the implant to the sclera. In this case, each needle of the double-armed 9-0 nylon suture has been passed through one of the fixation holes and then through superficial sclera before the two ends were tied together to secure the plate. Some surgeons will place an interrupted suture through each hole.

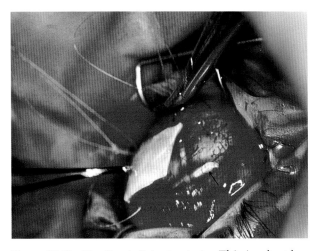

Figure 19.12 The Krupin Valve implant. This implant has a Silastic ridge, rather than fixation holes, through which the fixating sutures may be passed (arrow).

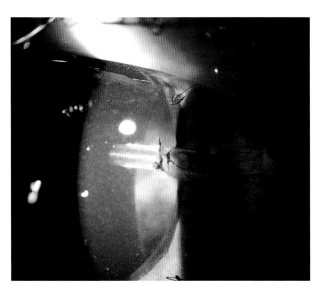

Figure 19.13 Methods to restrict the flow of aqueous humor through drainage devices without an internal valve. Many investigators have reported on methods to restrict the flow of aqueous through the tube when Molteno or Baerveldt implants are placed in a one-stage procedure. These methods include the use of an external suture ligature, an internal stent, or both. As shown here, one method is to occlude the proximal end of the tube with a polypropylene or nylon suture. This end of the tube is then inserted into the anterior chamber and may be lysed with a laser in the immediate postoperative period. Alternatively, a chromic, 5-0 nylon or 3-0 supramid suture can be threaded first through the tube and then through the episcleral plate where its distal end can be placed subconjunctivally, either over the plate or 90 to 180° away from the tube. This suture (also known as a rip-chord) can then be removed in the immediate postoperative period as needed. Another method of occlusion is to tie a vicryl, chromic, nylon, or silk suture around the tube posterior to the scleral flap or donor patch graft. This suture can later be cut with a laser or with scissors through a conjunctival incision if it does not dissolve or is not releasable. Sherwood and Smith reported on the placement of vertical slits in the tube anterior to an absorbable external suture ligature. These slits help prevent the intraocular pressure from being too high in the immediate postoperative period while the fibrotic capsule forms around the episcleral plate. Despite the restriction of flow through tubes with these methods, problems with ocular hypotony may occur. (Courtesy of Jeff Liebmann, MD, The New York Eye and Ear Infirmary.)

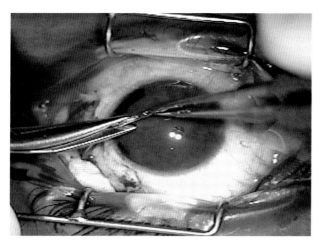

Figure 19.14 Tube trimming. After the episcleral plate is securely tied down to its quadrant, the end of the tube is cut with a bevel towards the corneal endothelium. A beveled tip makes insertion into the anterior chamber easier.

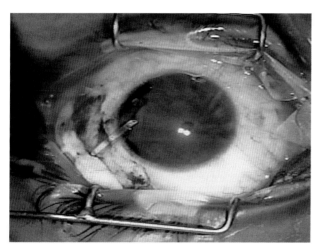

Figure 19.15 Trimming the tube. It is ideal to cut the tube so that it will extend 1–2 mm beyond the surgical limbus when placed into the anterior chamber, as illustrated here prior to insertion. After the tube has been trimmed to the correct length, a corneal paracentesis away from the surgical site may be done.

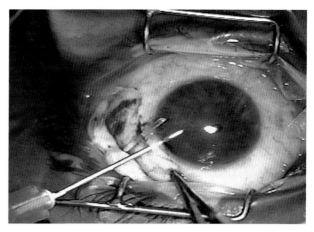

Figure 19.16 Tube insertion tract. The eye is entered with a 22- or 23-gauge needle. Viscoelastic may be attached to the needle and injected as the needle is withdrawn. This will focally deepen the chamber, push the iris away from the opening, and lubricate the tract for tube insertion. The tract should be parallel to the iris, well away from the cornea (particularly in patients who have had a penetrating keratoplasty) and slightly above the iris. Alternatively, the tube may be inserted into the posterior chamber through the pars plana in aphakic or pseudophakic patients, if a complete pars plana vitrectomy has been performed to prevent tube blockage with vitreous.

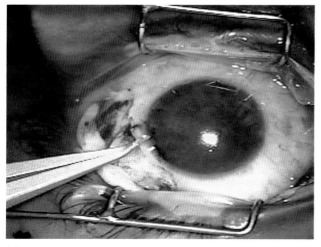

(a)

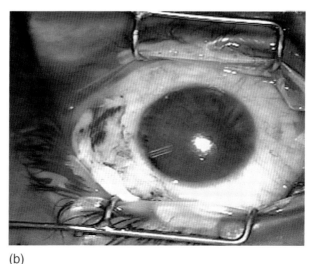

(b)

Figure 19.17 Inserting the tube. (a) The tube is inserted through the opening into the eye made with the 23-gauge needle. (b) The tube is properly positioned in the anterior chamber. The scleral portion of the tube may be secured to sclera with a non-absorbable suture. If this is done, care should be taken so that this suture does not constrict the tube.

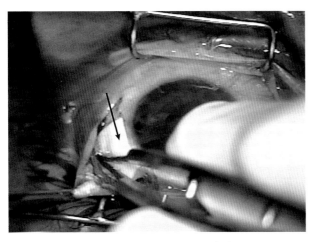

Figure 19.18 Coverage of the tube. To help prevent erosion of the tube through the conjunctiva, the tube is usually covered with a patch graft consisting of human donor sclera or cornea, dura mater, fascia lata, or pericardium. It may also be placed underneath a partial-thickness scleral flap created at the limbus. In this figure the tube is being covered with donor pericardium (arrow). The pericardium is secured to the sclera with absorbable or non-absorbable sutures. In this case, 8-0 vicryl sutures were placed through each anterior corner. Occasionally, sutures may be required posteriorly as well.

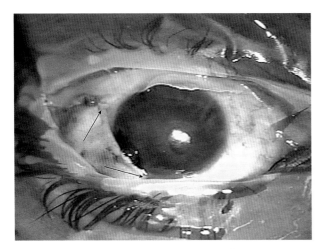

Figure 19.19 Closure of the peritomy. The conjunctiva should be closed over the implant and the patch graft with absorbable sutures. Since the implant is a foreign material, care should be taken to completely cover the implant and patch graft. Arrows point to the corners of the original peritomy where running sutures of 9-0 monofilament vicryl were placed to close each end of the radialized incision. Postoperatively the patient is treated with topical corticosteroids, antibiotics, and possibly cycloplegic agents.

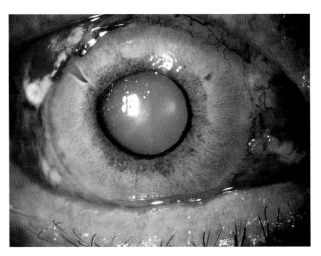

Figure 19.20 A flat anterior chamber secondary to malignant glaucoma. This eye has a flat anterior chamber secondary to malignant glaucoma and the tube is occluded by the surrounding iris. Flat anterior chamber has been reported following insertion of valved and non-valved aqueous shunts. When single-plate Molteno implants without modifications to restrict aqueous flow were inserted into 30 eyes in a one-stage procedure, seven (23%) of the eyes had flat anterior chambers the first postoperative week. Even when Molteno and Baerveldt implants have external suture ligation or internal stents placed to decrease aqueous egress, there are still cases of flat anterior chambers postoperatively, reported in up to 30% of cases. The incorporation of a valve into the shunt design dramatically reduces, but does not eliminate, the risk of flat anterior chamber. Flat anterior chambers may require re-formation of the anterior chamber with saline, viscoelastics, or gas after the determination and management of their etiology, e.g. wound leak, overfiltration, pupillary block, etc.

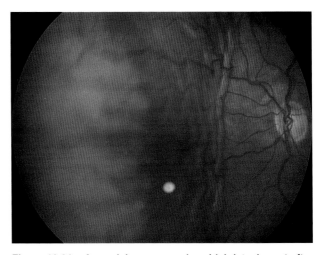

Figure 19.21 A resolving serous choroidal detachment after placement of a drainage device. Serous choroidal effusions occur in up to 32% of eyes following shunt placement. The presence of a valve in the device does not alter the risk of choroidal effusion, and most are probably due to ocular decompression. Drainage of the choroidal effusion may be necessary.

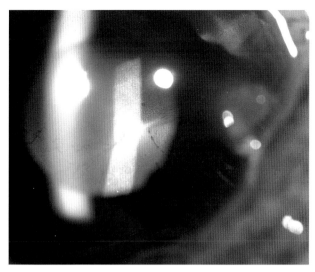

Figure 19.22 Kissing choroidal detachments. This eye with glaucoma due to the Sturge–Weber syndrome has kissing choroidal detachments that required surgical drainage. (Courtesy of Neil Choplin, MD.)

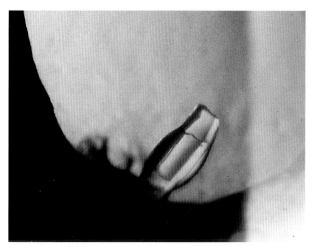

Figure 19.24 A tube blocked by silicone oil. This tube was blocked by a silicone oil that entered the tube despite the placement of the tube and implant inferiorly.

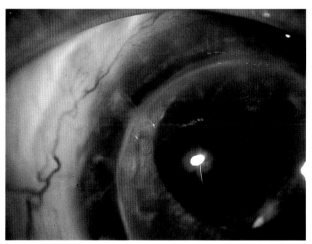

Figure 19.23 Blockage of drainage device tube by vitreous. This tube was blocked by a strand of vitreous after a Nd:YAG capsulotomy. The obstruction of tubes by vitreous, fibrin, blood, inflammatory debris, silicone oil, or iris has occurred in 0–20% of eyes with an aqueous shunt. The blockage of tubes seems to occur as frequently with non-valved implants as with valved implants. The Nd:YAG laser may be used to open a tube blocked with fibrin, blood, inflammatory debris, iris, or a vitreous strand. In addition, the tube may be irrigated intracamerally or may be removed from the eye prior to its being flushed.

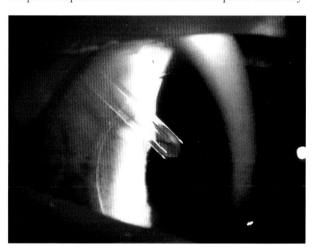

Figure 19.25 Tube malposition – here too long. This tube, which is anterior to an anterior chamber intraocular lens and extends beyond the pupillary margin, is too long, since it is in the pupillary space and may cause glare or visual disturbances. Tubes may also retract and become too short or require repositioning in 0–7% of eyes. Tubes may retract as intraocular pressure rises and the decompressed eye fills following recovery from surgery and the decompressed eye fills.

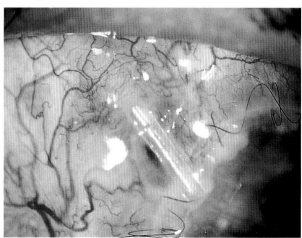

Figure 19.26 Tube erosion. This tube has eroded through the host cornea and corneal graft. It was repaired with a corneal patch graft.

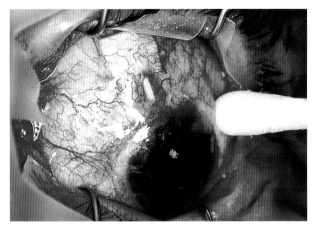

Figure 19.27 Tube erosion. This tube has eroded through the patch graft and conjunctiva. Erosion of the tube through the conjunctiva or cornea (as seen in Figure 19.26) may occur in 0–5% of eyes, despite the placement of a patch graft. Treatment of tube erosion through the conjunctiva includes re-grafting with a donor material while erosion through the cornea may require local corneal grafting. Foreign material such as tube shunts should not be left uncovered and exposed, because of the high risk of infection.

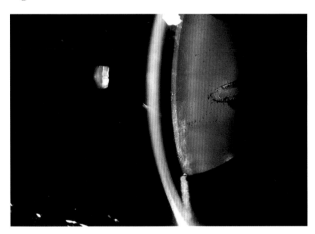

Figure 19.28 Tube–lens touch. This eye has a shallow anterior chamber and tube–lens touch. Intermittent or persistent tube–lens touch may be associated with the formation of a cataract in phakic eyes. The incidence of cataract may be as high as 25% even in the absence of lens–tube touch.

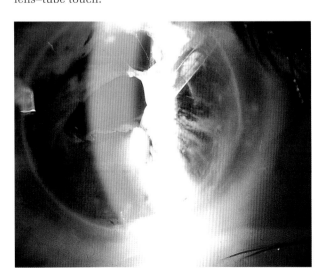

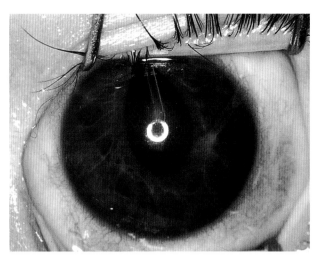

Figure 19.29 Intermittent tube–corneal touch. This eye with two Ahmed Glaucoma Valve implants has intermittent tube–corneal touch that has resulted in focal corneal edema and haze. Despite careful positioning of the tube, as many as 10% of eyes may have tube–corneal touch postoperatively. This tube–corneal touch may or may not result in corneal decompensation. Corneal decompensation following placement of a tube shunt has been reported in up to 18% of eyes. Although progressive corneal endothelial cell loss after uncomplicated implantations of Molteno drainage devices has been reported, it is not believed to be clinically significant.

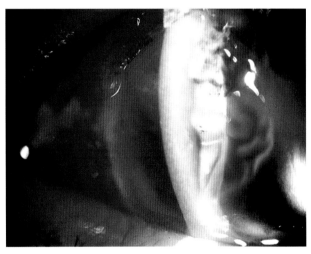

Figure 19.30 An eye with epithelial downgrowth. This eye has epithelial downgrowth, which is an indication for a glaucoma drainage device over a trabeculectomy. The tube was positioned posterior to the cornea and anterior to the sheet of epithelial cells.

Figure 19.31 Clear corneal graft after drainage device. This eye has Peter's anomaly with a clear corneal graft and Ahmed Glaucoma Valve implant.

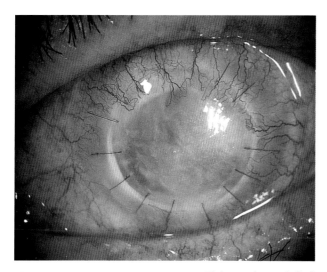

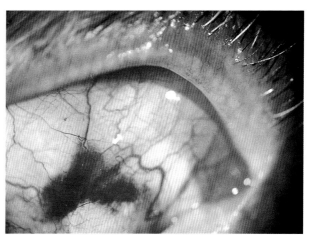

Figure 19.34 This eye has a normal-sized bleb over the Ahmed Glaucoma Valve implant.

Figure 19.32 A failed corneal graft. This eye has a failed corneal graft after the placement of an Ahmed Glaucoma Valve implant. In eyes with prior corneal grafts, corneal graft failure has been reported in up to 45% of cases following tube–shunt implantation.

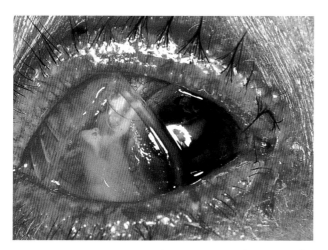

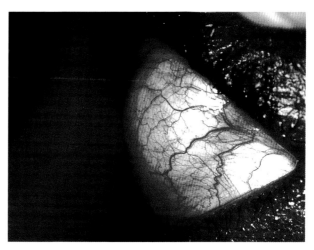

Figure 19.33 Extrusion of the plate. In this eye, the Ahmed Glaucoma Valve implant eroded through the conjunctiva. The tube remained secured to the sclera and inside the eye. Because of the risk of infection, this implant was removed. Implants may erode through the conjunctiva, with a reported incidence of about 3%. Anterior placement of the plate closer to the limbus increases the risk, as blinking causes the conjunctiva to be rubbed over the hard plastic. Securing the plate at least 8 mm from the limbus reduces the risk of plate erosion.

Figure 19.35 Tenon's cyst. When this patient looks straight ahead, the Tenon's cyst over the Ahmed Glaucoma Valve implant is quite prominent from the side. A rise in pressure following tube–shunt implantation commonly occurs 3–6 weeks postoperatively, and has been termed the 'hypertensive phase'. This phase can last 4–6 months. Bleb encapsulation or Tenon's cysts have been reported in 0–10% of eyes with aqueous shunts. Intraocular pressure may be quite high if encapsulation occurs. They are treated similarly to the high bleb phase seen after trabeculectomies and may or may not require surgical intervention. Some authors advocate needling of the bleb around the plate with or without antifibrotic agents.

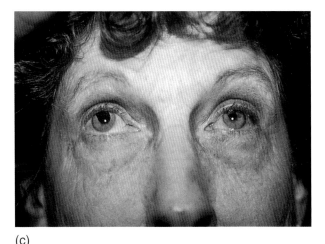

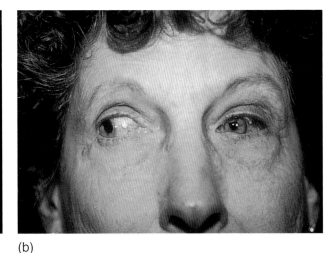

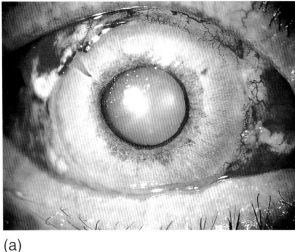

of the left eye. (a) Primary position shows exotropia and hypertropia. (b) Adduction of the left eye is restricted on attempted right gaze. (c) Upgaze of the left eye is similarly restricted. This patient required muscle surgery to correct horizontal and vertical diplopia. At surgery, the bleb capsule was found to be adherent to the intermuscular septum of the superior and lateral rectus muscles, restricting and fore-shortening the muscles. Following surgery, she has minimal diplopia in extreme positions of gaze, but is asymptomatic in most positions. (Courtesy of Neil Choplin, MD.) Motility disturbances have been reported with Molteno, Baerveldt, Krupin, and Ahmed implants. Acquired restrictive strabismus may occur from direct interference of muscle contraction by the plate or by involvement of the muscle sheath or tendon (superior oblique) within the bleb capsule. Placement of a shunt in the superonasal quadrant may produce an acquired Brown's syndrome with inability to look up and in. This quadrant should therefore not be used for primary shunts.

Figure 19.36 Motility disturbances. Restrictive strabismus developed in this patient following placement of an Ahmed Glaucoma Valve in the superotemporal quadrant

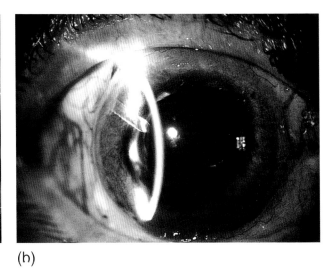

Figure 19.37 Malignant glaucoma. (a) This eye had malignant glaucoma after the placement of an Ahmed Glaucoma Valve implant for neovascular glaucoma. Aqueous misdirection occurs in 0–4% of eyes after the placement of an aqueous shunt. The presence of a valve-like mechanism does not protect an eye from developing malignant glaucoma. Malignant glaucoma may require surgical intervention if it does not respond to cycloplegic agents and aqueous suppressants. (b) After this eye had a lensectomy and vitrectomy, the chamber was formed and the intraocular pressure was controlled.

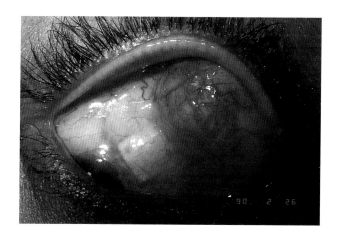

Figure 19.38 This eye has a mature, well-functioning bleb after the placement of a single-plate Molteno implant.

SUMMARY

Aqueous shunts have a role in the management of eyes with glaucoma. For most glaucoma drainage devices, the Kaplan–Meier estimated probability of success is approximately 70–80% at 12 months and 40–50% at 36–48 months following surgery.

Despite this success rate in eyes with usually poor surgical prognoses, aqueous shunts are no panacea. Their use in eyes may be fraught with serious complications. Appropriate case selection and excellent surgical technique and postoperative care may help prevent some but not all of these complications.

Further reading

Ayyala RS, Zurakowski D, Smith JA, et al. A clinical study of the Ahmed glaucoma valve implant in advanced glaucoma. Ophthalmology 1998; 105· 1968–76

Ayyala RS, Harman LE, Michelini-Norris B, et al. Comparison of different biomaterials for glaucoma drainage devices. Arch Ophthalmol 1999; 117: 233–36

Brandt JD. Patch grafts of dehydrated cadaveric dura mater for tube-shunt glaucoma surgery. Arch Ophthalmol 1993; 111: 1436–9

Brown RD, Cairns JE. Experience with the Molteno long tube implant. Trans Ophthal Soc UK 1983; 103: 297–308

Cantor L, Burgoyne J, Sanders S, et al. The effect of mitomycin C on Molteno implant surgery: a 1-year randomized, masked, prospective study. J Glaucoma 1998; 7: 240–6

Clayton D, Hills M. Statistical Models in Epidemiology. Oxford: Oxford University Press, 1993

Coleman AL, Hill R, Wilson MR, et al. Initial clinical experience with the Ahmed glaucoma valve implant. Am J Ophthalmol 1995; 120: 23–31

Coleman AL, Smyth RJ, Wilson MR, Tam M. Initial clinical experience with the Ahmed Glaucoma Valve implant in pediatric patients. Arch Ophthalmol 1996; 115: 186–91

Davidovski F, Stewart RH, Kimbrough RL. Long-term results with the White Glaucoma Pump-shunt. Ophthalmic Surg 1990; 21: 288–93

Egbert PR, Lieberman MF. Internal suture occlusion of the Molteno glaucoma implant for the prevention of postoperative hypotony. Ophthalmic Surg 1989; 20: 53–6

Ellis BD, Varley GA, Kalenak JW, et al. Bacterial endophthalmitis following cataract surgery in an eye with a preexisting Molteno implant. Ophthalmic Surg 1993; 24: 117–18

El-Sayad F, El-Maghraby A, Helal M, Amayem A. The use of releasable sutures in Molteno glaucoma implant procedures to reduce postoperative hypotony. Ophthalmic Surg 1991; 22: 82–4

Fellenbaum PS, Almeida AR, Minckler DS, et al. Krupin disk implantation for complicated glaucomas. Ophthalmology 1994; 101: 1178–82

Freedman J. Scleral patch grafts with Molteno setons. Ophthalmic Surg 1987; 18: 532–4

Heuer DK, Lloyd MA, Abrams DA, et al. Which is better? One or two? A randomized clinical trial of single plate versus double-plate Molteno implantation for glaucomas in aphakia and pseudophakia. Ophthalmology 1992; 99: 1512–19

Hill RA, Heuer DK, Baerveldt G, et al. Molteno implantation for glaucoma in young patients. Ophthalmology 1991; 98: 1042–6

Hill RA, Nguyen QH, Baerveldt G, et al. Trabeculectomy and Molteno implantation of glaucomas associated with uveitis. Ophthalmology 1993; 100: 903–8

Hitchings RA, Joseph NH, Sherwood MB, et al. Use of one-piece valved tube and variable surface area explant for glaucoma drainage surgery. Ophthalmology 1987; 94: 1079–84

Hoare-Nairne JEA, Sherwood D, Jacob JSH, Rich WJCC. Single stage insertion of the Molteno tube for glaucoma and modifications to reduce postoperative hypotony. Br J Ophthalmol 1988; 72: 846–51

Hodkin MJ, Goldblatt WS, Burgoyne CF, et al. Early clinical experience with the Baerveldt implant in complicated glaucomas. Am J Ophthalmol 1995; 120: 32–40

Honrubia FM, Grijalbo MP, Gomez ML, Lopez A. Surgical treatment of neovascular glaucoma. Trans Ophthalmol Soc UK 1979; 99: 89–91

Krupin T, Podos SM, Becker B, Newkirk JB. Valve implants in filtering surgery. Am J Ophthalmol 1976; 81: 232–5

The Krupin Eye Valve Filtering Surgery Study Group. Krupin eye valve with disk for filtration surgery. Ophthalmology 1994; 101: 651–8

Latina MA. Single stage Molteno implant with combination internal occlusion and external ligature. Ophthalmic Surg 1990; 21: 444–6

Liebmann JM, Ritch R. Intraocular suture ligature to reduce hypotony following Molteno seton implantation. Ophthalmic Surg 1992; 23: 51–2

Lloyd MA, Sedlak T, Heuer DK, et al. Clinical experience with the single-plate Molteno implant in complicated glaucomas: update of a pilot study. Ophthalmology 1992; 99: 679–87

Lloyd MAE, Baerveldt F, Heuer DK, et al. Initial clinical experience with the Baerveldt implant in complicated glaucomas. Ophthalmology 1994; 101: 640–50

Lloyd MA, Baerveldt F, Fellenbaum PS, et al. Intermediate-term results of a randomized clinical trial of the 350- versus the 500-square mm Baerveldt implant. Ophthalmology 1994; 101: 1456–64

Mascati NT. A new surgical approach for the control of a class of glaucomas. Int Surg 1967; 47: 10–15

McDermott ML, Swendris RP, Shin DH, et al. Corneal endothelial cell counts after Molteno implantation. Am J Ophthalmol 1993; 115: 93–6

Mermoud A, Salmon JF, Alexander P, et al. Molteno tube implantation for neovascular glaucoma: long-term results and factors influencing the outcome. Ophthalmology 1993; 100: 897–902

Mills RP, Reynolds A, Emond MJ, et al. Long-term survival of Molteno glaucoma drainage devices. Ophthalmology 1996; 103: 299–305

Minckler DS, Shammas A, Wilcox M, Ogden TE. Experimental studies of aqueous filtration using the Molteno implant. Trans Am Ophthalmol Soc 1987; 84: 368–92

Minckler DS, Heuer DK, Hasty B, et al. Clinical experience with the single-plate Molteno implant in complicated glaucomas. Ophthalmology 1988; 95: 1181–8

Molteno ACB. New implant for drainage in glaucoma: clinical trial. Br J Ophthalmol 1969; 53: 606–15

Molteno ACB. The dual chamber single plate implant – its use in neovascular glaucoma. Aust NZ J Ophthalmol 1990; 18: 431–6

Molteno ACB, Polkinghorne PJ, Bowbyes JA. The vicryl tie technique for inserting a draining implant in the treatment of secondary glaucoma. Aust NZ J Ophthalmol 1986; 14: 343–54

Noureddin BN, Wilson-Holt N, Lavin M, et al. Advanced uncontrolled glaucoma: Nd:YAG cyclophotocoagulation or tube surgery. Ophthalmology 1992; 99: 430–7

Perkins TW. Endophthalmitis after placement of a Molteno implant. Ophthalmic Surg 1990; 21: 733–4

Perkins TW, Gangnon R, Ladd W, et al. Molteno implant with Mitomycin C: intermediate-term results. J Glaucoma 1998; 7: 86–92

Prata JA, Mermoud A, LaBree L, Minckler DS. In vitro and in vivo flow characteristics of glaucoma drainage implants. Ophthalmology 1995; 102: 894–904

Rajah-Sivayoham ISS. Camero-venous shunt for secondary glaucoma following orbital venous obstruction. Br J Ophthalmol 1968; 52: 843–5

Rollett M, Moreau M. Traitement de le hypopyon par le drainage capillaire de la chambre antérieure. Rev Gen Ophthalmol 1906; 25: 481–9

Rubin B, Chan CC, Burnier M, et al. Histopathologic study of the Molteno glaucoma implant in three patients. Am J Ophthalmol 1990; 110: 371–9

Schocket SS, Lakhanpal V, Richards RD. Anterior chamber tube shunt to an encircling band in the treatment of neovascular glaucoma. Ophthalmology 1982; 89: 1188–94

Schocket SS, Nirankari VS, Lakhanpal V, et al. Anterior chamber tube shunt to an encircling band in the treatment of neovascular glaucoma and other refractory glaucomas: a long-term study. Ophthalmology 1985; 92: 553–62

Scott DR, Quigley HA. Medical management of a high bleb phase after trabeculectomies. Ophthalmology 1988; 95: 1169–73

Sherwood MB, Smith MF. Prevention of early hypotony associated with Molteno implants by a new occluding stent technique. Ophthalmology 1993; 100: 85–90

Siegner SW, Netland PA, Urban RC. Clinical experience with the Baerveldt glaucoma drainage implant. Ophthalmology 1995; 102: 1298 307

Smith MF, Sherwood MB, McGorray SP. Comparison of the double-plate Molteno drainage implant with the Schocket procedure. Arch Ophthalmol 1992; 110: 1246–50

Smith SL, Starita RJ, Fellman RL, Lynn JR. Early clinical experience with the Baerveldt 350-square mm glaucoma implant and associated extraocular muscle imbalance. Ophthalmology 1993; 100: 914–18

Spiegel D, Shrader RR, Wilson RP. Anterior chamber tube shunt to an encircling band (Schocket procedure) in the treatment of refractory glaucoma. Ophthalmic Surg 1992; 23: 804–7

Susanna R, Nicolela MT, Takahashi WY. Mitomycin C as adjunctive therapy with glaucoma implant surgery. Ophthalmic Surg 1994; 25: 458–62

White TC. Clinical results of glaucoma surgery using the White Glaucoma Pump Shunt. Ann Ophthalmol 1992; 24: 365–73

Wilson RP, Cantor L, Katz LJ, et al. Aqueous shunts: Molteno versus Schocket. Ophthalmology 1992; 99: 672–8

20 Combined cataract and glaucoma surgery

Arvind Neelakantan, Mary Fran Smith, James W Doyle,
Maher M Fanous, Mark B Sherwood

INTRODUCTION

Cataract and glaucoma frequently occur in the same patient, and there still remains a lack of consensus regarding the best surgical management of coexisting cataract and glaucoma. The options for an individual patient revolve around the ability of his or her optic nerve to withstand an intraocular pressure (IOP) spike and the likelihood of maintaining postoperative IOP control without further surgical intervention. In the 1980s, the procedure of choice for patients with a visually significant cataract was an extracapsular cataract extraction (ECCE). However, with the advent of phacoemulsification and foldable intraocular lenses, the way surgeons approach coexisting cataract and glaucoma has changed. There is some evidence to suggest that phacoemulsification by itself lowers long-term IOP by 2–4 mmHg. There is good evidence to suggest that long-term IOP is lowered better by a combined phacoemulsification and glaucoma surgery than by phacoemulsification alone. Small-incision cataract surgery combined with adjuvant intraoperative use of antimetabolites has improved the maintenance of long-term IOP control following the combined procedure, and a combined approach includes the advantage of patient convenience. Trabeculectomy alone, however, may lower IOP better than combined phacoemulsification and trabeculectomy surgery. Eyes with existing filtering blebs in general do well in terms of bleb survival after phacoemulsification cataract surgery, unlike ECCE.

Figure 20.1 illustrates our approach to the decision-making when choosing which procedure is most appropriate for a glaucoma patient with a cataract.

PHACOEMULSIFICATION

Technological advances in cataract removal techniques have greatly helped glaucoma patients. Phacoemulsification-style cataract removal does not appear to have as high an incidence of postoperative IOP spikes as did ECCE. Recent advances in glaucoma drop therapy such as topical carbonic anhydrase inhibitors and α_2-agonists have increased our ability to manage post-cataract surgery IOP spikes. Additionally, there is evidence that phacoemulsification lowers IOP by 2–4 mmHg, and possibly even more in patients with narrow-angle glaucoma. Therefore, many patients with cataracts and mild to even moderate glaucoma may do well with phacoemulsification cataract surgery alone.

Preoperative evaluation

During the preoperative evaluation of a patient with cataract and glaucoma, the question of whether to do phacoemulsification alone or a combined phacotrabeculectomy is considered. One approach is to make this decision based on the number of medications the patient requires preoperatively to control their glaucoma, modified by optic nerve and visual field appearance as well as by the patient's life expectancy. For example, a patient requiring few medications to control the glaucoma might do well with phacoemulsification alone, but if the patient is young and already has advanced nerve and field changes, a combined procedure might be the better choice. Close attention should be paid to the status of the corneal endothelium and the integrity of the zonules at this evaluation. This is particularly important in glaucoma patients such as those with iridocorneal endothelial syndrome,

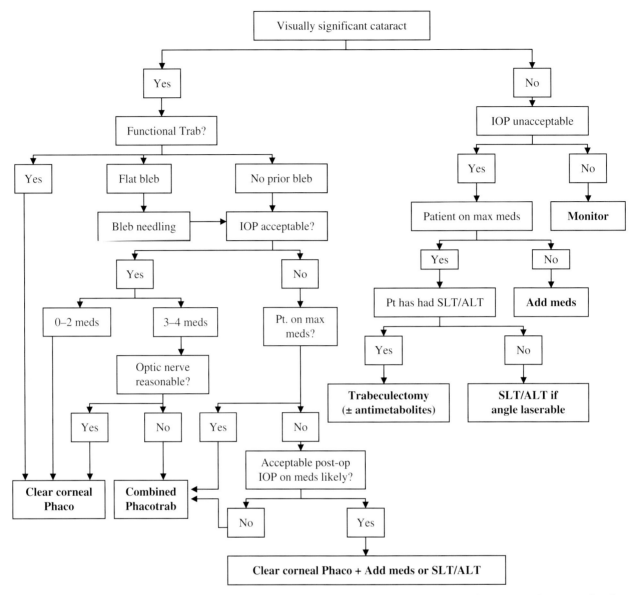

Figure 20.1 Choosing the appropriate surgical procedure. Flow chart illustrating the decision-making involved in choosing the appropriate surgical procedure for the glaucoma patient with a cataract.

Fuchs' dystrophy or pseudoexfoliation. Also, the preoperative evaluation is a good opportunity to judge the extent of pupillary dilatation. Eliciting a history of systemic α_1-blocker use for benign prostatic hypertrophy helps anticipate the possible occurrence of intraoperative floppy iris syndrome (IFIS).

Phacoemulsification alone

The options for phacoemulsification alone are a temporal or superior clear corneal approach or a superior scleral tunnel approach. The clear corneal temporal approach is the most popular technique and may be preferable to a scleral tunnel approach, because it leaves the superior conjunctiva undisturbed. This may enhance the success of trabeculectomy should it ever be needed in the future. Temporal clear corneal phacoemulsification should also be considered in patients with pre-existing filtering blebs to decrease

conjunctival manipulation and decrease the risk of scarring within the bleb. Recent advances in micro-incision cataract surgery (MICS) with two separate 1-mm incisions seem promising for the future of a glaucoma patient.

Figure 20.2 illustrates one approach to creating a clear corneal incision. The incision size is generally 3 mm or less, and single-use disposable blades are readily available in varied sizes (Figure 20.3). Development of newer dispersive and cohesive viscoelastic agents has increased our ability to perform phacoemulsification surgery in patients with crowded anterior segments and still protect the corneal endothelium.

Management of the pupil

Glaucoma patients frequently have pupils that dilate poorly, because of sphincter fibrosis from

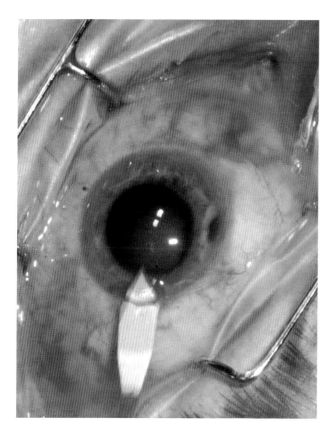

Figure 20.2 A 3-mm temporal incision. A standard 3-mm temporal incision was made temporally with a keratome. The bleb is to the surgeon's right.

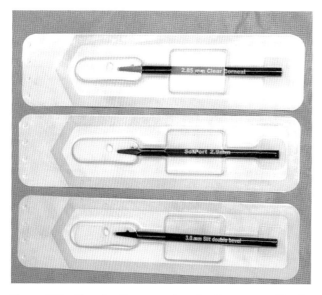

Figure 20.3 Choosing the appropriate-sized keratome. Single-use disposable metal keratomes are readily available in a variety of sizes.

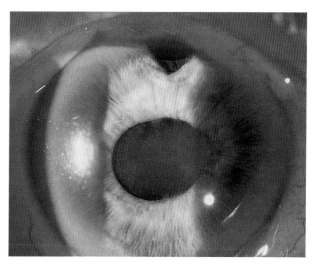

Figure 20.4 Pseudoexfoliation glaucoma. This 80-year-old woman with pseudoexfoliation glaucoma was status post successful trabeculectomy surgery performed 2 years previously. A bleb is present superiorly. She complained of glare and reading difficulties attributable to a cataract. Note poor pupillary dilatation.

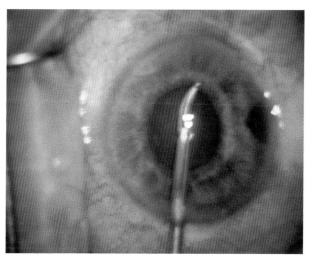

Figure 20.5 Multiple small sphincterotomies. Either Vannas or Rapazzo scissors or intraocular retinal scissors may be used for this procedure. Following 8–12 small cuts in the sphincter, viscoelastic can be used to open the pupil.

years of miotic therapy, from posterior synechiae, or from primary conditions such as exfoliation syndrome (Figure 20.4). The surgeon therefore may need to enlarge the pupil in order safely to perform phacoemulsification. Figures 20.5–20.10 show management options for a small pupil.

IFIS occurs in patients on systemic α_1 blockers, and has been known to occur even if these medications have been stopped weeks or months preoperatively. The lack of tone causes the iris to billow in response to the normal irrigation currents in the anterior chamber during phacoemulsification and these irides have a marked propensity to prolapse through the clear corneal incision sites. Progressive pupil constriction also occurs during surgery. IFIS is best managed by preoperative anticipation and employing methods of small pupil management described above prior to starting the capsulorrhexis.

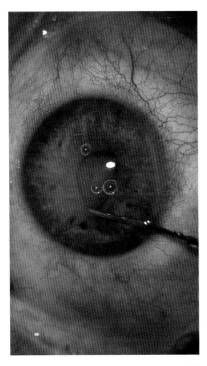

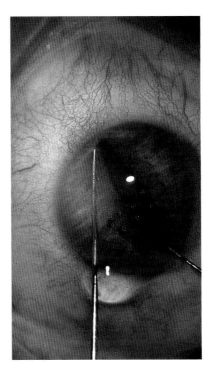

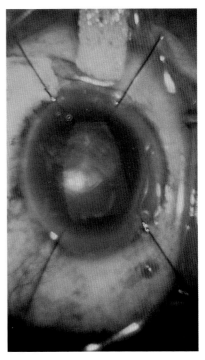

Figure 20.6   Posterior synechiae. If posterior synechiae are present they may be broken by injecting viscoelastic and sweeping with the cannula.

Figure 20.7   Enlarging the pupil. Another useful way to enlarge the pupil is by stretching using two hooks, first in the 6–12 o'clock direction and then at 3–9.

Figure 20.8   Dilating the pupil with disposable hooks. The pupil may also be dilated with disposable iris hooks, such as those available from Grieshaber, Switzerland. The hooks are inserted through limbal stab incisions approximately 90° apart. An adjustable silicone sleeve holds the hook (and the pupil) in place.

Zonules

Glaucoma patients, especially those with pseudo-exfoliation syndrome, are often at risk of weak zonules, and extra care must therefore be taken to avoid complications such as vitreous loss or loss of lens material posteriorly into the vitreous cavity. To avoid zonular stress, careful and thorough hydrodissection and hydrodelineation must be performed to free the nucleus from all its cortical attachments, allowing free rotation within the bag. The surgeon should avoid undue pushing of the nucleus with the tip of the phacoemulsification handpiece during sculpting, which could cause zonular disruption. A chopping or supracapsular technique as opposed to a traditional 'divide and conquer' technique might reduce intraoperative zonular stress. Figures 20.11–20.14 illustrate some of these points.

If zonular instability is suspected, pre- or intra-operative implantation of PMMA capsular tension rings or segments are helpful (Figure 20.15). These provide a circumferential expansile force to the capsule equator increasing intraoperative lens stability, enhancing IOL centration and reducing postoperative pseudophacodonesis. A Cionni-designed capsular tension ring can also be sutured to the sclera (Figure 20.16).

Completion of surgery

After quadrant removal and cortical clean-up, a foldable intraocular lens can be injected into the bag (Figures 20.17–20.19). Current foldable IOL materials include acrylic, silicone and hydrogel, all of which can be injected through sub-3-mm incisions. The acrylic platform appears to be best suited for the glaucoma patient, as it best prevents posterior capsule opacification as well as anterior capsule problems such as capsular contracture, phimosis and in-the-bag IOL decentration. The newer presbyopia-correcting intraocular lenses are not contraindicated in the glaucoma patient and they may in fact offer some visual advantages (Figure 20.20).

If there has been a disruption in the capsular bag or torn zonules, the lens may be placed in the ciliary sulcus, provided the surgeon is able to determine that there is sufficient capsular support. The injectable single-piece acrylic IOL is not suited for sulcus fixation; inadvertent sulcus placement has been associated with a secondary pigment dispersion syndrome. A three-piece acrylic-design foldable IOL (Figure 20.21) is preferred for sulcus fixation, as the optic is vaulted posteriorly keeping the optic away from posterior iris pigment epithelium.

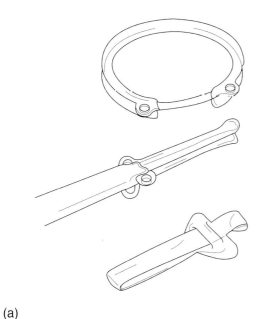

(a)

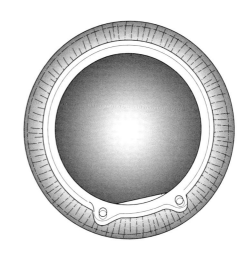

(b)

Figure 20.9 The Graether Pupil Expander. The Graether Pupil Expander offers another alternative for enlarging a small pupil. (a) The device inserter. (b) Drawing of the device in place. (c) Clinical photograph.

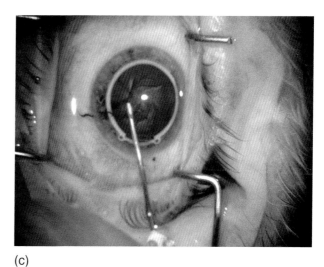

(c)

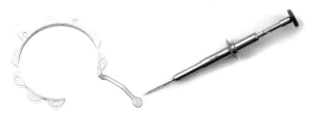

Figure 20.10 Perfect Pupil™. The Perfect Pupil™ is a flexible polyurethane iris expansion ring that can be injected under viscoelastic to securely hold a billowing, floppy iris through 315° and dilates the pupil to 7 mm.

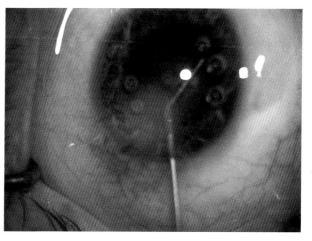

Figure 20.11 Hydrodissection and hydrodelineation. Hydrodissection and hydrodelineation is performed with balanced salt solution using a 27- or 30-gauge blunt cannula.

These lenses may require slight wound enlargement prior to insertion.

If a bleb is overfunctioning at the time of phacoemulsification, viscoelastic may be left in the eye postoperatively to maintain IOP and slow aqueous flow through the fistula, to allow some time for bleb healing. If no bleb is present or bleb function is

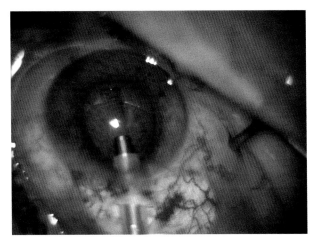

Figure 20.12 Initial nuclear grooving. During the 'divide and conquer' stage of phacoemulsification in glaucomatous eyes, suboptimal pupil dilatation (even after manual pupillary enlargement) may limit groove extension into the peripheral nucleus.

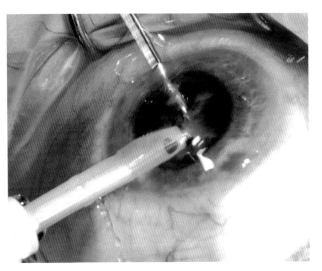

Figure 20.13 Chopping technique. Chopping maneuvers exploit the natural fracture planes within the nucleus segment, thereby replacing ultrasound power needed to sculpt grooves. Zonular stress is reduced as, in the chopping technique, the opposing forces of the two mechanical instruments break the nucleus into smaller bits without transferring the forces to the capsular bag.

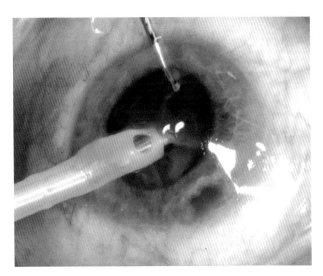

Figure 20.14 Quadrant removal. Once the nucleus has been segmented the quadrants are removed using high-vacuum low-ultrasound energy settings. The second instrument protects the posterior capsule from coming up into the phaco tip and also can be used to further chop the segment into smaller bits.

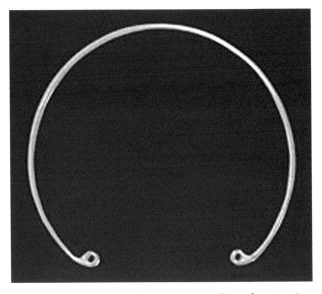

Figure 20.15 Capsular tension ring. Capsular tension rings are designed to stabilize the capsule by exerting circumferential expansile forces to the capsule equator in cases of zonular instability. These are available in 3–4 sizes (12–14.5 mm) and one can choose a size based on a horizontal white-to-white measurement.

COMBINED PHACOTRABECULECTOMY

Small incision size and the potential for less postoperative inflammation than that seen with ECCE are two advantages of phacoemulsification, which make it the procedure of choice for combination with filtering surgery in the co-management of cataract and glaucoma. As compared with combined extracapsular cataract extraction and trabeculectomy surgery, combined phacoemulsification/trabeculectomy surgery is associated with earlier visual rehabilitation, less postoperative astigmatism,

appropriate, extra care should be taken to remove all viscoelastic from these eyes to prevent an early postoperative pressure rise. Insertion of the injectable IOL is preferred, with a cohesive viscoelastic in the cartridge and capsular bag, as this permits a more complete removal at the end of surgery. If advanced nerve damage is noted preoperatively, it may be prudent to check IOP 3–6 hours after surgery, and treat if there is a significant spike. Burping the corneal wound to release retained viscoelastic combined with the use of aqueous suppressants helps in the management of postoperative IOP spikes.

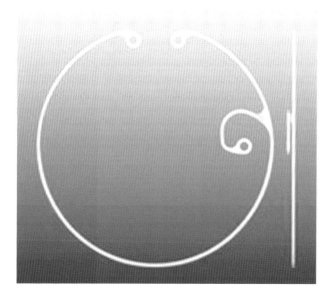

Figure 20.16 Cionni capsular tension ring. The Cionni design of the CTR is suitable for suture fixation to the sclera and helps achieve better capsular and IOL centration.

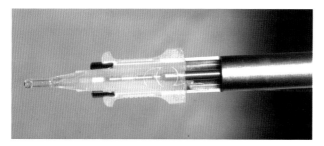

Figure 20.18 Injectable IOL. Single-piece acrylic IOL loaded on injector ready for endocapsular placement.

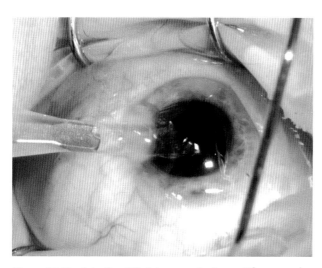

Figure 20.19 Injecting IOL into capsular bag. The capsular bag is filled with a cohesive viscoelastic and the injector is inserted through the clear corneal wound. The IOL is then slowly injected into the bag. A second instrument helps place the trailing haptic edge under the capsular lip.

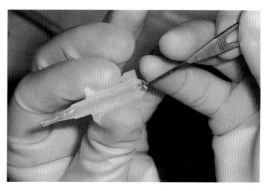

Figure 20.17 IOL injector cartridge. The cartridge is filled with viscoelastic and the IOL is loaded.

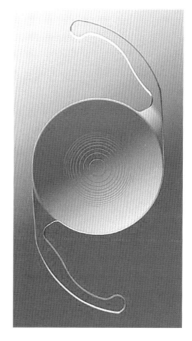

Figure 20.20 Presbyopia-correcting IOL. Using apodized diffractive and refractive optics these newer design IOLs achieve good unaided postoperative visual acuity – distant and near.

higher blebs, and improved long-term IOP control. Equally important, antimetabolite use to modulate wound healing following filtering surgery has made combined phacotrabeculectomy a better option for many patients.

One- or two-site approach

Combined surgery may be performed either with two separate incisions (one temporally for cataract extraction, and a superior trabeculectomy flap) or through one incision superiorly, through which phacoemulsification is performed, with subsequent conversion of the scleral tunnel to a trabeculectomy flap. In two-incision surgery, phacoemulsification is performed temporally first, followed by routine trabeculectomy superiorly. The advantages of a single incision include greater ease of surgery and

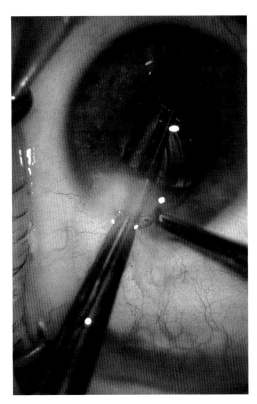

Figure 20.21 Foldable sulcus-fixated IOL. The wound is slightly enlarged permitting insertion of a three-piece foldable sulcus-fixated PCIOL in front of the anterior capsule.

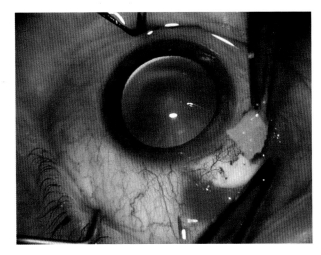

Figure 20.22 Application of mitomycin C. Intraoperative low-dose mitomycin C (200 μg/ml × 5 minutes) on a cellulose sponge is applied following development of a fornix-based conjunctival flap.

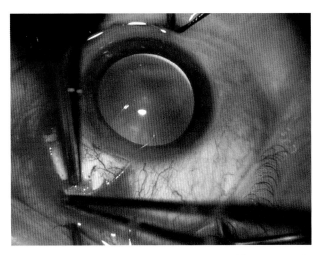

Figure 20.23 Application of mitomycin C. The sponge is inserted underneath the conjunctival flap.

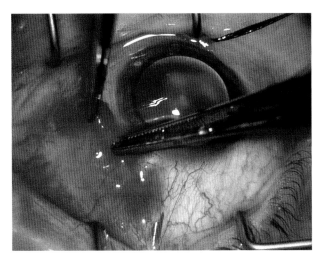

Figure 20.24 Application of mitomycin C. The conjunctiva is draped over the sponge, care being taken to avoid contact between the sponge and the conjunctival wound edge. After the 3–5-minute application, the site should be thoroughly irrigated with balanced salt solution.

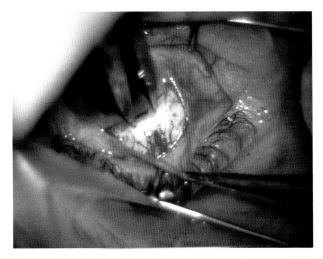

Figure 20.25 Creation of scleral tunnel. Phacoemulsification may be performed through a 2 mm long by 3 mm wide tunnel. The width of the incision is determined by the width of the tip being used and that of the keratome used to create the opening into the anterior chamber.

decreased operating time. One incision phacotrabeculectomy begins with a conjunctival incision superiorly. A fornix-based conjunctival flap allows for better visualization during surgery and, in one prospective study, was associated with equally successful final outcomes compared to eyes having a limbus-based conjunctival flap (although this study did not use adjunctive antimetabolites). It is

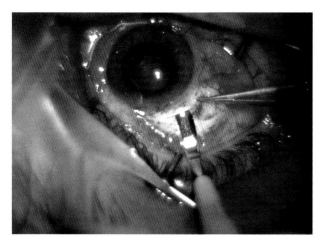

Figure 20.26 Creation of scleral tunnel. A crescent-type blade is used to create the scleral tunnel.

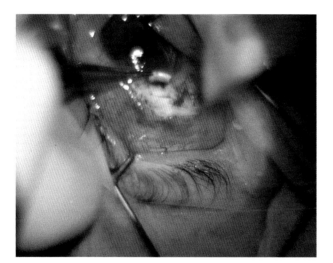

Figure 20.27 Insertion of intraocular lens. Lens insertion may be simplified by first converting the scleral tunnel to a flap with Vannas scissors. If the surgeon prefers, the lens may be inserted and the tunnel converted afterwards. Some surgeons perform the filtering portion of the procedure without radializing the flap, using a punch under the roof of the tunnel to remove a piece of the inner wall, thus creating a 'no-stitch phacotrabeculectomy' which requires no flap sutures.

important to ensure secure watertight closure of the conjunctival wound after a combined procedure to avoid postoperative bleb leaks and hypotony. This can be more difficult to achieve with a fornix-based conjunctival flap and newer techniques of closure include either a continuous vertical mattress suture described by Wise or an interrupted suture technique, where the knots are buried into small partial-thickness corneal incisions (Khaw).

It is generally accepted that intraoperative antimetabolite application with mitomycin C augments postoperative filter function in combined surgeries. A prospective study looking at 5-fluorouracil (5-FU) augmentation noted no

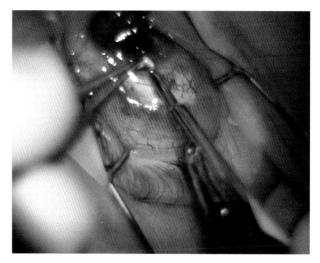

Figure 20.28 Removing a block of inner tissue. A block of inner tissue beneath the converted trabeculectomy flap is removed with a punch. Some surgeons prefer to remove the block of tissue by free-hand dissection.

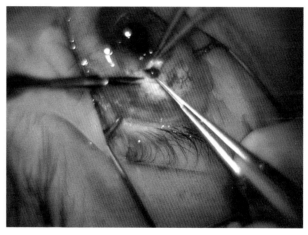

Figure 20.29 A peripheral iridectomy is performed.

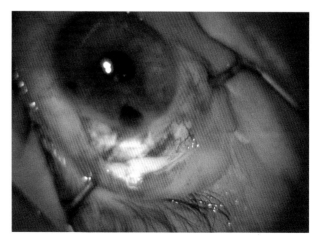

Figure 20.30 Appearance following peripheral iridectomy. In this case, viscoelastic has been left in the eye for stabilization purposes.

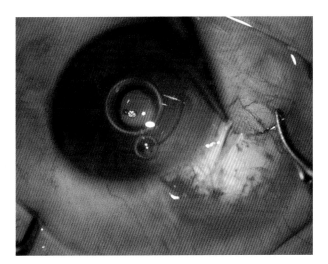

Figure 20.31 Closing the flap. The flap is securely closed with a combination of releasable and 'permanent' 10-0 nylon sutures.

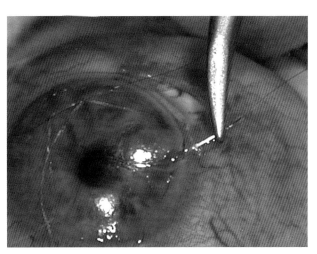

Figure 20.33 Closure of fornix-based conjunctival flap. Partial-thickness slits are made in clear cornea just anterior to the limbal conjunctival incision. The conjunctiva is brought forward to the limbus and sutured to clear cornea using 10-0 nylon mattress sutures.

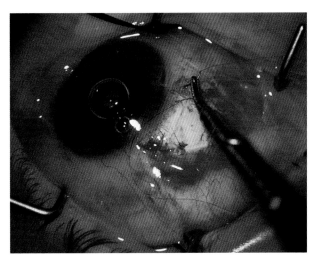

Figure 20.32 The releasable suture technique. The releasable suture technique involves a three- or four-throw slip knot formation, with externalization of the suture beyond the anticipated conjunctival 'hood'. Releasable sutures are useful in these cases, because laser suture lysis may cause conjunctival wound disruption when a fornix-based conjunctival flap has been used.

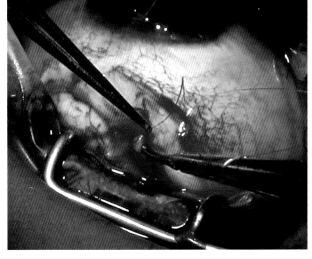

Figure 20.34 Closure of limbus-based conjunctival flap. A two-layer closure technique is used. The Tenon's capsule is first closed with interrupted sutures using 8-0 Vicryl on a BV needle. The conjunctiva is then closed with a running suture. The wound is checked for a leak on completion of closure.

difference between patients receiving and not receiving 5-FU. Following phacotrabeculectomy with mitomycin C, success rates as high as 90% for IOP control, and visual acuity better than 20/40 in 80% of patients have been reported. Possible complications, often secondary to either bleb leak or simple overfiltration, may include shallow anterior chambers, fibrin formation (associated with chronic use of miotics, exfoliation syndrome, iris manipulation such as stretching), hyphema, choroidal effusions, and hypotony maculopathy. Figures 20.22–20.24 illustrate the application of low-dose mitomycin C to the surgery site. Figures 20.25–20.34 illustrate

the remaining steps in performing a phacotrabeculectomy. There is some discussion regarding the necessity of performing a peripheral iridectomy in patients undergoing combined phacotrabeculectomy.

ALTERNATIVE GLAUCOMA PROCEDURES COMBINED WITH PHACOEMULSIFICATION

Goniosynechiolysis

In patients with relatively recent synechial angle closure (less than 6–12 months) it may be possible at the time of phacoemulsification surgery to break the adhesions between iris and trabecular meshwork mechanically by overinflating the anterior chamber with viscoelastic or by gently pushing the peripheral iris posteriorly with an iris or cyclodialysis spatula, thereby re-opening the conventional outflow pathway (Figure 20.35).

Combined phacoemulsification and non-penetrating glaucoma surgery

Phacoemulsification can be combined with either deep sclerectomy or viscocanalostomy using a two-site technique. The external wall of Schlemm's canal is exposed when the deep scleral flap is dissected and a thin intact Descemet's window allows aqueous to egress. This technique can be enhanced by use of mitomycin C. Some patients may require YAG laser goniopuncture months or years postoperatively.

Phacoemulsification and glaucoma drainage implant surgery

This technique is particularly helpful in patients with previously failed mitomycin trabeculectomies or in patients with uveitic, neovascular or other secondary glaucomas. The episcleral plate of the glaucoma drainage implant is sutured to the eye generally before the phacoemulsification procedure. After IOL implantation the tube is inserted into the eye via a needle track and the external part of the tube is covered with donor sclera or pericardium. In patients with valved implants the viscoelastic is sometimes not removed, but in stented, non-valved tubes it should be thoroughly

removed. A newer, small, stainless-steel, FDA-approved implant (ExPress® shunt) can be used with phacoemulsification surgery and is inserted under the standard trabeculectomy scleral flap (Figure 20.36). The scleral flap is sutured in the usual manner to prevent early postoperative hypotony and the sutures can be released or lasered in the usual manner.

Phacoemulsification with endoscopic cyclophotocoagulation

Endoscopic cyclophotocoagulation (ECP) at the time of phacoemulsification surgery is an evolving technique for postoperative IOP control. A 20-gauge fiberoptic probe is inserted through the phacoemulsification incision and this allows direct

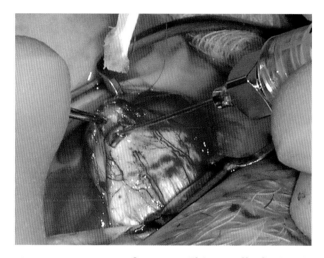

Figure 20.36 ExPress® shunt. This small device is inserted into the anterior chamber beneath the scleral flap through a needle track incision.

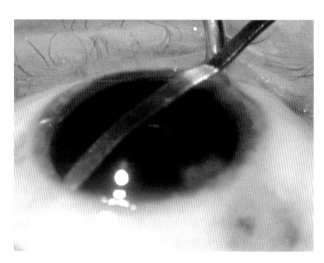

Figure 20.35 Goniosynechiolysis. In patients with relatively recent synechial angle closure, the angle adhesions can be broken mechanically with use of an iris or cyclodialysis spatula. The peripheral iris is gently pushed posteriorly with the flat edge of the spatula. This may also be done with viscodissection. Some prefer to do this under gonioscopic control.

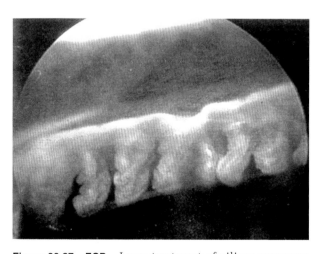

Figure 20.37 ECP. Laser treatment of ciliary processes with the 810-nm diode laser under direct visualization delivered through an endoscope. This can be done on completion of phacoemulsification before or after IOL implantation with the anterior chamber full of viscoelastic. The end point of treatment is whitening of the ciliary processes.

visualization and treatment of the ciliary processes with an 810-nm diode laser to reduce aqueous production (Figure 20.37).

New techniques under investigation

Glaucoma techniques currently under investigation include implants that drain aqueous from the anterior chamber into Schlemm's canal (Eyepass® and Glaukos iStent), new instruments that remove the inner wall of Schlemm's canal (Trabectome™ and Tuilaser Excimer laser trabeculostomy) and an implant that directs fluid into the suprachoroidal space (SOLX gold microshunt).

Further reading

Allan BD, Barrett GD. Combined small incision phacoemulsification and trabeculectomy. J Cataract Refract Surg 1993; 19: 97–102

Arnold PN. No-stitch phacotrabeculectomy. J Cataract Refract Surg 1996; 22: 253–60

Colin J. Exfoliative syndrome and phacoemulsification. J Fr Ophthalmol 1994; 17: 465–9

Costa VP, Moster MR, Wilson RP, et al. Effects of topical mitomycin-C on primary trabeculectomies and combined procedures. Br J Ophthalmol 1993; 77: 693–7

Friedman DS, Jampel HD, Lubomski LH, et al. Surgical strategies for coexisiting glaucoma and cataract – an evidence-based update. Ophthalmology 2002; 109: 1902–15

Gimbel HV, Meyer D. Small incision trabeculectomy combined with phacoemulsification and intraocular lens implantation. J Cataract Refract Surg 1993; 19: 92–6

Hughes BA, Song MS, Shin DH, et al. Primary glaucoma triple procedure with or without adjunctive subconjunctival mitomycin and risk factors for failure. Invest Ophthalmol Vis Sci 1995; 36: 876

Hurvitz LM. 5-FU-supplemented phacoemulsification, posterior chamber intraocular lens implantation, and trabeculectomy. Ophthalmic Surg 1993; 24: 674–80

Kim DD, Doyle JW, Smith MF. Intraocular pressure reduction following phacoemulsification cataract extraction with posterior chamber intraocular lens implantation in glaucoma. Ophthalmic Surg Lasers 1999; 30: 37–40

Lederer CM. Combined cataract extraction with intraocular lens implant and mitomycin-C augmented trabeculectomy. Ophthalmology 1996; 103: 1025–34

Lyle WA, Jin JC. Comparison of a 3 and 6-mm incision in combined phacoemulsification and trabeculectomy. Am J Ophthalmol 1991; 111: 189–96

Munden PM, Alward WL. Combined phacoemulsification, posterior chamber intraocular lens implantation, and trabeculectomy with mitomycin-C. Am J Ophthalmol 1995; 119: 20–9

O'Grady JM, Juzych MS, Shin DH, et al. Trabeculectomy, phacoemulsification, and posterior chamber lens implantation with and without 5-fluorouracil. Am J Ophthalmol 1993; 116: 594–9

Smith MF, Doyle JW. Cataract surgery in the glaucoma patient: advances and modifications. Semin Ophthalmol 1999; 14: 124–9

Shields MB. Textbook of Glaucoma. Baltimore, MD: Williams & Wilkins, 1992

Stewart WC, Crinkley CM, Carlson AN. Results of trabeculectomy combined with phacoemulsification versus trabeculectomy combined with extracapsular cataract extraction in patients with advanced glaucoma. Ophthalmic Surg 1994; 25: 621–7

Stewart WC, Crinkley CM, Carlson AN. Fornix- vs limbus-based flaps in combined phacoemulsification and trabeculectomy. Doc Ophthalmol 1994; 88: 141–51

Wedrich A, Menapace R, Radax U, et al. Combined small incision cataract surgery and trabeculectomy – technique and results. Int Ophthalmol 1992; 16: 409–14

Wells AP, Cordeiro MF, Bunce C, Khaw PT. Cystic bleb formation and related complications in limbus- versus fornix-based conjunctival flaps in pediatric and young adult trabeculectomy with mitomycin C. Ophthalmology 2003; 110: 2192–7

Wise J. Mitomycin compatible suture technique for fornix-based conjunctival flaps in glaucoma filteration surgery. Arch Ophthalmol 1993; 111: 992–7

Wishart PK, Austin MW. Combined cataract extraction and trabeculectomy: phacoemulsification compared with extracapsular technique. Ophthalmic Surg 1993; 24: 814–21

21 Treatment of developmental glaucoma

Carlo E Traverso, Graciano Bricola

MEDICAL MANAGEMENT BEFORE SURGERY

Medical treatment of developmental glaucoma is used mostly as a temporizing measure pending surgical treatment, as it has little chance to obtain and maintain the target IOP in most cases. Topical beta blockers and other aqueous suppressants, such as acetazolamide and other carbonic anhydrase inhibitors are commonly used in preparation for surgery with the hope of improving corneal transparency, thus facilitating gonioscopy and funduscopy. Caution must be exercised with infants and small children when using medical therapy, as the relatively small blood volume may lead to high systemic levels of many medications if used in adult dosages, leading to significant side-effects. For example, there is an increased risk of apnea in children under 2 years of age on topical α agonists such as apraclonidine.

SURGICAL MANAGEMENT

The purpose of surgery is to preserve vision. Since visual disability in developmental glaucoma seems to be related to pressure-induced optic nerve atrophy and to surgical complications, a balance must be struck between surgical risks and the maintenance of the target intraocular pressure. A team approach may be necessary in many cases to treat anisometropia, amblyopia, strabismus, corneal opacity, and cataract. Prompt lowering of the intraocular pressure can be helpful to clear cornea edema, which can rapidly cause irreversible amblyopia.

Surgical treatment can be divided into the following categories: angle surgery, filtration surgery, cyclodestructive procedures, and aqueous shunts.

Angle surgery

Since angle surgery is rarely performed in adults, most surgeons have little experience with these types of procedure. However, success rates can be very high. Poor prognostic factors include larger corneal diameters, longer intervals from diagnosis to treatment, and newborn developmental glaucoma. Various methods have been described, and each surgeon develops his/her own modifications. The techniques described below are illustrative.

Goniotomy

This technique, nowadays facilitated by the availability of viscoelastics, is recommended when the cornea is sufficiently clear to allow good intraoperative visualization of the angle. In some cases the removal of edematous epithelium can be necessary.

Goniotomy technique   After positioning the operating microscope with a 40° tilt, the globe is exposed with a speculum and rotated with a bridle suture. A goniolens with an irrigating handle is then positioned over the cornea. After obtaining a clear view of the angle sectors to be incised, the goniolens is removed. A small paracentesis tract is performed in the opposite quadrant, i.e. on the surgeon's side, and a viscoelastic is introduced into the anterior chamber. The tip of the goniotomy knife is then introduced and brought forward (Figure 21.1). As soon as the knife is pushed safely across the anterior chamber beyond the pupil, the goniolens is again positioned. The tip of the knife is then pushed to incise the trabecular tissue right above the scleral spur or the apparent iris insertion, whichever is the most anterior. The knife is then swept from side to side. During the cut it is often possible to see the iris tissue fall posteriorly.

The site of the incision will appear strikingly white in contrast to the grayish surrounding tissue (Figure 21.2). In order to reach around 150° of the angle, some rotation of the globe and goniolens is usually necessary. The knife is withdrawn, the anterior chamber is irrigated, and the viscoelastic aspirated. A single 10-0 nylon suture is placed at the entry site to prevent leakage and iris incarceration; the knot should be carefully buried. Blood *ex-vacuo* and from direct damage to the angle vessels is commonly observed at the end of the procedure (Figure 21.3).

Trabeculotomy

The principle of trabeculotomy is to open Schlemm's canal to the anterior chamber by cutting in towards the dysgenetic trabecular tissue after probing Schlemm's canal from an external approach. Since the procedure is based on the *ab-externo* recognition of the Schlemm's canal area, it can be difficult in buphthalmic eyes with abnormal and distorted limbal anatomy. The main advantage of trabeculotomy is its applicability in cases with corneal edema that prevents a gonioscopic view of the anterior chamber, thus precluding goniotomy.

Trabeculotomy technique After positioning the microscope with a 20° tilt, the eye is exposed with a speculum and a fornix-based conjunctival flap is dissected (Figure 21.4). A bridle suture is then passed under the superior rectus muscle. The globe is rotated downwards and a limbus-based, two-thirds thickness scleral flap dissected. A small paracentesis is made 120° away. At maximum microscope magnification, radial, layer-by-layer incisions are made, centered on the corneoscleral transition zone at the limbus, in the bottom of the scleral bed. As the cutting proceeds very slowly, the

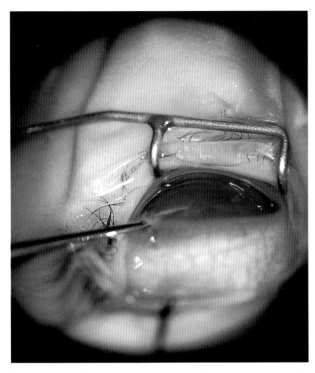

Figure 21.1 Goniotomy technique. The goniotomy knife is introduced into the anterior chamber.

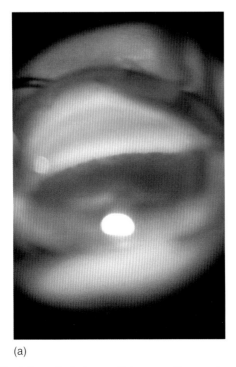
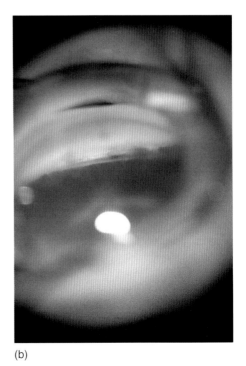

(a)   (b)

Figure 21.2 Goniotomy technique. Intraoperative gonioscopic view before (a) and immediately after goniotomy (b). The incised site appears strikingly white in contrast to the surrounding tissue. Some blood is also seen.

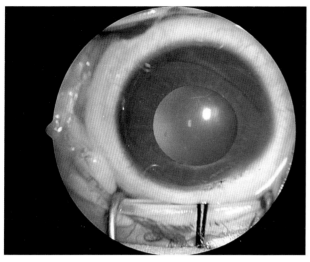

Figure 21.3 Goniotomy technique. At the conclusion of the procedure, a moderate amount of blood is frequently seen in the anterior chamber.

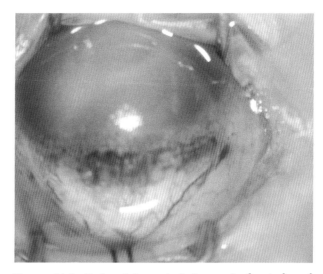

Figure 21.4 Trabeculotomy technique. A fornix-based conjunctival flap is prepared.

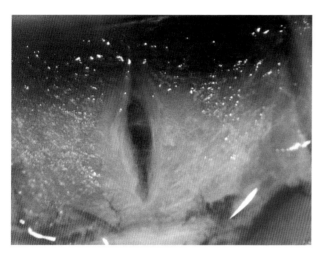

Figure 21.5 Trabeculotomy technique. Underneath a scleral flap, a radial incision is made until a change in the pattern of the connective fibers is seen, indicating the location of Schlemm's canal.

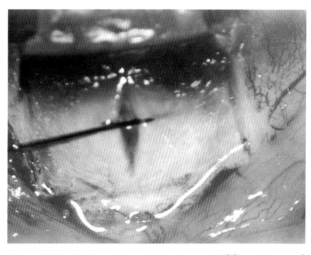

Figure 21.6 Trabeculotomy technique. Schlemm's canal is probed with a 6-0 nylon suture.

assistant continuously dries the incision site with sponges. As soon as minimal amounts of aqueous begin to percolate from the bottom, the incision is halted. With the help of sponges the exact origin of the aqueous ooze is identified. A change in the pattern of the connective fibers is typical. A few very delicate radial cuts are then sufficient to open the outer wall of Schlemm's canal (Figure 21.5). Aqueous leakage will be evident. Care must be taken not to enter the anterior chamber. Schlemm's canal is then probed with a piece of 6-0 nylon suture (Figure 21.6), the cut end of which has been blunted with mild cautery to facilitate a smooth movement, decreasing the chances of creating false routes. Using two tying forceps, the nylon probe is held parallel to the limbus and introduced into Schlemm's canal with a gentle push. It should advance for at least 1 cm on each side, meeting some resistance. If the tip appears in the anterior

chamber, a conversion to trabeculectomy should be considered. The introduction of the probe can be facilitated by snipping the walls of the radial incision with a 15 blade, right over the Schlemm's canal area. A double-armed Harms' trabeculotome is then introduced on one side. Its lower arm is pushed forward, parallel to the limbus, keeping a mild constant outward pressure to mantain it against the sclera (Figure 21.7); if the anterior chamber is inadvertently entered, again conversion to trabeculectomy should be considered. When the arm is introduced fully, the handle is very gently rotated in both directions by 10°. A slight alternate bulging and depression of the sclera over the tip of the trabeculotome should be observed, confirming its correct positioning. If, during this maneuver, the anterior chamber is entered without resistance, once again conversion to trabeculectomy should be considered. Trabeculotomy is performed by

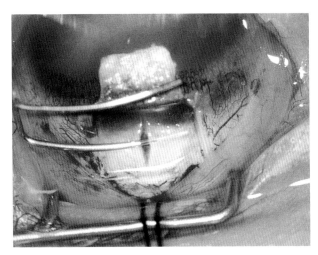

Figure 21.7 Trabeculotomy technique. The lower arm of a Harms' trabeculotome is introduced into Schlemm's canal.

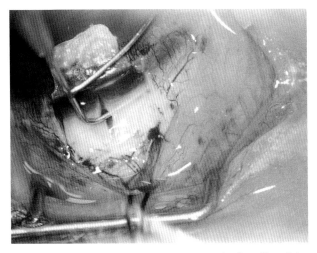

Figure 21.8 Trabeculotomy technique. The handle of the trabeculotome is rotated and the lower arm is pushed forward through the trabecular tissue into the anterior chamber.

rotating the handle of the instrument so as to move the distal part of its arm towards the pupil (Figure 21.8); the sweep should be aimed between the iris plane and the corneal endothelium, to avoid damage to either of these or to the lens. The trabeculotome is then quickly withdrawn and the procedure repeated on the other side. If the anterior chamber is shallow or flat after the first sweep, it must be deepened with viscoelastic injected through the paracentesis. The second sweep is not to be attempted with a shallow anterior chamber. The scleral flap and conjunctiva are then closed. Although trabeculotomy can be performed without first preparing a scleral flap, there are advantages in using one. From a deeper scleral bed the radial, layer-by-layer incisions are less difficult to make and the approach for the nylon probe is less angled. In addition, a scleral flap allows a prompt conversion to trabeculectomy

should it be necessary. As an alternative technique, Schlemm's canal can be probed for 360° with a polypropylene suture which is then pulled to rip open the trabecular tissue.

Filtration surgery

Trabeculectomy is the filtration procedure of choice, and is detailed in Chapter 17. Variable success rates have been reported in developmental glaucomas, and many factors must be considered when evaluating the options. Since these eyes are at high risk for failure due to episcleral fibrosis, antimetabolites are often necessary. Considering the difficulty of administering 5-fluorouracil injections in the pediatric age group without general anesthesia, intraoperative mitomycin is the most practical choice in this age group. A combination of trabeculotomy and trabeculectomy has also been used.

For the application of mitomycin it is convenient to use filter paper rather than sponges. Filter paper is easily cut to a shape fitting the contour of the limbus; it does not swell after being soaked with the solution, and the solution is not easily squeezed out of the paper. The conjunctiva can be easily draped over a thin piece of filter paper, keeping the edges of the incision away from the antimetabolite (Figure 21.9). Larger areas of exposure to antimetabolites decrease late antiproliferation-related bleb complications, such as rupture, leakage, and infection. Consideration of the long-term risk/benefit ratio of the use of antimetabolites in the pediatric age group must be realistically weighed against the chances of sight-threatening complications in such patients. The use of combined trabeculotomy–trabeculectomy is also an option, reported to obtain good IOP control in infants with congenital glaucoma. All complications described for filtration surgery in Chapter 17 can occur in developmental glaucoma, including delayed massive suprachoroidal hemorrage (Figure 21.10).

Cyclodestruction

In developmental glaucomas, cyclodestructive procedures such as cyclocryotherapy and transscleral laser cyclophotocoagulation (see Chapter 16) can be performed with the same modalities used for adults. Special attention should be paid to the localization of the ciliary body, since the anterior segment anatomy can be distorted. In most cases, transpupillary retroillumination with a penlight will be sufficient (Figure 21.11). Postoperative pain following cyclocryotherapy (Figure 21.12) can be excruciating; therefore, when the procedure is performed under general anesthesia, a retrobulbar block with a long-acting anesthetic such as bupivacaine is advisable to blunt the pain when the patient awakens. Postoperative chemosis can be

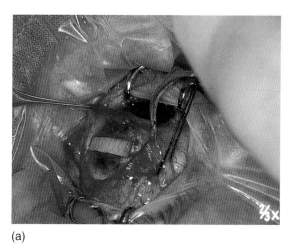

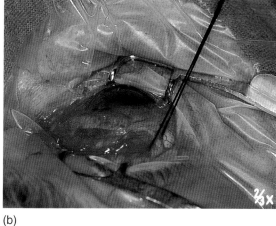

(a) (b)

Figure 21.9 Trabeculectomy for developmental glaucoma. Mitomycin is applied with a filter paper (a). The conjunctival flap can be easily draped over the paper, keeping the incision margins away from the antimetabolite (b).

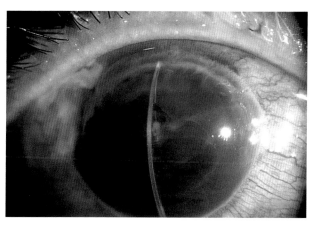

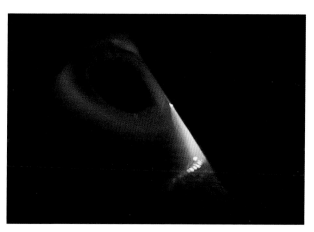

Figure 21.10 Trabeculectomy for developmental glaucoma. Massive postoperative suprachoroidal hemorrhage. This hemorrhage occurred 2 days after uneventful trabeculectomy. The eye had undergone multiple previous procedures, was buphthalmic and aphakic. Blood and retinal membranes can be seen in the anterior chamber.

Figure 21.11 Ciliodestructive procedures. Transpupillary retroillumination to localize the ciliary body.

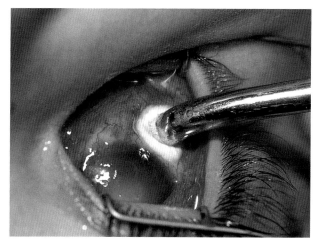

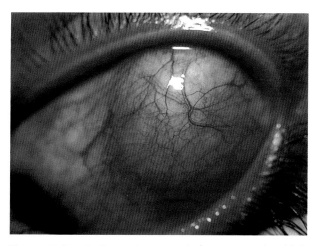

Figure 21.12 Ciliodestructive procedures. Application of a cryo probe for cyclocryotherapy. Exposure time should be reduced from standard adult settings (e.g. 1 minute freeze at −60 °C) in cases with thin sclera.

Figure 21.13 Drainage devices. A large posterior bleb may interfere with extraocular muscle contraction, leading to strabismus. Amblyopia is of concern in the pediatric age group.

severe in children; a peritomy can avoid the freezing of conjunctiva and aspirin pre-treatment can decrease the swelling.

Drainage devices (aqueous shunts)

Draining implants are detailed in Chapter 19. All types of implant have been tried in children with varying degrees of success and some frustration. In the long term, failure due to occlusion, fibrosis, and dislocation of the tube and/or plate are of concern. Oversized blebs can cause muscle imbalance (Figure 21.13). Even minor additional procedures, such as the removal of releasable sutures, in this age group might need general anesthesia. In order to prevent corneal decompensation, iris atrophy, and cataract formation, the tube should be appropriately positioned in the anterior chamber (Figure 21.14).

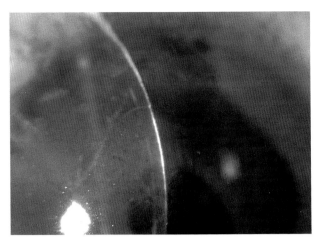

Figure 21.14 Drainage device. Localized corneal decompensation over an anterior chamber tube. The tube is positioned too anteriorly and is touching the cornea.

Further reading

Akimoto M, Tanihara H, Negi A, Nagata M. Surgical results of trabeculotomy ab externo for developmental glaucoma. Arch Ophthalmol 1994; 112: 1540–4

Beck AD, Lynch MG. 360 trabeculotomy for primary congenital glaucoma. Arch Ophthalmol 1995; 113: 1200–2

Costa VP, Katz LJ, Spaeth GL. Primary trabeculectomy in young adults. Ophthalmology 1993; 100: 1071–6

Elder MJ. Combined trabeculotomy–trabeculectomy compared with primary trabeculotomy for congenital glaucoma. Br J Ophthalmol 1994; 78: 745–8

Mandal AK, Bhatia PG, Bhaskar A, Nutheti R. Long-term surgical and visual outcomes in Indian children with developmental glaucoma operated on within 6 months of birth. Ophthalmology 2004; 111: 283–90

Munoz M, Tomey KF, Traverso CE, et al. Clinical experience with the Molteno implant in advanced infantile glaucoma. J Pediatr Ophthalmol Strabismus 1991; 28: 68–72

Quigley H. Childhood glaucoma: results with trabeculotomy and study of reversible cupping. Ophthalmology 1982; 89: 219–23

Rabiah PK. Frequency and predictors of glaucoma after pediatric cataract surgery. Am J Ophthalmol 2004; 137: 30–7

Susanna R Jr, Oltregge EW, Carani JCE. Mitomycin as an adjunct chemotheraphy with trabeculectomy in congenital and developmental glaucomas. J Glaucoma 1995; 4: 151–7

Traverso CE, Tomey KF, Al-Kaff A. The long-tube single plate Molteno implant for the treatment of recalcitrant glaucoma. Int Ophthalmol 1989; 13: 159–62

Traverso CE, Tomey KF, Day SF, et al. Surgical treatment of primary congenital glaucoma. Analysis of prognostic factors on 519 cases. Boll Oculist 1990; 69 (Suppl 2): 255–62

Index

(Page numbers in italic refer to figures and tables)